NEGOTIATING PARTNERSHIPS WITH OLDER PEOPLE

W0234765

To the memory of my father who made me believe in my abilities and myself. He waited in anticipation for the completion of this work, but sadly was unable to wait until the end. His memory lives on through my memories of this journey.

Negotiating Partnerships with Older People

A person centred approach

BRENDAN McCORMACK
University of Ulster/Royal Hospitals Trust, Belfast, Northern Ireland

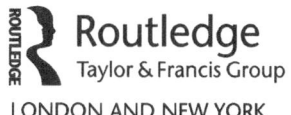

Routledge
Taylor & Francis Group

LONDON AND NEW YORK

First published 2001 by Ashgate Publishing

2 Park Square, Milton Park, Abingdon, Oxon OX14 4RN
605 Third Avenue, New York, NY 10017

Routledge is an imprint of the Taylor & Francis Group, an informa business

First issued in paperback 2021

Publisher's Note
The publisher has gone to great lengths to ensure the quality of this reprint but points out that some imperfections in the original copies may be apparent.

Disclaimer
The publisher has made every effort to trace copyright holders and welcomes correspondence from those they have been unable to contact.

A Library of Congress record exists under LC control number: 00111396

ISBN 13: 978-1-138-71958-3 (hbk)
ISBN 13: 978-0-367-24963-2 (pbk)

Contents

Acknowledgements

This work has been a journey of discovery. A journey of growth in personal understanding and a journey that has challenged my beliefs and values as a gerontological nurse. One that has required much self-exploration and reflection as a means of achieving a coherent thesis. As John O' Donohue (1997) reminds us, '*there is such an intimate connection between the way we look at things and what we actually discover*'. In undertaking this work, my journey of discovery has been a shared journey - shared with many people who have helped me to choose the right route in times of conflict, encouraged me when I did not wish to carry on and celebrated with me when new insights were discovered.

Over the life of this work many people have participated in this journey and while there are far too many to name, each of them know how much their company has been appreciated. However, a number of people have been particularly influential on my growth and development:

- The people who agreed to participate in this research. For many of them it was a venture into the unknown, but through their commitment to the process has my own growth and development arisen.
- Mary, my wife and partner throughout the journey. Her selfless attention to creating an environment and circumstances that enabled my work has been unrelenting.
- Richard Pring and Alison Kitson, who provided me with the appropriate help, support, encouragement and challenge.
- My colleagues Pauline, Angie, Brigid and Jan who also provided help, support, encouragement and challenge, but in addition, they provided me with a belief in myself that the completion of this work was possible.
- Kaye, whose attention to detail in the initial transcribing of recorded conversations made my subsequent work less arduous.
- To my various employers, who provided me with the time to complete this work.

1 Introduction

This book explores the issue of autonomy and older people. In particular it explores autonomy in the relationship between nurses and older people in hospital settings developed through a primary research study. The focus of the book is the use of language and the way autonomy is presented through the language of health care practice.

While this research focuses on a particular concept in practice, i.e. autonomy, it also reflects my own personal journey towards understanding my motivations for working with older people. This book is both an attempt to understand through academic work many of the challenges that face nurses who work with older people and a personal reflection about my own practice as a nurse. In doing this I see this research as a mirror image of my practice world - by standing back and viewing others' practice I hope to understand my own practice more. For as Gadamer (1975, cited in Dunne, 1993) suggests - 'The horizon of the present cannot be formed without the past ...'. My particular drive is to explore ways in which nurses can more effectively work with older people, confirm their value as citizens of society and find ways of working that respect personhood (Kitwood, 1997).

Book Structure

The book begins with a detailed account of my reasons for focusing on the issue of autonomy and older people in hospital, which includes a reflective account of my practice experiences. The exploration of practice in this way raises issues about the organisation of health care practice and the development of health care practitioners as professionals. An exploration of the development of health services and of the meaning of professional practice is undertaken, prior to engaging in a philosophical analysis of the concept of autonomy. The intention is to make explicit those factors that may have influenced my understanding of autonomy in my research work.

Chapters 2 and 3 address these issues and highlight the need for universal moral principles to be placed in the context of an individual relationship based on principles of partnership.

What emerges from these chapters is the complexity of the concept of autonomy and the multifaceted understandings that exist in both philosophical and applied literature. It is argued in Chapter 4 that attempts at measuring the existence of the concept in practice are fruitless unless the conceptual underpinnings are made clear at the outset. However, the problems of 'seeing' autonomy in practice represent one of the greatest methodological challenges to understanding the way the concept of autonomy is operationalised. Chapter 4 addresses this issue and presents an approach to 'seeing' the concept based on an integrated methodology of Gadamer's Hermeneutics (Gadamer, 1993) and Conversation Analysis (Drew and Heritage, 1992).

Chapters 5 to 7 will present a detailed analysis of the research data using the methodology previously described. These chapters are based on the major themes that emerged from data analysis. Chapter 5 describes the communication style adopted between nurses, older patients and other health care practitioners. It is from the analysis of this communication style that further themes in the research emerged - the first and significant one of these being that of 'Power and Control' in the nurse-patient relationship. In the context of this research, power and control in the nurse-patient relationship are seen as significant factors in enhancing or limiting the autonomy of older people in hospital. However, the manifestation of power in the relationship was complex and related to other factors such as the interplay in interactions and the use of language between nurses, patients, their families and other professionals. This interplay has been captured in this book through the phrase 'speaking for you or speaking for me?' and in Chapter 7 the three themes that capture the essence of this interplay are presented - constraints on autonomous actions; socialisation and enculturation of nurses and older people, and the roles that families play in influencing decision-making. At the end of each chapter (Chapters 5 to 7), 'Principles for Action' have been identified. These represent particular issues that may require changes in attitudes, organisations and practice frameworks, should a person-centred approach be realised. No attempt was made in this research to test these principles out in practice and as such they are 'tentative' in nature.

The identified principles for action were grouped according to their common focus and formed into five themes. As the question of 'expertise' and 'context of care' were important to this work, that is, could patient autonomy be enhanced according to the degree of clinical expertise demonstrated by the nurse and/or by the removal of institutional barriers?, then the themes emerging from Chapters 5 to 7 were used to analyse the data collected in a community setting and by a recognised expert practitioner. Chapter 8 presents the results of this data analysis and concludes that the issue of expertise and context are important factors in the enhancement of autonomy with older people as the discourse in these data was considered to be significantly different from that presented in other chapters.

Using the themes generated from the 'principles for action', an alternative presentation of autonomy is presented in Chapter 9 based on Heidegger's (1990) theory of 'authentic consciousness'. This chapter proposes that an understanding of autonomy as authentic consciousness represents a values based understanding of the concept, whereby the patient's values are held central to all decision-making. It is also proposed in this chapter that, autonomy, as authentic consciousness is best articulated through the concept of a life plan. When autonomy is understood as authentic consciousness and articulated through a life plan, it is argued that the potential for a person to be reduced to a 'thing' is minimised and personhood is maintained. However, the barriers to making this approach a reality given the internal and external constraining factors identified in earlier chapters, are significant. Therefore Chapter 10 addresses key issues for nursing practice that would need to be considered if autonomy as authentic consciousness is to be realised.

Chapter 10 presents an approach to practice that views the nurse as a 'facilitator of authentic consciousness'. The themes derived from the principles for action will be presented in the form of 'Imperfect Duties' as described by Immanuel Kant (Sullivan, 1990), i.e. maxims that guide action, but account for contextual issues, individual preferences and individual values. It will be proposed that these imperfect duties can form the basis of an approach to person-centred practice that enables the facilitation of an older person's authentic consciousness.

The final chapter of the book (Chapter 11) will discuss some implications of the findings of this research and 'next steps' in testing out the approach to practice recommended.

Why Autonomy?

Autonomy is a significantly relevant concept for nurses, because it is argued that autonomous nurses are not only autonomous persons, but also advocates for clients and professionals able to function independently yet collaboratively in a complex health care environment (Wood *et al*, 1986). Watson (1988) argues that at the core of nursing's philosophy is the humanity of the patient. Nursing addresses the unique needs of patients or clients as persons and this acts as the central ethical concern for nurses. Indeed van Hooft (1990) argues that it is the day to day events in the relationship between the nurse and the patient that is of greatest ethical concern for nurses. The foundation of the nurse-patient relationship is based on a mutual humanity of the participants with its nature rooted in the determination of the patient's human needs and the nurse's response to them (Curtin and Flaherty, 1982).

Contemporary nursing practice emphasises the importance of the nurse/patient relationship set within an individualistic presentation of nursing practice. This has been referred to in the literature as 'New Nursing' (Salvage, 1990; Porter, 1994), but is more often referred to as 'professional nursing practice'. The essence of new nursing, lies in the nature of the nurse/patient relationship. The approach emphasises the acceptance of patients as whole human beings with wants, needs and fears that need to be addressed if health care is going to be effective. It includes the explicit rejection of a dominant biomedical approach that is seen as unable to take account of the phenomenological aspects of ill health (Porter, 1996). It emphasises the importance of the autonomy of the nurse and supports organisational practices that encourage individual nursing decision making and the exercise of individual accountability.

Emphasis on the nurse-patient relationship has brought about a 'softening' of the distinction between person (both patient and nurse) and professional (Gadow, 1990). Professionals are encouraged, and in many cases expected to 'get involved with' patients as individuals, i.e. to remove some of the professional barriers and behave more like persons. Research by Taylor (1992; 1994) suggests that nurses and patients share a common humanity, a humanity so ordinary that it is often overlooked by attempts to professionalise nursing. Professional caring is far greater than simply providing nursing care (Dewing, 1994), but involves deep emotional involvement; self-awareness and the purposeful use of self; inter subjectivity and aesthetic qualities. It is this conceptualisation of care that has achieved a significant change in thinking about the moral and ethical dimension of the nurse-patient relationship. In any relationship there are periods of intensity; periods of withdrawal; activities based on partnership and times of individual decision-making and action. But whatever the focus, a caring relationship exists because of the unconditional regard for the other person's intrinsic values.

It is here that challenges for nurses emerge. The focus on individuality has resulted on a movement away from the recognition of universal principles that guide practice. Instead clinical decision-making has shifted towards a 'contextualised' position, whereby each decision is unique to the particular patient's situation and hence needs to be explored from that individual's perspective. In shifting to this position, it has been argued that nurses have rejected universal moral values (Bradshaw, 1995) and replaced them with an ideology of patient autonomy, patient-centredness and individuality. However, despite this ideology, everyday practice still requires nurses to balance the individual needs of patients with universal moral principles and the needs and aspirations of an organisation. Commitment to patients must be carefully contained within the managerial ideology of productivity, efficiency, cost-containment and organisational loyalty. As Yarling and McElmurry (1990) argue, professional nursing practice is conceived in moral contradictions and borne in practice through daily compromise. Decisions concerning an appropriate ethical position continue to be dominated by professional ideology, and while the patient's perspective may be taken into account in moral deliberations it is the professional who predominantly does the deliberating and the professional's concerns that are seen to prevail.

The current changes to the NHS and the consideration of 'market forces' set within a consumerist ideology places health care within a market economy. This political force, coupled with an individualistic approach to nursing practice, whereby the individuality of the patient is central to practice decisions, requires nurses to re-evaluate the nature of their professional practice and redefine their interpretation of key concepts. Autonomy represents one such concept, as the consumerist ideology and patient-centred individualised practice sometimes find themselves in opposition (Savage, 1995). The nature of professional nursing practice has been subjected to much debate (for example, distinctions between the role of registered nurses and nursing assistants, the advocacy role of nurses and the need for registered nursing in the continuing care of older people) and the nursing profession has needed to adopt new ways of working in order to meet consumer demand; new ways that mean making knowledge and expertise more accessible, a drive towards a greater sense of openness and the requirement for nurses to define the nature of their professional work (Watkins *et al*, 1992). In the development of professional nursing practice, the moral principle of paternalism is often rejected by nursing, as it is viewed as being detrimental to the nurse/patient relationship and replaced with other concepts such as partnership, reciprocity and intimacy (Muetzel, 1988). It can be argued that this position has been a necessary one for nursing to take in its transition towards establishing its own unique professional identity (Manthey, 1980). While this transition can be applauded for the profession of nursing, there is little evidence to suggest that as a result of this movement, patients themselves have gained greater autonomy. It has been indicated that when nurses are explicitly allowed to practice in an autonomous way, the concept of 'ownership' becomes a problem (Pearson, 1985). One form of imperialism [medicine] appears to have been replaced by another [nursing] (Pearson, 1985). Other studies have indicated the emergence of similar problems (Johns, 1989; McCormack, 1992). Indeed Bradshaw (1995) arguing from a Judeo-Christian perspective, suggests that in contemporary nursing theory, the interpretation of patient and nursing autonomy as 'individualism' has lead to a destruction of nursing's fundamental caring principles.

Contemporary nursing theory suggests that the essence of nursing is the relationship with the patient (*for example* Watson, 1988; Johns, 1994; Boykin and Schoenhofer, 1993). Therefore nurses must understand the appropriate rules of behaviour in such a relationship, in order to meet the demands of the informed consumer.

Why Older People?

> I felt glad to fit in so comfortably with young people. In fact, most of the time I don't feel any different in age to them. That's one of the reasons why ageing is so hard. The ageless, eternal child in me - the youthful spirit - has remained unchanged but the body gets creaky and the humours get cranky. Traitors both! I was lucky this time and felt pathetically grateful but I have already experienced the terror of invisibility. One day you're an attractive alluring woman and the next day you become one of the faceless group of old ladies who sit alone in cafes and on park benches. One of the wrinklies, shrinklies, crumblies, old bags, old bats - bewildered at the speed of the descent - dismissed as irrelevant, dying of loneliness. With no recognized rites of passage, we grope uneasily in the frightening tunnel of transition, unsure of what lies ahead, afraid to relinquish what has gone before (Taylor, 1993).

Taylor (1993) presents a biographical account of the meaning of ageing in Western society. Through an anthropological comparison, she identifies the problems that Western society has with dealing with issues of ageing. The media images of older age reinforce the stereotypical image of decline and lacking productivity. The often derogatory language associated with media perceptions of ageing perpetuate such attitudes (Dalley *et al*, 1997).

Slater (1995) suggests that the separation of groups of people through the use of common descriptive terms is an attempt by society to create an 'us' and 'them' culture. In creating such a culture, behaviour enacted by one of 'us' may be seen as situationally caused and the context of the behaviour will be taken into consideration. But similar behaviour in one of 'them' is taken as a disposition. Such attitudes are not exclusive to older people, as essentially this attitude prevails in all prejudicial thinking (Hewstone *et al*, 1989). Nurses, as members of society hold no less negative views of older people than society at large (Ebersole and Hess, 1990). The majority of studies into the attitudes of nurses towards older people demonstrate that indeed nurses are likely to hold extreme negative views of older age because of their continual involvement with frailty and disability. For example, Baker (1978) identified that attitudes held by society were manifested in nursing practice through 'the routine geriatric approach' to practice. More recently, studies of loneliness experienced by older people in communities (*for example* Ryan and Patterson, 1987) have demonstrated that such loneliness can continue in institutional care because of limited communication patterns between older residents and nursing staff (Coupland *et al*, 1991).

The use of the phrase 'older person/older people' is an attempt therefore to dispel ageist language from my vocabulary. Challenges to the use of the 'older person' phrase, are often made from the anecdotal basis of 'the elderly don't mind being called elderly'. This would not appear to be correct. Only five percent of those retired and over 55 in a British Gas survey (1991) said they would like to be called that, presumably because such words produce a knee-jerk response about decrepitude (Slater, 1995). Thirty six percent of the people in this survey preferred the term 'senior citizen' and the same number preferred the term 'retired'.

Why Autonomy and Older People? - A Personal Journey

The relevance of ageism, prejudice, stereotypes and stigma have been identified from a broad socio-political and professional perspective. While these perspectives raise significant challenges for the autonomy of older people, my experience as a nurse and, in particular, my personal journey towards appreciating a humanistic approach to working with older people are also significant to this book.

In 1980 I began my nursing career as a student psychiatric nurse in Ireland. The hospital had 1100 patients and was divided into a male and female section. Male nurses only cared for male patients and the 'male side' of the hospital was totally separated from the 'female side'. In the hospital, male and female staff and patients only integrated during social events and in the staff dining room.

My initial reaction to the world that I had entered was one of shock and abhorrence. Although I had previously been a visitor to the hospital in which I was a student nurse, I had no understanding of the culture of psychiatric nursing. My initial twelve-week preparation course did not prepare me for the realities of the ward culture. Practice was in general, traditional, routinised and ritualistic and a culture of neglect and abuse existed (Biggs *et al*, 1995). The degree to which this culture existed varied according to the profile of the particular ward. The 'acute admissions ward' had little overt demonstration of this culture because of its high profile with the general public.

It was on the 'continuing elderly care ward' that the culture was most obvious and it is here that I spent time as both a student and staff nurse. The 40 patients all had a dementing illness of some kind or were too physically frail to be cared for on another ward. The culture of this ward (and significant other parts of the hospital) is best articulated using Goffman's (1961) notion of 'total institution'. Goffman suggests that:

> Total institutions disrupt or defile precisely those actions that in civil society have the role of attesting to the actor and those in his presence that he has some command over his world - that he is a person with 'adult' self-determination, autonomy and freedom of action (Goffman, 1961: 43).

Lidz and Arnold (1990) have developed a framework (from the work of Goffman (1961) for analysing institutional behaviour. The use of an adapted form of this framework in this chapter has enabled a thorough reflection of the culture and its impact on my beliefs and values as a nurse.

Entry rituals, such as history taking and removal of items of identity functioned to strip people of their individuality Once patients entered the continuing care ward, they had any remaining personal belongings that were considered to be of value removed and placed in 'safe keeping'. Patients had a medical examination undertaken and a 'care prescription' made. Patients had a bath on their day of arrival, serving to symbolise the removal of previous identities. They were allocated a bed in a 20 bedded dormitory. All clothes were part of a communal wardrobe and patients usually had ill-fitting or inappropriate clothing.

Non-differentiation of location - all aspects of life take part in the same place Patients rarely left the ward except those who were physically mobile and those who were allocated hospital 'tasks'. The completion of these tasks was rewarded with sweets or cigarettes. Patients ate, slept and spent their waking hours in the same place. The more physically disabled the person was, the more limiting the space was. Those with incontinence problems were 'not allowed' in the day room and therefore were prevented from taking part in the few social activities that did take place including music and television viewing. Patients with severe physical disabilities spent their waking hours in a chair, tipped backwards and restrained, sitting at one end of a twenty bedded dormitory around a single-bar electric fire.

Non-differentiation of authority - there was a single unspecialised hierarchy of authority Each part of the day was set within a strict routine dictated by the charge nurse. Students, staff nurses and patients had little say in decisions made. Interaction consisted of patients seeking permission from students and staff nurses and staff nurses seeking permission from the charge nurse. The charge nurse was always the final arbiter of decisions.

Individuals had to request staff permission for even routine activities Because of their level of physical and mental disability, patients needed to request help from staff for most aspects of their daily life. However, such control extended beyond such needs and included permission for access to 'luxury' items such as jam, soap and cigarettes. Such items were used as a means of controlling behaviour or for punishment of 'bad' behaviour such as incontinence, screaming and shouting, refusal to take medications or failure to comply with an order. When these items were refused for a period of time as a punishment, the nurse decided when the punishment would end.

Each phase of the person's daily activity was carried on in the immediate company of a large batch of others, all of whom were treated alike Patients were required to conform to a rigid set of institutional rules. These rules were not written down, but all staff and 'astute' patients knew them. These rules rather than individual needs, guided staff behaviour with the principal aim of achieving institutional efficiency. The dominance of the institutional rules served to develop covert and subversive behaviours among student nurses in particular. Students developed creative methods of 'rule breaking' and in assisting patients with the breaking of the rules.

Daily activities were tightly scheduled by staff, with little individual variation permitted The routine of the ward dictated all daily activities. Patients who were independent with their washing and dressing needs were required to be up by 8.00 am. Failure to do so resulted in 'punishment'. It was not unusual for 'protesting' patients to be physically removed from their bed. All other patients were required to be up before 10.00 am prior to the charge nurse doing a 'round' and inspecting the quality of the bedmaking and the tidiness of the dormitory. Meals, drinks, elimination, socialising and bedtime all occurred within a set routine. Only physically fit patients were allowed to stay up past 6.00pm.

Individuals were excluded from making plans about themselves Patients did not take part in discussions or case conferences. There were no nursing care prescriptions and a predominant medical focus of care existed. Care 'tasks' were prescribed by the consultant or 'duty doctor'. The predominant therapy used was drug therapy, which was used as a 'chemical restraint' and means of controlling behaviour. Patients had little say in their care and refusal to comply with treatment resulted in punishment.

Individuals and staff viewed each other through narrow hostile stereotypes Staff generally viewed patients as demented, demanding and 'less than human'. These ageist and inhumane attitudes towards patients dominated the daily care regime, including making practical jokes at the patients' expense, laughing at patients' inability to perform particular activities and through verbal and physical abuse. Patients however treated staff as their 'keepers', i.e. the people who controlled their life and this attitude perpetuated the dominant culture. Both sides viewed each other in the collective and there were few positive individual staff/patient relationships. Some patients and staff were 'liked' more than others - usually patients who were physically fit and able to participate in the 'work' of the ward and staff who positively assisted with the maintenance of the ward regime.

Violations of privacy were common Privacy for personal aspects of care was not considered. Thence there were no curtains around beds, toilets had no doors and bathrooms had no locks. Patients were regularly stripped naked in open wards and multiple commodes were 'lined up' in the communal toilets at set times for patients to attend to their toileting needs.

All activities were brought together into a single rational plan designed to fulfill the official aims of the institution Most institutions possess some kind of organisational plan. Such plans endeavour to enable members of the organisation to contribute positively to the goals of the organisation. Therefore the content of the plan enables positive action. In this case however, the organisation was set within a 'medical model' - the practice emphasis was on maintaining a safe environment and ensuring that medical prescriptions were administered. Nursing knowledge was set within biological and psychological systems and behaviours. Student nurses were taught by doctors or by nurses who used a medical model. Nursing care was taught through tasks and treatments and there was no philosophy of 'nursing as a therapy' in itself. Therefore the nurse's main role was in telling patients what to do within a predetermined boundary of acceptable behaviours, rather than enabling them to develop their own potential and individuality.

Reflections on the Journey

It was widely recognised by both hospital management and nurse teachers that this culture existed, but I was unaware of any significant attempts to change it. A staff rotation system was seen as the solution by managers who did not understand that the culture was so strong that all newly appointed staff to the ward adopted the previous staffs' culture. In my early days as a student, I questioned some of these practices, resulting in my alienation from the ward team and the allocation of domestic duties as punishment. I was considered to be an idealist who didn't understand the realities of life in a psychiatric hospital. I was however considered to be good at 'physical' care and for that reason was requested back to the ward by the charge nurse when student placements were being devised. By the third year of my training I had realised that I did not want to be a psychiatric nurse in such an institution but felt driven by the caring aspects of my role. I knew I made a difference to the lives of individual patients on that ward by adopting a paternalistic approach that protected patients from the punitive approaches of other 'institutionalised' staff. On completing my training I recognised that I would never properly 'fit in' and that I should develop my career elsewhere - a decision I actively pursued.

It was not until twelve years later, having completed my training as a general nurse and developing my career further that I realised the impact that this experience had on me. Although my career choices had not always taken me to work with older people, I knew I held very strong values about their care. While undertaking further nursing studies, I began to understand more fully issues about organisational culture, abuse, the meaning of 'care', psychosocial motivational factors and power. My dissertation towards the award of a degree in nursing identified the issue of 'ownership' as being significant among the practice of nurses (McCormack, 1992). In a ward that had adopted a culture of professional and practice development, and where nurses had considerable autonomy over their practice, nurses felt a sense of ownership over patients. This ownership manifested itself in a number of ways including, nurses not willing to 'let go' of the relationship they had with their patients, maintaining control over decision-making, possessiveness of the relationship with patients and seeing other nurses' input as 'interference'.

In 1991 I was appointed to a position where my principal responsibility was the development of practice with older people in a community hospital setting. Again on commencing this post, I was struck by the ageist attitudes and routinised approaches to care. While the unit did not have all the trappings of the 'total institution' that I had previously experienced, I was sensitive to the potential situations that could occur if some practices did not change. I had however, underestimated the emotional effects my previous student nurse experience had on me, including guilt and regret for not having tried harder to change the culture. I also questioned my credibility as a nurse. However, changing an organisation such as this requires a philosophical shift in the organisational culture and a collective approach to its implementation (Handy, 1985). I have learned not to feel guilty and to recognise the importance of the experience in the development of my caring values. I believe the experience has largely shaped my beliefs and values about 'good' care, including the meaning of caring, the importance of the nurse/patient relationship, the importance of a humanistic approach to care and a belief in the worth of persons throughout their life. In addition it created a passion for the development of practice 'in practice' as a means of enabling individuals to change the culture and to be empowered to create a caring environment that respects and acknowledges the self-worth of older people. The importance of these values can never be underestimated, as the reduction of persons to objects is a serious moral problem. The destructive outcomes of such occurrences, in terms of the individual losing connection with themselves and the outside world, is indeed something to be avoided. Sacks (1991) suggests that our bodies are personal, defined by how we appear to the outside world, how we inwardly feel about ourselves and the totality of our life experiences. As we age, we need to be able to adapt to the different demands made upon us.

Older people move through a journey of dependence while seeking their own individuality and identity. This sense of 'seeking the individual', brings with them their past in order to create a future. Being hospitalised may be a new experience, assimilated by the influence of their past and their aspirations for the future. However, the depersonalisation of the individual that occurs in institutional settings is well documented (e.g.: Goffman, 1961; Miller and Gwynne, 1972; Kenny, 1990). As described in the earlier practice experience, Goffman's work eloquently describes how this process occurs, with the chief cause being the breakdown of the barriers normally separating the three spheres of life, i.e. sleep, play and work. Instead all aspects of life are conducted in the same surroundings, in the public eye of the same authority, with others who are pursuing the same thing at the same time. The activities of the day are tightly scheduled within an explicit set of rules and boundaries. Having entered the institution with certain conceptions of himself made possible by certain social arrangements in the social world of his home (Kenny, 1990), the person is stripped of the support provided by such arrangements. Or as Goffman (1961) asserts 'he begins a series of abasements, degradations, humiliations and profanations of self'. When older people realise that they are no longer part of their human world, they experience despair (RCN, 1993). These feelings of such despair may be manifested through non-specific complaints of physical or psychological distress and the person may be stereotyped as hypochondriacal, mentally unstable, depressed or just a 'complainer' (RCN, 1993). Kastenbaum (1983) demonstrated how older people in residential care may subsequently be ignored by staff, neglected, ridiculed or given drugs - the symptoms are treated rather than the emotional distress. The ensuing dependence on others creates a form of learned helplessness (Abramson *et al*, 1982) whereby loss of control over particular aspects of their lives results in ensuing beliefs that the events or outcomes in their lives are independent of their actions (Robertson, 1986).

Assisting the individual to find meaning in their lives may help them to tolerate the incongruity of their situation and help create a future. As Moody (1991) asserts, if my life is intelligible, my life has purpose and my hopes and desires ultimately can be satisfied, then happiness can be found:

> At first we want life to be romantic; later, to be bearable; finally, to be understandable (Moody, 1991).

The meaning of life for older people is not demonstrated through the tedium of superficial daily life. Current approaches to reminiscence and life review attempt to aid an understanding of the meaning of life through a wish to find in the experience of older people elements of strength and positive affirmation (Moody, 1991). Even though life around the person may have little meaning or significance, through individual life review, the person may discover meaning in his or her own life.

It is these values that shape my personal philosophy of care as articulated through the following set of beliefs and values:

- An objective understanding of the ageing body, coupled with an understanding of the individual's subjective interpretation of their own ageing journey, contribute a sense of wholeness and enables the nurse to enter the subjective world of the older person in meeting care needs.
- Respecting the older person's ways of life is perhaps one of the most humanistic qualities shown in nursing care.
- The older person is mindful of the many roles played during life and the losses suffered over the years. To have a nurse show through respect, an empathic understanding of their losses and present limitations, enables the achievement of effective outcomes from care that are centred on the person's needs and life perspectives.
- An understanding of the person's self-worth directs the nurse towards flexibility in nursing care that seeks to preserve the integrity of the person. Through the appreciation of the individual's uniqueness, it makes explicit to the nurse, the limits beyond which the person cannot be taken, and prevents the setting of unrealistic objectives.
- The according of humanistic respect to the older person can in itself offer an approach to the 'healing' of the body and the restoration of individual self-worth.

Conclusions

In introducing this book, the 'prejudices' (Gadamer, 1993) that I hold have been made explicit through the articulation of my own philosophy of care. It has been suggested that the essence of nursing is a humanistic relationship between the nurse and the patient and that it is within such a relationship that patient autonomy is manifested (*for example* Singleton and Nail, 1984; Yarling and McElmurry, 1990). Through this reflection, issues about the organisation of health care practice, approaches to care delivery and the role of the nurse when working with older people have been identified as significant factors in the creation of a practice culture that values the autonomy of the patient in decision-making.

2 Autonomy - A Health Care Perspective

Introduction

The concept of patient autonomy itself is not a 'new' concept in health care. Indeed it is one that health care practitioners have considered throughout the development of the health services. It is generally considered that a major goal of health care is the restoration of autonomy in individuals who for varying reasons may have their autonomy compromised or diminished. A lack of information, lack of understanding about one's circumstances, inability to make rational choices due to disease or illness and lack of power to act on the choices made, are all contributing factors to the patient autonomy debate (Norman, 1993; Oddi, 1994; Seedhouse, 1988). Yet, even in situations where the patient is reliant on the health care practitioner, it is often argued that if people are considered to be autonomous, then this autonomy should be respected (Seedhouse, 1988). The challenges and conflicts in operationalising this principle, are evident in the literature (*for example* Scoccia, 1990; Pollard, 1993; Ridley, 1989; Abramson, 1990; Langslow, 1992). For some commentators, the centralising of the concept of autonomy in health care practice merely reduces the practitioner's role to that of 'servant of the patient' (McKinstry, 1992). While for others (Fulford, 1996; Hope, 1992; Agich, 1993; Judge, 1996) such a position makes explicit the role of the professional in the context of patient decision making.

However, throughout the development of health services, the validity of autonomy as a 'central' concept of health care practice (Fulford, 1996) is continuously challenged. For some it represents the core of bioethics (Seedhouse, 1988) while for others it is an unnecessary unattainable ideal in contemporary health care (Johns, 1995). Such debates about the value of autonomy are evident in health services, professional and clinical practice developments.

While it is not contended in this book that autonomy is the central concept underpinning health care developments and decision-making, the conclusion drawn by Fulford (1996: 2) is central to the focus of this work:

... as a principle, autonomy has been and remains an important bulwark against the worst excesses of medical paternalism. And as a principle supporting patient power, it is one to which a wide range of disciplines have subscribed.

Therefore autonomy is seen as an essential guiding principle in ethical health care, but not the only guiding principle. Contemporary health care practice emphasises such concepts as equality, partnership, power, collegiality and holism (Fulford, 1996; Porter, 1996; Emanuel, 1991). The explication of such principles can be seen through the history of health service reforms since 1948.

This chapter will present an overview of the development of health services and the way these developments have influenced the current focus on issues of autonomy, and in particular those of patient choice. The chapter will present an analysis of four phases of health care development - consumerism, managerialism, nursing developments and patient-centred care. The development of consumerism alongside an organisational philosophy of managerialism in health care will be considered. These philosophical shifts in health care will then be discussed in the context of the professionalisation of nursing and the more recent emphasis on 'patient-centred practice'. Whilst highlighting these as important developments in health care organisation and practice, it will be argued that consumerism and patient-centredness can find themselves in opposition with a subsequent impact on patient autonomy.

A Focus on Consumerism

Since the inception of the National Health Service in the United Kingdom, the conflict between patient need based on an ethics of 'rights' (Emanuel, 1991), and professional autonomy based on an ethic of professional 'independence'(Seedhouse, 1992) has been an issue. The idealist unification policy as originally planned (Klein, 1989) never came into existence as medical power proved too great for the planners of the service. It was not until the Griffiths Report of 1984 (DHSS, 1984) that any significant reforms to health care delivery began, with the introduction of 'General Management' into the NHS as a means of creating clear lines of accountability and responsibility. It also, for the first time recognised the need for the health service to be responsive to the needs of the patient and began to use the language of the 'consumer'.

To most people, being a consumer means being able to make informed decisions about the product or service bought. In order to do so, access to reliable information and freedom of choice are required (Hope, 1996). In the 'old' National Health Service, it would be unrealistic to use the word 'consumer', as choice was restricted to the services immediately available and quality of service varied from area to area (Townsend, 1974) with little controls or monitoring programmes in place. In the 'new' National Health Service the concepts of equality, partnership, power, collegiality and holism were subsumed under the 'umbrella concept' of consumerism. Autonomy within this ideology would usually mean that people who understand the implications of what they are doing should have the final say about the kind of treatment or care that they undergo (Seedhouse and Cribb, 1989). However, this general rule poses difficulties for health care practice and challenges assumptions about the role of the patient in health care decision-making. The consumerist philosophy can be seen to alter the patient career and critical commentators of the changes in the National Health Service (NHS) usually challenge the relevance of consumer terminology in health care (*for example* Klein, 1989). Whether consuming health care is similar or different to other consumer decisions about choosing a particular product or service is often the focus of such debates. Commentators such as Klein (1989) argue that health care is different from other consumer purchases because the consumer does not know best. This paternalistic approach to health care provision was manifested in many of the dissatisfactions highlighted in consumer surveys (Jones *et al*, 1987).

Judge (1996) suggests that for 'the interested layman' barriers to making choices about treatment options are beginning to be removed and people are being encouraged to make choices about their own treatment with as much help as they need. She suggests that there is more openness about service provision, changes in public expectation and recognition of the different roles that consumers of health care play (for example, patient, carer and potential users). The success of such an aim however, is in part dependent on the readiness of the health care practitioner to accept the informed consumer. Evidence continues to exist that highlights the common problems of patients being uninvolved, uninformed, dissatisfied and disassociated with much of what happens to them (Brown *et al*, 1992;

The Health Advisory Service 2000, 1998). In a critique of the National Health Service reforms, Holliday (1992) argues that as far as the individual patient is concerned, the new NHS represents a partial but incomplete move from paternalism to autonomy.

A complete introduction of consumer choice highlights an inherent conflict of values for the NHS. The full-scale shift of values towards consumer autonomy could result in eroding the NHS itself and thus decreasing and not increasing autonomy for large sections of the population, as it would reduce freedom of choice. It is clear from other Government initiatives, that this outcome was never intended. Reports, such as *Health of the Nation* (Department of Health, 1991 [i]) and *The Patient's Charter* (Department of Health, 1991 [ii]) clearly signified the government's intention to retain control over the planning of health care and indeed set the limits on individual choice. Indeed, the introduction to *Health of the Nation* clearly outlined the Government's intentions to ensure that the provision of health care would not be completely led by 'the market', but would be based on a balance between individual responsibility and Government action. In contrast to Holliday's (1992) argument, Fulford (1996) suggests that a complete autonomous focus, represented as 'patient power' is too narrow a focus for health care delivery and reduces professional practice to being only responsive to patients' wishes irrespective of presenting 'facts'.

Perhaps it is inevitable that all health care systems will contain elements of conflict between paternalism and individual freedom of choice. Without sufficiently widespread information systems, to provide the necessary information that allows people to take for themselves the health care decisions that confront them, individual autonomy can never be the prevailing health care value system. Equally, it must be considered how far the public is prepared to make their own decisions considering, in most cases, the brevity of these decisions. For that reason one needs to consider if the language of consumerism is appropriate for the health care arena, as making decisions about one's health may not be equivalent to those decisions about buying a new car, or repairing a household appliance. Consumerism requires a service whose prime concern is the needs of the individual patient, rather than the protection of bureaucratic structures.

The Older Person as a Consumer of Health Care

For older people, the challenges of the consumerist ideology are greater than for other sections of the population (Dalley *et al*, 1997). Current health and social care policy omits reference to older people and Victor (1991) highlights the importance of this omission, given a prevailing culture whereby older people have decisions made on their behalf without consultation with them.

The growing number of older people in society is widely reported (House of Commons Health Select Committee, 1996; Falkingham, 1986; Laing and Buisson, 1996). One argument is that the increasing number of older people results in a corresponding rise in the number of dependent older people on a diminishing working population. Currently, there exists much debate concerning the validity of this generally held belief. Falkingham (1986) argues 'it is not necessarily the case that a change in the age profile of the population will lead to a greater burden of dependency'. The Health Select Committee (House of Commons Health Select Committee, 1996) concluded that there is little conclusive evidence to suggest that the rise in the number of older people results in a corresponding rise in dependency due to illness or disability. Victor (1991) argues that the main assumptions underpinning dependency ratios are that all those aged 0-15 and 65+ are dependent, all those aged 16-64 are gainfully employed and supporting those who are dependent, and that all members of the 'dependent population' are equally dependent, and do not present varying social costs of support.

Such a collective attitude to the dependency of older people perpetuates ageism and reduces older persons' capacity to exercise their rights as health care consumers. Agich (1993) however argues that viewing older people as being dependent on the state in this way reduces them to 'objects' that need to be managed and contained within economic pressures. It is generally assumed that an increasing number of older people results in greater demands for health care. Certainly the process of ageing places greater demands on an individual's health status with a corresponding need for more support from health and social care resources (Grimley-Evans, 1991). Whether it is the increasing number of older people or the shrinking availability of health care resources that has resulted in the increasing demands on resources is widely debated (House of Commons Health Select Committee, 1996; Laing and Buisson, 1996).

There are those that see an ageing population as 'a problem' because of the demands they make on health and social care resources (Callahan, 1991). From this perspective such language as 'bed blocking' becomes commonplace with the older person, rather than their health status being seen as a problem. For others, an increasing ageing population is indicative of success - increasing effectiveness in medical practice, health promotion, improved housing, sanitation and diet are all seen as important public health advances that have enabled people to live healthier for longer (Dalley, 1997; Seedhouse, 1986). From this perspective society has a responsibility to both support and maximise life potential through its health and social care policies.

The achievement of such an ideal has been hindered in the UK by a number of factors, including an emphasis on individual as opposed to a societal responsibility for health, the division between health and social care provision and the fragmentation of providers with an emphasis on competition rather than collaboration/cooperation (Traynor, 1996). Most policy analysts recognise that the health and social care divide is a false one, and indeed it has been argued that it is an untenable division that results in the loss of nursing services to older people (*for example*, RCN, 1997; CSAG, 1998). Nursing has traditionally developed from both health and social care perspectives with its role established in the maintenance and re establishment of health set within the context of the individual's social circumstances. The health and social care divide has enabled the reduction of NHS' commitment to the support of older people throughout their life and in particular the erosion of continuing [residential] and continuous [community] care services (RCN, 1994; RCN, 1995).

The erosion of the NHS' continuing care services has coexisted with the reduction of secondary care facilities through an emphasis on a Primary Care Led NHS and the loss of specialist gerontology units. Reduced lengths of stay, day case treatment and a focus on the effective management of medical emergencies has meant that secondary care facilities are more stringently targeted at acute care episodes and the expectation that follow up care would take place in a community based facility. For older people in particular, this policy has resulted in significant changes to the organisation of their care services. For the majority of older people, acute illness is not 'packaged' in the same way as it may be for the rest of the adult population. Physiological, psychological and sociological changes as a result of ageing, and an increasingly fragile health status demands that services for older people focus not just on the acute episode and its symptoms, but also on the overall effects of such illness on the person's homeostasis. Average lengths of stay in secondary care of between 7.7 and 10.2 days (CSAG, 1998) do not allow for such considerations. It is not surprising therefore that the language of 'bed-blocking' is pervasive as older people 'fail' to comply with average lengths of stay that do not accommodate longer recovery periods. The pressures on secondary care services to discharge people quickly in order to maximise throughput and reduce average lengths of stay (key NHS indicators used for monitoring efficiency and effectiveness) have been highlighted as factors contributing to the quality of care delivered to older people in hospital (Bright and Durham, 1997). Bright and Durham's 'Dignity on the Ward' campaign in *The Observer* newspaper and supported by consumer organisations such as 'Help the Aged' and 'Age Concern England' - highlighted a lack of dignity in care delivered to older people in hospital. The campaign resulted in the Government commissioning a review of the quality of care delivered to older people in hospital (The Health Advisory Service 2000, 1998).

Coupled with this situation is the increasing pressures placed on Primary Health Care Teams (PHCTs) to provide more 'acute' care, with many PHCTs reporting a differing focus in their work from one of continuous care to that of disease management and treatment (CSAG, 1998). The role of the community nurse has changed significantly and is no longer a resource immediately available to support the continuing care of older people in the community (CSAG, 1998). The introduction of a market economy in the NHS and the increasing role of PHCTs as purchasers of health care for populations, have further threatened the position of older people as consumers of health care. This further serves to reinforce Holliday's (1992) argument that changes to the NHS represent a partial but incomplete move from paternalism to autonomy. For older people the 'multiple-pathology' associated with ageing, often means that their health care needs are more complex and often more expensive than those that can be reasonably provided by individual primary health care teams. Dalley (1997; 99) suggests that:

> Issues of equity, subjectivity, priority and fairness in decision-making will be played out in the privacy of the consulting room. The need for transparency and accountability is clear, but so far little concern has been expressed about these issues.

The White Paper, 'The New NHS - Modern and Dependable' (Department of Health, 1997), offered proposals to make health care purchasing decision more transparent with an emphasis on greater openness in decision-making. However, it remains unclear as to whether these changes will significantly effect the provision of continuing care for older people. The continuous debate about the provision of continuing care services resulted in the establishment of a 'Royal Commission' to investigate its provision and funding arrangements (Royal Commission on Long Term Care, 1999). However, one year since the completion of this work, a government response to the findings is still awaited.

The principle of people living for as long as possible in their own homes or a home of their choice was a central principle of The NHS Community Care Act (Department of Health, 1990), but the reality is very different and it is estimated that, although 43 percent of all continuing care is provided in residential care settings, only 3 percent of older people would choose such an option for themselves (Bernard and Phillips, 1998). In addition, older people requiring support with long term care, unlike other sections of the population, have these needs 'means tested' and are required to pay for their care should their financial assets exceed a given amount. Such barriers to the exercise of consumer choice by older people has resulted in the emergence of advocacy organisations (Dunning, 1995) with the power to speak on behalf of older people. Indeed it has been argued (McCormack and Ford, 1999) that the history of nursing older people has taken a similar path to that of services for older people in general, resulting in significant challenges to the development of its professional identity.

Nursing Developments

The changing status of nursing in society is widely documented in historical and sociological nursing texts (e.g. Dingwall *et al*, 1988; Dingwall and McIntosh, 1978; Baly, 1980). Nursing's inevitable tensions often arise as a result of its search for its autonomy in bureaucratic organisations that sometimes fail to understand the reality of nursing practice (Davies, 1976). Since the introduction of primary nursing - an organisation method based on the principle of one nurse being accountable for the care of an individual patient (Manthey, 1980) the issue of autonomy in nursing practice has come to the fore. The concept of primary nursing is often used as the focus for professional nursing practice and consequently the notion of autonomy has been widely discussed *(for example*, Pearson, 1985; Johns, 1995, 1989; Wright, 1990). Using the medium of primary nursing, nurses have striven to develop a body of knowledge and divorce themselves from medical dominance. Manthey (1980) describes authority, autonomy and accountability as three of the fundamental principles of the role of the primary nurse. However, even such a dynamic structure, can impose internal organisational limits on the practice of professional practitioners. The fact that one nurse is accountable for the care of a patient 24 hours per day, limits the self-direction of professional colleagues. The primary nurse in making all the decisions about the patient's care reduces the decision-making capacity of other nurses in the team. Many references *(for example* Bailey and Mayer, 1980; Binnie, 1988; MacGuire, 1989; Burns, 1988) have highlighted this issue as problematic within the organisation of primary nursing. Further, many references can be found in the literature, describing problems experienced by nurses in attempting to function as an autonomous practitioner while at the same time respecting the autonomy of the individual patient (Brown *et al*, 1992; Lanceley, 1985). Other studies (Pearson, 1985; Johns, 1989) found that when nurses were explicitly allowed to practice in an autonomous way through the medium of primary nursing, for many the concept of 'ownership' became a problem. Pearson (1985) eloquently described the effects of this problem when he stated that ... 'one form of imperialism (medicine) appeared to have been replaced by another (nursing)'. These studies describe the inherent problems experienced by nurses in attempting to integrate organisational autonomy for the profession and individual autonomy in the nurse/patient relationship.

But the two could be integrated, with the practice of the latter becoming the foundation stone on which to build the former. It is argued that the essence of nursing lies in the nature of the nurse/patient relationship (Singleton and Nail, 1984; Yarling and McElmurry, 1990; Johns, 1994). Singleton and Nail (1984) argue that the nurse can achieve considerable autonomy through her interactions and relationship with the patient. They suggest that the freedom to control one's practice is directly correlated with the responsibility one takes in initiating nursing actions. They outline such practices as the therapeutic use of self, therapeutic questioning, being available for the patient, explaining care, dealing with intimate aspects of care in a sensitive and individualised manner and observing expressions that infer a need, as practices for which nurses can exercise considerable autonomy.

This focus on the essence of nursing autonomy being located in the nurse-patient relationship is evident in contemporary nursing literature, with the view that the foundation of this relationship is a commitment to humanistic caring (*for example*, Watson, 1988; Johns, 1994; Newman, 1994; Boykin and Schoenhofer, 1993). The dominant philosophical shift has been away from traditional notions of 'care as service' (Bradshaw, 1994), dominated by Nightingale's notion of the character of the nurse. In contrast, it is argued that contemporary nursing theory is dominated by a humanistic existentialist philosophy (Conway, 1996).

The move towards such a humanistic ideal in health care represents a rejection of previously accepted behaviourist approaches. Previous passive deterministic views of the patient as expressed by such theorists as Parsons (1954) are rejected within a humanistic caring philosophy. Humanism represents a philosophy that emphasises an individual's uniqueness and freedom to choose a particular course of action. Behaviour is not a response to unconscious forces or to external stimuli, but to the individual's perception, interpretation and comprehension of external stimuli. Humanism suggests that as we are the only ones who can know our perceptions, we are therefore the best experts on ourselves (Rogers, 1961). We each have first hand experience of ourselves as persons and therefore have the ability to understand our own self-concept. Such an ideal is evident in much of the nursing literature and is manifested through discussion of concepts such as partnership (Christensen, 1993), empowerment (Connelly *et al*, 1993), friendship (Trygstad, 1986) and intimacy (Savage, 1995). Campbell (1984) on challenging the representation of nursing as mothering suggests that if the analogy of nursing as mothering is allowed to go unchallenged, then the autonomy of the patient quickly suffers. Campbell suggests that given such a representation, instead of nursing offering a means of appropriate support at a time of need, it can become a subtle means of control and the perpetuation of helplessness, with the patient being treated as a baby who can never grow up and gain any kind of independence. Bradshaw (1995) argues that despite talk of 'patient-centredness', contemporary nursing development relies on personal and professional self-fulfillment and advancement.

Indeed Johns (1995; 262) argues that autonomy is not a helpful concept within a humanistic perspective of care as 'commitment to another person'. He questions how an individualistic notion of autonomy can be helpful in a nurse-patient relationship that is based on principles of connectedness and partnership (Gilligan, 1982). Whilst Johns' arguments perpetuate an individualistic and rights based understanding of autonomy as manifested in consumer ideology, he does highlight the importance of organisational structures and roles supporting a person-centred approach to practice that empowers individual nurses to practice in this way. Indeed Kitson (1996) argues that:

> nursing needs to demonstrate its commitment through innovative schemes that bring together its essential ingredients - empowering, enabling and educating people to take control of their lives.

Fulford's (1996) holistic notion of 'patient-centredness' offers one approach to bringing such an ideal alive through the balancing of patient autonomy (patient-power model) and the professional's understanding of their needs. However, in adopting such a position, Fulford and others (*for example*, Johns, 1995) assume a position that autonomy has a universalised meaning in health care and that health care practitioners understand approaches to its operationalisation. While autonomy appears to be a constant variable within professional-client relationships, which helps to define trust and self-respect, it would appear that nurses (and others) need to be sufficiently astute to recognise the subtle changes in behaviour, emotion and feeling that emerge when working in a patient-centred way, in order to be able to initiate appropriate action. The current emphasis on patient-centred care however, can be seen to represent a shift in emphasis from individualistic and economically driven health care agendas, to a position where the humanity of the patient is given greater emphasis (Department of Health, 1997; CSAG, 1998).

Patient-Centred Practice

The political force of consumerism, coupled with emerging philosophies among practitioners that people should be valued as individuals, has led to the contemporary 'speak' of patient-centred practice (Fulford, Ersser and Hope, 1996). Central to the notions of consumerism and its presentation in health care as patient centredness, are issues of rights and social justice. Indeed it could be asserted that it was the recognition of these values as fundamental to health care and the rejection of paternalism that began the movement towards health care having an explicit 'patient' orientation. This may seem like a paradoxical assertion, but the historical development of health care clearly demonstrates a closed professional orientation, rather than one that focuses on the particular needs of the patient (Bradshaw, 1995; Judge, 1996). Indeed Downie (1986) argues that it is not necessarily a commitment to ethical education in medicine that has resulted in the raising of standards of professional practice, but it is as a result of consumer pressures, internal competition, a better éducated public, journalistic investigations and other 'market oriented' devices. The collectivist notion of 'patient', where needs were met in accordance with general principles of behaviour, has been the prevailing practice norm.

Both Judge (1996) and Fulford (1996) highlight the contradiction inherent in the term 'patient-centred health care'. If health care is not aimed at benefiting patients, then what is its central purpose? Fulford suggests that the change is one of philosophy and a shift of focus on the power relationship between the professional and patient. Respect for persons is central to the notion of patient-centredness and is rooted in a Kantian ideal of mutual respect and sympathetic benevolence (Richards, 1989). Therefore, the rights of individuals as persons would be the driving force behind patient-centred health care. It represents an attitude of respect for ordinary individuals to make rational decisions and determine their own ends. The idea of respecting the patient's right to self-determination has resulted in a shift in thinking about the role of the patient in health care decision making. Fulford (1996) suggests that this philosophical shift requires health care to think beyond concepts of 'cure' based on scientific 'facts', to the adoption of a more holistic approach that also incorporates 'values'. In such an approach, values as well as facts 'are woven together into the very fabric of every aspect of health care' (Fulford, 1996: 13). The approach acknowledges the complementarity of science and the humanities, disease categories and patient's experiences, technological care and primary care and the patient's wishes with the professional's understanding of their needs.

Yet in a complex relationship between professionals and consumers, competing demands on health care resources can violate the principle of autonomy, or at best, make it difficult to follow. The nature of professional health care practice has subsequently been questioned and the professions have needed to assert themselves in order to meet consumer demand and adopt 'new' ways of working - new ways, that mean less control over knowledge and expertise and a drive towards a greater sense of 'openness' (Hugman, 1991). As a result, the assumption that respect for patient autonomy is implicit in professional practice has been exposed and the nature of professional power challenged (Porter, 1996; Hugman, 1991). Consumer politics has demanded such a change to occur in the professions, with the ability to demonstrate professional accountability to the customer, consumer and statutory bodies, being one of the main concerns of the contemporary professional. Coles (1993) cites examples from health care, education and law, to illustrate the growing dissatisfaction among professionals at the process of change in professional practice:

> A midwife told me that she had been informed she was now a profit centre and her unit would be closed down if she hadn't a throughput of so many babies.

This conflict of values, from one of 'care' an one hand to one of 'profit margins' on the other permeates the professions collectively and is one of the predominant catalysts of change to the present social order. All these changes have required professionals to re-evaluate their practice and the meaning of professional autonomy. The prevailing culture of paternalism in health care has led critics to ask if indeed it is the nature of professional training to inoculate practitioners from patients' real needs and prey on the rhetoric of thinking and believing that they know better than people themselves what is good for them (Brown *et al*, 1992).

Conclusions

This chapter has traced the development of patient-centred health care in the United Kingdom's National Health Service. It has highlighted the way autonomy has been considered in such developments and although autonomy is not the only important concept in the organisation and delivery of health care, it is considered to be central to the prevention of paternalism. It is apparent throughout the consumerist and patient-centred literature that an implicit assumption concerning autonomy as 'individualism' prevails and it is from this approach that much of the debate about service provision and clinical practice emerge. However, in determining the philosophical basis of autonomy in a health care context, it is necessary to explore the concept through an analysis of the philosophical literature.

3 Philosophical Foundations

Introduction

There is a large and diverse literature relating to the concept of autonomy. But while this may be so, it is evident from the previous analysis of current issues in the organisation of health services and in health care practice that a prevailing understanding of the concept of autonomy as 'individualism' exists - an understanding that appears to be based on the rights of individuals to make decisions about their health care needs, but with interference by health care practitioners being seen as paternalistic practice. However, it has been identified that if an aim of professional nursing practice is to develop therapeutic relationships with patients then a 'rights based' approach to autonomy is unworkable, as it results in the inevitable tension between nurses' professional autonomy to make independent decisions and the rights of individual patients to be the final arbiters of decisions about their care needs. Autonomy from this perspective is therefore understood as 'independence or self-determination', i.e. the freedom to do what one wants to do.

This chapter challenges this perception of autonomy, through an analysis of the concept from a number of philosophical perspectives. The chapter begins with a discussion about the relationship between autonomy and freedom. The discussion concerning the concept of freedom is used as the basis for exploring the various conceptual understandings of autonomy that exist, as it is argued that autonomy is a desirable attribute of persons (*for example* Beauchamp and Childress, 1983). It is through an exploration of the concept of a person that two perspectives of autonomy are identified:

contextualised perspectives understandings of the concept that consider 'context' as an important factor in determining a person's capacity to be autonomous.

universalist perspectives understandings of the concept based on universal principles or laws that are applied in all cases irrespective of context.

It is from these two perspectives that the concept of autonomy will be explored later in this chapter.

The Concept of a Person and Freedom of the 'Will'

There is a sense in which the word 'person' is merely the singular form of 'people' and in which both terms represent no more than membership of a certain biological species. However the word 'person' is of greater interest than this, and instead it aims to capture those attributes of persons which represent our humanness and the factors which we regard as the most important and the most challenging in our lives. Kant's second formula of the Categorical Imperative presents a doctrine of the supreme and equal value of persons, with moral, political and religious principles. To be a person requires an understanding of one's own state of consciousness and experiences and, in having such, one is able to ascribe similar states of consciousness to others (Ayer, 1964).

Frankfurt (1989) argues that it is not enough to claim that human beings are different from other species on the basis of a collection of physical and psychological attributes. It is conceptually possible that members of another species could lay claim to personhood. If attributes such as sight, taste, smell, sexuality, memory, desires, motives etcetera, were to be used as a means of classifying persons from animals, then we could easily provide a list of members of other species who would possess similar attributes. Indeed even such higher order attributes as 'thought' and decision-making fail to distinguish persons from other creatures. Human beings are not alone in having desires and preferences. Members of other species share these attributes with human beings and some species could even be seen to base action on deliberation and even prior thought.

Indeed Frankfurt (1989) argues that this kind of higher order thinking is not unique to human beings and he postulates that it is indeed an assumption on the part of humans to believe that the uniqueness of persons is found in a set of characteristics that are generally supposed to be uniquely human. Frankfurt suggests that this may not be the case, and in the case of some animal species, higher order thinking involving deliberation and sophisticated decision making can be seen (language and rational deliberation, for example). This of course can be seen to be the basis of the arguments put forward by 'animal lovers' who would argue that animals have the same rights to life as humans. As a result, Frankfurt (1989; 64) is led to assert that:

> It is my view that one essential difference between persons and other creatures is to be found in the structure of a person's will.

But it is not the 'will' in the Kantian tradition that Frankfurt describes, as many of the higher order characteristics of persons can be found in other creatures. What distinguishes persons from other creatures is the:

> ... peculiarly characteristic of humans, .. that they are able to form what I shall call 'second-order desires' or 'desires of the second order' (Frankfurt, 1989,64).

It is the ability to engage in reflective evaluation of action that according to this theory distinguishes persons from other creatures. Other creatures are able to have the capacity for 'first order desires', i.e. 'desires to do or not to do one thing or another'. But according to Frankfurt's theory, it is a peculiar human trait to not just *want*, choose or be moved to action, but to also *want* to have (or not to have) certain desires and motives. Persons are capable of wanting to be different in their preferences and purposes from what they are, i.e. 'second-order desires' or 'desires of the second order' (Frankfurt, 1989). Through this reflection, an individual is able to derive a set of principles which guide one through life and determine what one should do in particular situations. In this way the individual is able to see life as a whole.

Frankfurt addresses the elusive notion of *wanting* to do this or that. Being free and acting autonomously is often seen as being able to do what one wants to do. While this position goes some way towards describing freedom, it would be quite easy to describe other species in this way too. What this description misses is the notion of the *will*. Animals (who are free) can run in whatever direction they wish. Therefore having the freedom to act is a sufficient condition of being free, but not a necessary one. The freedom to make a free choice would be seen as 'negative freedom' by Berlin (1992). Berlin outlines two differing concepts of 'freedom' - *negative freedom*: being free to do what one wants to do or 'freedom from' (suppression, *for example*) and *positive freedom*: the freedom to live a prescribed form of life or 'freedom to' make decisions as a thinking, willing, active being, bearing responsibility for one's own choices and being able to explain them through reference to one's own ideas and purposes:

> I wish to be an instrument of my own, not other men's acts of will. I wish to be a subject, not an object .... deciding, not being decided for, self-directed and not acted upon by external nature or by other men as if I were a thing, or an animal, or a slave incapable of playing a human role, that is, of conceiving goals and policies of my own and realising them (Berlin, 1992, 131).

Berlin presents the individual in society as a self-determined actor, contributing to and creating the social world, through the making of rational choices and the recognition of authentic desires. Even though a person may be no longer free to do what he wants to do (because of a disabling illness *for example)* his *'will'* may remain as free as he was before. Although the person cannot turn his desires into actions, he is still free to form those desires and determine possible actions as freely as if his freedom of action had not been impaired (Frankfurt, 1989: 70). Therefore having a free will is not about the relationship between what one does and what one wants to do, but rather it is about having the desires that one wants - 'positive freedom'. Autonomy in this sense refers to more than the actual psychological condition of self-determination, but instead is a right to be treated in certain ways - the right to be treated as a person, as a master of one's own body, as a master of one's own decisions and as the maker of choices.

But is it ever possible to have such total freedom, considering Feinberg's assertion that individual autonomy is commensurate with the freedom one is accorded as a member of a community? As Feinberg (1989, 45) asserts:

> the ideal of the autonomous person is that of an authentic individual whose self determination is as complete as is consistent with the requirement that he is, of course, a member of a community.

In this statement, Feinberg invokes the 'no man [sic] is an island' analogy and argues against the idea of the autonomous person being equated with having 'negative freedom'. He argues that it is impossible for a human being to live in such isolation that they are free from any kind of socialisation or influence from society. Later in this chapter autonomy as a 'competency' (Meyers, 1989) will be discussed and will be seen to further develop Feinberg's rejection of the self-ruling individual who is free from external influence. However, throughout Feinberg's descriptions of the various manifestations of the concept of autonomy, the claim that there is an important *core* idea of individual independence remains undisturbed.

When formulating his second formula, Kant appeared to be quite clear about the notion of 'person':

> Act in such a way that you always treat humanity, whether in your own person or in the person of any other, never simply as a means, but always at the same time as an end (Paton, 1964).

In differentiating between persons and things, Kant suggests that if things have any value at all, then it is merely extrinsic value. That is, things (whether of natural or artificial origin) are only regarded as artificially good, insofar as someone happens to desire them and regard them as valuable. It follows that things have a price, i.e. their value is determined by the price that someone is willing to pay for them; and as artifacts can be exchanged for things of equal or relative value then it clearly has no unique, absolute, intrinsic worth. If things can be measured in terms of money, then money is regarded as the ultimate standard of value (Sullivan, 1990). What though, does it mean for persons to exist 'as an end in themselves'? As Kant explains, things and animals are only contingently desired (or feared) by and so possibly valued (or given a negative value) by someone. Kant argues that while persons have conditional value, such as being nice, good, likeable, loveable or useful, persons should always be regarded as having objective, absolute and intrinsic worth, whether or not they also happen to be valued because they contribute to another's happiness. But one can imagine situations where people are not treated as their own end - treatment decisions based on cost rather than on effects on individual quality of life, the attribution of salary to particular work roles and social class division, are examples of people not being treated as their own end. In the context of this book, the potential for older people to be treated as a 'thing' is great, given the potential impact of institutionalisation (Goffman, 1961). The reflections on my early practice experiences (Chapter 1) can be seen to represent an example of people not being treated as their own end. It is the 'moral personality' that gives persons status and it is this *humanity* that distinguishes persons from other species:

> It is because of being under the moral law that each and every person has an intrinsic, inalienable, unconditional, objective worth or dignity as a person. By virtue of that law we are elevated above being merely part of the natural world. We have an absolute and irreplaceable worth for our value is not dependent on our usefulness or desirability. It has no price or no equivalent for which the object of esteem could be exchanged. We may never renounce our right to respect, and we ought never act in such a way as to reduce either ourselves or others to the status of mere things (Sullivan, 1990, 197).

This plea to the intrinsic moral good of personhood represents a universal moral principle that extends beyond politics, religion, wealth or privilege. Everyone desires to lead a good life and therefore has the capacity to reason morally. Possessing such an ideal is central to Kantian autonomy. Freedom of the will does not mean the freedom to do whatever one wants as a free agent. Instead, moral considerations need to be made. Freedom of the will is a moral freedom, based on a worldview where the person can:

> ... identify with his motivating influences, assimilates them to himself, views himself as a kind of person who wishes to be moved in particular ways and that these influences are the ones he wishes to be identified with (Dworkin, 1989).

So far in this discussion, freedom (and *ipso facto* autonomy) has been discussed from an 'either - or' perspective, i.e., the individual either being free or not and thence the individual being autonomous or not. But what happens to autonomy if I do not wish to exercise the full range of my freedom? Autonomy can be seen as one such desire in a range of human desires. For example, when making a difficult decision I may choose not to exercise the full extent of my freedom to decide, because I may not want to accept full responsibility for the outcome of the decision, thus limiting my autonomy in choosing courses of action. Therefore I may vary in different periods of my life, how much autonomy I may wish to exercise and in some cases may only exercise partial autonomy. So, in this sense the concept of autonomy has something to do with the notion of preferences and whether or not the whole person is autonomous is dependent on the freedom of the individual to make independent, rational choices. Young (1980) argues that a person who may be free to perform a particular action, may fail to do so because of a desire to do some alternative action of lesser importance that may ultimately interfere with and frustrate his pursuit of what he would acknowledge to be more significant and more authentically 'him'. To Young (1980), this situation represents weakness of the will and he suggests that before the individual can lay claim to autonomy the chosen desire must be part of a 'unified life plan':

> Where there is no inner unity because the self is divided and torn over which projects to engage in or what order to engage in them there will be no unified life.

The importance of a life plan in the context of autonomy will be discussed later in this chapter. The view that autonomy might be understood in terms of 'the degree' to which it exists in any situation rather than the view that a person either is autonomous or is not is important to this research and the care of older people in hospital. For a variety of reasons (such as, physical disability, mental confusion, disorientation, ignorance or fear) older people may not choose to exercise their full capacity for decision-making. However, they may exercise autonomy in some situations and not others or may feel more autonomous about some decisions than others. The context of the relationship between the patient and the health care team would impact on the way such degrees of autonomy were facilitated and enabled. These perspectives will be developed later.

It has been argued so far, that the word 'person' is of greater significance than the mere possession of a set of physiological and psychological characteristics. Persons are seen as possessing a will that enables rational deliberation on action. However, a distinction has also been made between 'negative' and 'positive' freedom (Berlin, 1992). A complete concept of freedom includes not only the right to do something, but also the ability to take responsibility for rational choices in a way that contributes to and creates the social world. The contrasting themes of 'individual freedom' to do 'what one wants' as a self-governing agent, and 'moral freedom' based on universal principles, are central to the various manifestations of the concept of autonomy and these will be developed in the remaining sections of this chapter. What is clear from the various theoretical perspectives is that there is a core idea of freedom in the concept of autonomy.

Autonomy: Contextualised Perspectives

This notion of personal autonomy derives from an understanding of the concept as one's capacity for self-determination or self-governance. Originating in the Greek word *autos* (meaning 'self') and *nomos* (meaning 'rule' 'governance' or 'law') with the literal meaning of 'the having or making of one's own laws', the concept of autonomy has been translated from a term that was originally used to describe a state's ability to self-govern and be independent of another's laws, to one that refers to an individual's ability and capacity to make self-determined decisions. Approaches to this understanding of personal autonomy include:

- autonomy as second order reflection (Dworkin, 1989, 1991);
- autonomy as an end state or a side constraint (Childress, 1982);
- autonomy as 'competency' (Meyers, 1989);
- autonomy as 'care' (Gilligan, 1977, 1979, 1982).

All of these perspectives are considered under the broad heading of 'contextualised perspectives' as there is a consideration of 'context' as an important factor in determining a person's capacity to be autonomous.

Autonomy as Second-Order Reflection

Dworkin (1989, 1991), building on the work of Frankfurt (1989) and his understanding of the concept of a person (i.e. freedom of the will and the ability to engage in second-order reflection on action), has taken a hierarchical approach to autonomy and defines it as:

> ... a second-order capacity to reflect critically upon one's first-order preferences and desires, and the ability either to identify with these or to change them in the light of higher-order preferences and values (Dworkin, 1991, 108).

The autonomous person is one who cares about his 'will' to the extent that he examines whether or not a first order desire (lower-order) would be appropriate. In this way a person exercises freedom of the will when he acts upon the first-order desires that he wants to have. If however, there exists some discrepancy between the first and second order desires then he lacks such freedom.

The approach to self-evaluation needs to be independent in order to constitute personal autonomy. This independence must occur on two fronts - independence from manipulative forces (coercive persuasion and strong prudential desire for example) and from the impact of others (for example, being manipulated into a particular action by another person). When a person acts autonomously, he doesn't act upon a desire that he rejects or would reject nor does he act vicariously. Instead, the autonomous person identifies with his desires, goals, beliefs and values and that the process of identification must be one that can be defended by the individual and based on universal principles (procedural independence) - principles that enable persons to see their life as a whole and evaluate a whole way of living one's life (critical reflection). In this way the person acts on authentic desires that are based on universal principles that have been critically reflected upon and integrated into one's life. It requires the person to distinguish those conditions that restrict and subvert their critical and reflective faculties from those that enhance and improve them. In this sense autonomy is extracted from the narrow view of being free to do what one wants to do at particular points in time to a more global view of life as a whole. Therefore Dworkin's full formula for autonomy is

AUTONOMY = Authenticity + Procedural Independence

The notion of procedural independence as described by Dworkin is criticised for being vague (Thalberg, 1989; Watson, 1989; Christman, 1989). Critical reflection takes place when an agent reflects on a desire and, at the higher level, approves of having the desire. Watson (1989) highlights how the having of a higher-order desire to have another lower-order desire is not sufficient to pick out the special character of autonomous desires. For example a patient whom, although having a desire to stay in hospital for necessary treatment and care, may have another desire to be at home. Such a person has higher-order disapproval of his lower-order desire, resulting in a conflict of desires, at different levels. Watson (1989) argues that this is an unsatisfactory position, as it amounts to nothing more than a conflict of desires without clarification of their autonomy. Christman (1989) suggests that the process of critical reflection has to be seen either as simple acknowledgement of one's desires, or an evaluation of the desires one finds oneself with. Neither position clarifies whether an action was autonomous or not and therefore Christman is led to conclude that the only way identification can be a useful concept is if it includes an endorsement of the desire. This then would rule out the possibility of having an autonomous desire one doesn't approve of (Christman, 1989).

Authenticity in Dworkin's model requires persons to have desires that can be identified as their own. Christman (1989) identifies what he refers to as the 'threat to regress' as a potential problem within the model. He suggests that it is unclear how one can approve one's second-order desires without drawing on further desires and therefore creating a hierarchy of desires, that is, third-order desires, fourth-order desires, etcetera. Childress (1982) suggests that such arguments as this are fruitless unless attention is paid to differences that result from viewing autonomy as *an end state* (or goal) as opposed to *a side constraint* (or restraining factor).

Autonomy as 'End State' or 'Side Constraint'

Drawing on the work of Nozick (1974), Childress (1982) argues that if autonomy is a side constraint (that is a concept that restrains action), then it limits the pursuit of goals such as health and survival and autonomy itself. In pursuing goals for ourselves or for others we are not permitted to violate others' autonomy. Given this approach one could not take life saving action on an unconscious patient without violating the person's autonomy and all action would be paternalistic in nature. In contrast, when autonomy is viewed as an end state to be realised it has a very different function:

> Autonomy is a condition, not a constraint, and the goal might be to minimise damage to autonomy whether that damage results from nature, disease, or other persons (Childress, 1982, 65).

Taking this approach, some violations of autonomy (such as resuscitating an unconscious patient) would be justified because overall more autonomy would result and that is the desired end state. The confusion that Childress refers to is evident in health care literature and results in a misunderstanding of the concept of autonomy as self-governance and the ensuing suggestion that the concept of autonomy itself is not particularly useful (Johns, 1991) in health care practice because of its emphasis on individual independence. This understanding of autonomy appears to view autonomy as implicitly selfish based on prudential wants or desires, rather than a universal desire to lead a good life.

However, Childress (1982) does not agree that autonomy should be pursued as *the ideal* end state. Patients may autonomously choose not to pursue autonomy as an end state and while pursuit of another's autonomy as an end state may be an important goal of altruistic beneficence, it is the patient who should determine how important it is. What is unclear from Childress' argument however, is how health care workers deal with situations where an individual's autonomy is reduced, e.g. the unconscious, the delirious or the dementing patient. Further, the complexity of many health care decisions (as is often presented as the argument against consumerism, patients' access to their health records and patient participation in decision-making), coupled with the stresses and fears of illness, with their related anxiety, dependency and regressive tendencies, means that a patient's ordinary decision-making abilities are often significantly diminished. Lindley (1986) argues for treating autonomy as a 'goal' rather than a constraint, on the grounds that there are situations (such as the dementing patient) where it would seem implausible not to be justified in violating autonomy in order to avoid adverse consequences.

It is precisely from this position that Weiss (1985) argues for the notion of paternalism in health care and Buchanan and Brock (1989) argue that if patients hold the ultimate responsibility for their health care decisions, then their treatment choices may fail to serve their well-being as conceived by patients. Thus they argue, the same value of patient well-being that requires patients' participation in their own health care decisions may sometimes also require persons to be protected from the harmful consequences to them of their own choices. When considered in practice, the risk to autonomous decision-making by patients from paternalistic health care workers is significant. Both Weiss (1985) and Buchanan and Brock (1989) fail to recognise the issue of partnership in decision-making. Siegler (1977) and Szasz and Hollander (1956) assert that the means of preventing such action is by having a clear picture of what the patient really values about their life and how they make sense of the things happening to them. Pellegrino (1979) refers to this as the patient's *value history*, where decisions regarding the diagnosis and treatment are made consistent with their value history.

In considering such a 'value history' the health care practitioner takes into account 'quality of life judgements'. Whether a particular treatment is in the patient's best interest depends on how it affects the patient's life. The choices that the patient makes regarding a particular course of action or treatment depend upon whether life under the conditions that would exist if the care in question were provided would be worth living for the patient:

> Quality of life judgements are unavoidable because whether life would be worth living for the patient depends not only upon the length of time that life would be extended but also upon the character of the life for the patient during that period (Buchanan and Brock, 1989; 123).

In such cases it would appear more desirable to work towards the ideal of autonomy as an end state as the patient may not have the capacity to exercise their right to autonomy. It is from such a position that Meyers (1989) develops her understanding of autonomy as 'competency'.

Autonomy as 'Competency'

Through the adoption of a feminist perspective Meyers (1989) argues that approaches to understanding autonomy such as that of Dworkin (1991), Childress (1982) and Lindley (1986) are sterile because they treat autonomy as a special case of free will:

> Construing autonomy as a form of free will implies that the problem of autonomy is primarily an ontological question that raises subsidiary procedural questions. On this understanding, autonomy will be unintelligible unless a free agent can be found (Meyers, 1989; 42).

Meyers argues that in this sense, a free agent is one who hasn't been 'tainted by socialisation'. In the adoption of a psychoanalytic perspective of personal growth and development, Meyers (1989) argues that persons are not free from influences of socialisation and that therefore the notion of a free will can only exist if an individual is able to transcend the influences of socialisation. The expectation that autonomous people are not people who 'do what they want' but people who 'do what they *really* want' is daunting.

Instead, Meyers (1989) suggests that autonomous people have 'autonomous life plans'. A life plan is a 'comprehensive projection of intent', i.e. a conception of what a person wants to do in life (Meyers, 1989: 49). A life plan must include at least one activity that the person wants to pursue, or a value that the person wants to advance or an emotional bond that the person wants to sustain. As most people have a variety of activities, values and emotions that they would wish to be identified with, then typically a life plan would consist of an ordering of assorted desires and concerns and some ordering of their priority, so that they can invest time and energy appropriately:

> Typically a life plan couples an ordering of assorted concerns and objectives with some notion of how to initiate progress toward fulfilling some of them and detailed schemes for ensuring the successful realization of others (Meyers, 1989: 49).

The approach adopted by Meyers, starts from the position that everyone possesses autonomy as an 'inborn potential', but that individuals learn how to exercise it through social experience. Autonomy as a competency then is the securing of an 'integrated personality', i.e. an authentic personality that is not imposed. A life plan is not merely a list of objectives with a plan and strategies for carrying them out. Instead a life plan enables reflection on life goals within the context of achieving an integrated personality. Being autonomous is to live in harmony with one's authentic self without one's life projects persistently violating one's current life plan. Life plans evolve over time, with new experiences that are consistent with one's life plan being integrated into one's personality in order to create future goals and projects. It is through the possession of such a life plan that Holmes and Lindley (1991) adopt a view of autonomy that has been described by Hope (1992) as the 'Russian Doll' model of autonomy. On the outside there is the obvious person, with one's overt desires and choices. But this outer self is not necessarily free as it is constrained by hidden emotions. The outer doll must be chipped away to bring the inner emotions into view and one will then locate the inner doll, the authentic self. It is the choices made by the authentic self that must be realised if autonomy is to be respected. As Hope (1992; 9) identifies, the implications of such a representation of autonomy are important for patient care. It suggests that the nurse cannot take at face value the choices made by the patient:

> For, normally, when it is said that patients' wishes should be respected (even if this is apparently not in their interests) what is being considered is what patients say they want. To ensure maximum autonomy, the patient should not be constrained by external factors, and the patient should be properly informed about the consequences of the various possible choices (Hope, 1992, 9).

Holmes and Lindley (1991) argue for a type of partnership in autonomous decision making that is based on the guiding principle of neither what the nurse thinks is best for the patient, nor what the patient at first seems to want, but whatever will help the patient to minimise factors that would reduce real autonomy (*for example*, emotional state, lack of knowledge, conflict of interests and motives). It further reinforces autonomy as seeing life as a whole and the role of the nurse in helping the patient to be properly and sufficiently informed, identifying with his desires, goals, beliefs and values in order to make the most appropriate choices in care. The concept of a life plan as described by Meyers (1989) can be seen to facilitate the achievement of such a partnership between the nurse and patient.

Autonomous people must be able to pose and answer the question 'What do I really want, need, care about, believe, value etc'. To do this Meyers (1989) describes a complex process of self-reflection in the formation and re-evaluation of life plans. Drawing on the work of Rawls (1971) she suggests that the two processes of 'rational choice' and 'deliberative rationality' are utilised as the means of reflecting on one's life plan and deciding on a course of conduct that best fits with that plan. This rational approach requires individuals to know what things are important to them, estimate the relative intensity of their desires, order their preferences consistently and envisage alternative plans of action. The account of the authentic self that emerges from this account of autonomy is one that is shaped by social experience as well as individual choice (Meyers, 1989).

Autonomy as 'Care'

Gilligan (1977, 1979, 1982) appears to support such a view when she argues for an approach to autonomy based on principles of 'care' rather than 'rights'. Gilligan's theory of moral development has been formulated through her research into the differences between women and men's approach to moral decision-making and her rejection of Kohlberg's (1981) 'rights based' theory of moral development, because of its misunderstanding of women's psychological development. She sees the psychology of women as being distinctive in its orientation towards relationships and interdependence whereas rights, justice and fairness dominate the psychology of men. The moral position that emerges according to Gilligan (1982; 100) is that women have a dominant injunction to care, a responsibility to alleviate the real and recognisable trouble of the world. For men the dominant injunction is to respect the rights of others and thus to protect from interference the rights to life and self-fulfillment. In terms of autonomy then, Gilligan argues for a 'responsibility-based' approach as contrasted with an individualistic, rights based approach as described by Kohlberg. She suggests that instead of pursuing autonomy from a universalist position where the emphasis is on the rights of the individuals involved, that a position of 'attachment' should be achieved where the emphasis is on an 'ethic of care' (Gilligan, 1982; 164):

> The morality of rights is predicated on equality and centred on the understanding of fairness, while the ethic of responsibility relies on the concept of equity, the recognition of differences in need. While the ethic of right is a manifestation of equal respect, balancing the claims of other and self, the ethic of responsibility rests on an understanding that gives rise to compassion and care.

In the context of a relationship, moral problems arise because of conflicting responsibilities rather than competing rights. Moral problems require an approach to problem solving that considers the context of the problem and the individual's narrative - that is, their beliefs and values, rather than 'formal and abstract' (that is, based on universal principles and rules).

Gilligan (1982; 147) views a 'rights based' approach to moral decision making with its emphasis on the protection of individual rights as a simplistic approach to understanding complex problem solving, and a failure to recognise the dynamics of relationships:

> Since moral problems arise in situations of conflict where either way I go, something or someone will not be served, their resolution is not just a simple yes or no decision ...

Effective decision-making comes from working through everything one thinks is involved and important in the situation, and taking responsibility for the choice made. This approach by Gilligan can be seen to be similar to Dworkin's (1991) notion of 'critical-reflection' in autonomous decision-making. In seeing individual lives as connected and embedded in relationship to others, Gilligan suggests the notion of 'collective life' (p147) whereby responsibility includes both self and other, viewed as different but connected rather than as separate and opposed.

When applied to the context of patient care, Gilligan's approach emphasises the importance of attachment between the nurse and the patient and a relationship that enables patients to fulfil their true potential based on their unique value system. Gilligan's theory of autonomy based on a morality of responsibility is supported in a number of theories of 'caring' (Noddings, 1984; Mayeroff, 1971). Noddings argues that in a caring relationship, 'motivational displacement' (p16) is necessary, whereby the carer views the objectives of care from the viewpoint of the one being cared for and adopts these objectives as her own. Heidegger (1990) refers to this approach to care as 'engagement', whereby the carer and the one being cared for are in harmony through a mutual agreement about the motives for care. Noddings (1984; 25) however, does address the problem of the caring relationship moving from a position of attachment to one based on rights with an emphasis on abstract problem solving. In the latter position, the focus is not on the person being cared for, but on the problem. An objective attitude prevails where decisions are made against competing rights. Noddings argues that in such a relationship, only an illusion of care exists because the connectedness between the carer and the one being cared for is missing due to the neglect of the context and the individual's narrative.

In contrast to a universalist perspective of autonomy, contextual accounts consider such factors as individual relationships, emotional state, knowledge and decision making capacity in determining appropriate courses of action. The individual is not viewed as existing in isolation from others, but instead there is a consideration of the importance of interpersonal relationships, thus challenging the idea of autonomy as an individual right 'to do what I want to do'. Contextual accounts of autonomy consider universal principles in moral deliberation as an important element in deciding on the meaning of 'doing good', but only in the context in which such principles are applied. This is a key distinction between contextual accounts and universalist perspectives that view the operationalisation of universal principles as being central to being a moral agent.

Autonomy: A Universalist Perspective

In contrast to considering contextual influences on autonomy, universalist accounts require that all relevant similar cases be treated in a similar way (Beauchamp and Childress, 1983). The works of Immanuel Kant represent a major influence on current understandings of autonomy and the person as a moral agent from a universalist perspective. Kant claimed that if we really are moral agents, then we must be aware of what that means. However, unlike Plato's idea of *the Philosopher King*, Kant does not expect a high degree of articulation and recognises that most of us may only be able to articulate our knowledge in a somewhat disorganised and unclear way. Therefore, he viewed our everyday convictions as the ultimate data for the analysis of morality.

Bradshaw (1994) however, argues that Kant's ethical position relied on the Protestant tradition of the eighteenth-century in which he grew up. She demonstrates how the Kantian tradition that draws on a Judeo-Christian ethic has been highly influential on contemporary nursing theory and practice. Such influence is seen in the focus on the humanity of the patient (Gadow,1990: Watson, 1988; Boykin and Schoenhofer, 1993 *for example*) as the central tenet of the nurse-patient relationship. Nursing addresses the unique needs of patients as persons and this acts as the central ethical concern of nurses (Johns, 1994; Watson, 1988 *for example*). It is this 'everyday' focus of moral decision making that is central to ethical nursing practice and it is argued that the day to day events in this relationship between the nurse and the patient are of greatest ethical concern for nurses (*for example* Carper, 1978; Benner, 1984).

Kant's concept of autonomy considers individualistic ideas of 'doing what I want to do' as untenable in the absence of universalised moral principles. It is important to consider the Kantian position in view of the prevailing health care drive towards consumerism, based on an individualistic notion of 'rights'. The previous section has highlighted the importance of context to the concept of autonomy and has argued against an individualistic rights based position. A further argument against this individualistic position will be presented here, from the perspective of universal moral laws.

Kantian Moral Reasoning and Objectivity

Kant's approach to moral decision-making is founded on his theory of knowledge as articulated in the *Critique of Pure Reason* (Kemp-Smith, 1962). Moral reasoning is objective and therefore is overriding, i.e. has rightful priority over all other interests of individuals and groups (Beck, 1956). The route to deciding on principles for action lies in the central question of Kantian moral deliberation: 'what are the necessary conditions of the moral decisions that we make?'. In order to answer this question, Kant focuses on the word 'ought'.

Reason, according to Kant lies beyond all possible sensory experience and therefore can only originate in our own reason. Unlike prudential principles and actions, autonomous practical reasoning is not based on desire. Therefore reasoning such as, 'I ought not strike a patient because I might get caught', would not be considered as moral reasoning in the Kantian view, as it is based on the selfish desire of not being caught, irrespective of the greater harm caused by the actions. Moral (practical) reasoning concerns what 'ought' to happen, and its objects are those actions that should be performed and ends that should be adopted (categorical ought). It is objective reasoning that determines ethical freedom. It is not the same as what Kant calls 'psychological freedom', which is based on internal and external impediments to doing what one wants to do (hypothetical ought) or what Berlin refers to as 'negative freedom' (Berlin, 1992). Such freedom, according to Kant is inadequate, as it is based on experience and describes only prudential, not moral conduct. To be free means that one must be able to act from moral reason (which must be independent of desire) and independently determine how one should act without relying on desire. Autonomy is much more than thinking for oneself, but requires the moral agent to think from the standpoint of every other person and to think consistently.

In the context of health care consumerism, this is an important assertion. It has been identified in Chapter 2 that health care consumerism is based on the individual's right to make choices about their health care and to be the final arbiter of decisions. However, from a universalist perspective, such a position would be inappropriate unless the choices and decisions made could be accorded to similar cases. Conflicts between the rights of the individual and the need for universal principles in health care decision-making are prevalent in debates about state provision of long-term care (Darton and Wright, 1993), rationing of care provision (Callahan, 1991) and reforms to the provision of community care (Loxley, 1997; Hunter, 1993).

For Kant the moral law does not obtain its objective character by being chosen or willed by a person, but demands the person to act on that maxim which can be willed as a universal law. While one ought to act morally according to universal principles, it is difficult to ascertain from Kant what the outcome for persons is, should one's actions not match the moral intention. The ultimate test of objectivity in moral reasoning is the test of universalisability of maxims. According to Kant, the law of autonomy is a universal law stated as:

> act only on that maxim through which you can at the same time will that it should become a universal law.

Kant calls this the supreme principle of right, as it obligates recognition and respect for the right of every other person to choose and act autonomously. When acting as an autonomous practitioner within the Kantian view, the law of autonomy is both the ultimate law of morality and the ultimate law of pure practical rationality. Therefore what Kant is proposing is an *a priori law* of autonomy, that everyone can know and the obligations it generates. The making of *bad* moral decisions is seen as resulting from unscrupulous decision-making and bad moral character. Kant did not wish to rule out the possibility of a person making an 'honest mistake' in moral reasoning, without being an evil person. Therefore errors in Kantian ethics are seen as errors in reasoning, as a result of a 'crude and unpracticed judgement' (White Beck, 1956). The *categorical imperative* acts as the test by which to judge the universalisability of moral maxims.

The Categorical Imperative

Kant presents the categorical imperative as a means of telling people what *not* to do, e.g. not to tell lies, break promises, commit suicide. But MacIntyre (1992) argues that the categorical imperative appears to be silent when it comes to telling us what we *ought* to do. From where are moral maxims derived in the first instance? From where does the nurse derive her view of humanity, justice, and truth, in order to guide moral deliberations? An example of a lack of clear direction for action in Kantian ethics arises in relation to the nurse's motives for caring. What does motivate the nurse to care for the patient? Factors such as 'respect for persons' beneficence, justice or non-maleficence could all motivate the nurse to care. Within the Kantian position, altruistic motives are unreliable as moral motives, for they are transitory and changeable. Blum (1982) argues that one acts according to how one feels - one's moods, impulses and inclinations - and not according to the moral requirements of the situation. Blum raises the important question of the influence of emotion on moral agency. He recognises that feelings for different people differ, sometimes independently of moral action. Such a position is also articulated in theories of caring (Noddings, 1984; Graham, 1991) where the importance of life experience and emotion in the caring relationship are emphasised. The Kantian view would suggest that a moral motive couldn't be unreliable in this way. It adopts the position that moral motives must consistently be available to an individual in order to provide a careful guide to morally right action.

Kant suggests that when a maxim is stated as a universal, it must be stated so that it can apply to all moral agents, in the kinds of circumstances to which it is meant to apply, and not merely promote the interests of particular individuals or groups. This requirement presents particular difficulties for nurses' and patients' autonomy. Although Kant allows for the universality of principles to be applied in particular circumstances, even then it is difficult to see how nurses can do this. For example, how can all patients be expected to participate in their care programmes without considering contextual factors? How can the nurse treat each patient as an individual under the umbrella of a universal law, without considering the idiosyncrasies of each particular case? Cartwright *et al* (1992) argue, that the objective of moral education should be the promotion of the development of an individually endorsed, or autonomously held, normative ethic comprised of a set of well understood and thought-through universal moral principles. Principles relating to preserving the patient's dignity, respecting the patient as a person, allowing the patient access to information and access to appropriate treatments are all seen as universalisable. However, even such 'obvious' humanistic principles as these are fraught with difficulty in practice and each situation presents a new set of dilemmas for the nurse, dilemmas that Gilligan (1982) suggests can only be addressed through the 'connected' relationship between the nurse and patient.

Once the context of decision-making is considered, then the notion of universality becomes problematic. Kant repeatedly suggests that judgements about anyone's actual motivation in moral reasoning are inherently beset by uncertainty. Sullivan (1990) argues that one can never be sure of one's own motives and aims in any particular instance, much less those of others. He goes on to suggest that the best that can be done is to make inferences on the basis of one's own genuine efforts or the behaviour of others, and the best one can hope to achieve is a high degree of probability, or what is referred to as moral certainty. It is from this position that contextualised concepts of autonomy are derived (Dworkin, 1991 *for example*) and leads Meyers (1989) to assert that the important consideration is the way moral decisions concur with one's overall life-plan.

If the best one can hope for is a degree of moral certainty, then this raises particular problems for the nurse who is trying to decide on a course of action 'here and now'. What sort of behaviour is morally required or permissible, given that it is her own reasoning from which her judgement is based and she can never be sure of her aims or motives? Unlike prudential thought moral reasoning is inextricably linked to recognising the existence and thus the autonomy of the other person. The nurse seeks to offer general principles of behaviour that apply to everyone as independent and rational moral agents. The ultimate test of the proposed principle or action is that it could be universalised, that is, it would be acceptable not just to the proposer of the action but also to everyone whom it effected.

Summary

Two perspectives of autonomy have been presented in this chapter - universalised and contextualised positions. The work of Kant offers a comprehensive account of autonomy as a universal principle. Kant reinforces the idea that autonomy is not transient, but represents the supreme principle of morally right action. The central tenet of the Kantian argument is that of the universality of principles that guide morally right action. The categorical imperative determines those principles that should be universalised. However, the Kantian principle of autonomy (namely, being able to engage in moral reasoning on the basis of universalising one's principles) takes one only so far in moral deliberation. For example, a universal position of equality of access to health care on the basis of need rather than ability to pay would be widely supported. However, such a universal principle does not illuminate the moral reasoning needed to operationalise such a universal principle. Further, it does not illuminate the moral dimension that is based on the kind of deliberation relating to highly contextualised interpersonal relationships where 'caring' and 'respect for persons' become very 'concrete' and where it can be seen that a different kind of moral deliberation is needed. For nursing, this can be seen as the nurse achieving a balance between objective moral reasoning and particularising such reasoning to an individual context.

It is from this perspective that contextualised accounts of autonomy arise. Persons are viewed as socialised beings, existing in a community and interacting through complex relationships. Therefore, the simple application of 'right' to complex decisions is seen as inappropriate and misunderstands the interconnectedness of persons. The complexities of human nature and the subtle (and not so subtle) differences in individual circumstances means that such an all-encompassing law as the categorical imperative may not provide the solution to the complexities of interactions in the nurse-patient relationship. Indeed, Penticuff (1991) and Davis (1989) argue that universal principles have failed to help nurses deal with value conflicts in a practice world that is constantly changing and challenging.

Implications for Nursing Practice, Patient Autonomy and Older People in Hospital

It would appear that two opposing decision-making positions are possible. Firstly, as in Rawls' (1992) 'veil of ignorance', the nurse could be expected to act impartially and separate her moral deliberations from her knowledge of the situation. She would be obliged to evaluate the merits of particular actions solely on the basis of general considerations and the law of universality. On the other hand, the nurse could adopt a contextualised position and believe that there is no objective reality on which to base decisions, and that each situation is unique, thus requiring the adoption of a unique set of principles.

Alternatively, a 'compromise position' could be adopted - a position that acknowledges the presence of universal principles that are interpreted to suit the particular decision making context. Such a position would incorporate reflective approaches to deliberation, as highlighted by Dworkin (1991) and values based approaches as articulated by Meyers (1989), Holmes and Lindley (1991) and Hope (1992). Such a position would consider the rights, feelings and views of the other in the context of the nurse-patient relationship.

In the development of his theory of autonomy in the context of long-term care for older people, Agich (1993) argues that the concept of autonomy properly understood requires that individuals be seen in an essential interrelationship with others and the world. Agich argues against a liberal concept of autonomy as independence and noninterference because it fails to address the ethical responsibilities of persons in the everyday world. Agich argues that a focus on independence means that older people are obliged to view any dependence on another as failure and as best avoided. This is further perpetuated in a policy context, through the lack of provision of state-funded long-term care. Older people who have valued independence through the acquiring of financial assets are expected by the state to retain this independence through an expectation that they will pay for their long-term care needs. As Agich (1993; 162) argues:

> long-term care is required precisely because elders experience to some degree a practical loss of functional abilities that we routinely associate with autonomy.

Drawing on the work of Agich, Capitman and Sciegaj (1995) argue that in the context of the care of older people, a 'contextual approach' to autonomy (i.e. an approach that focuses on the relationships among individuals within particular social/institutional contexts) is more consistent with current understandings of how people make moral decisions. It acknowledges that patients and health care professionals are distinctive psychological, social cultural and moral individuals who are in a particular relationship with one another and the care environment. Capitman and Sciegaj (1995) articulate this position when they argue that in order to adequately assess individual autonomy, one must also assess the relationship and context between the individual, other persons and the social institution. In support of Gilligan (1982), Hardwig (1984; 443) argues that there are differences in approaches to morality in the context of relationships. He suggests that an ethic of close personal relations is one of responsibility:

> Rights are impersonally defined ...Rights are general or universal in the sense that anyone in a similar situation can claim the same rights, whereas my relationship to those I am close to is not general or universal, and it cannot be impersonally defined. Rather, my relationship to you, if we are close, is a relationship to you, dependent on and defined by your unique individuality and mine.

Kitson (1993) in supporting a 'compromise position' describes such an approach as '*caring - as ethical - position*'. Kitson (1993; 41) suggests that such an approach demands individual accountability for independent judgements on each case based on the context of where the care is carried out:

> This level of ethical decision making is seen as the most advanced and requires experience and the ability to learn from that experience.

This approach, which is similar to that of Gilligan (1982), acknowledges the need for guiding principles that are interpreted in the context of the particular relationship. It highlights the important place of emotions in decision making, by highlighting the importance of emotional factors being made explicit and acknowledged as influences on the process and outcome of decision-making. Issues such as how much the nurse 'likes' the patient, the individual nurse's personal experiences and the behaviour of the patient are seen as significant. The approach offered by Kitson, explicitly raises the importance of an interpretive decision-making approach that acknowledges universality. Indeed it could be argued that without universality such an individualised approach to decision-making could be seen as normative and fatalistic from the patient's perspective.

Holmes and Lindley (1991) warn against normative approaches in caring situations where the patient is in a potentially weak state and the nurse in a position of power. While Holmes and Lindley's work was directed at therapists, it is clear that a similar argument could be posed for nursing. They argue that the more powerful the nurse's personal qualities, the more the patient may be attracted to them. This power can create a state of dependency to the extent that the patient's autonomy really is put at risk. They suggest that:

> ... there is always the danger that therapeutic dependency may provide opportunities which bad therapists [or nurses] can exploit.

In respect of older people, Haug and Ory (1987) provide a comprehensive list of factors that can contribute to a weakening of the patient's position in patient-provider interactions - including the attitude of the clinician (ageism), social class differences, the care setting, clinicians' focus on the family rather than the patient themselves, communication skill and style, control of information and the older person's socialised view of their 'patient role'. While, in ideal circumstances, the rights of the older patient should be no different from those of younger adults, in reality inequalities prevail in health care provision, in terms of the availability of choices and the ability of the older person to exercise their choice (BMA/RCN, 1995). In the development of their 'consent and care' guidelines for older people, the BMA/RCN acknowledge the need for such guidelines because in the day-to-day reality of working with older people, many situations arise, in which older people, to varying degrees, may be unable to understand, make or express choices. In addition, it is acknowledged that in health care settings, the rights of older people are often ignored and the ability of the older person to dictate the quality of their life overlooked by 'well-intentioned' clinicians. Research by Lanceley (1985) and Koch and Webb (1996) clearly demonstrated the dominance of professional control in care settings.

Doyle (1993) addresses the benefits of universalising human needs/rights and knowledge to nursing in particular. He argues for two essential principles in ethical decision making - the universal duty of good clinical care, using expertise to protect the life and health of the patient to an acceptable standard; and secondly the universal duty to respect patient autonomy. Doyle (1993; 9) suggests:

> ... some beliefs about moral duties are not based on emotion or simply the preference of one from many cultural traditions. Rather, they follow from rational argument, of the sort which is our only hope in ordering our personal and international affairs in ways that do not arbitrarily harm others, including the patients for whom we are professionally responsible. What is at stake in not recognising this, is the relativizing of human suffering for the sake of the false emotional comfort of thinking that we are being tolerant.

If nursing is to be based on a close personal relationship with the patient that is espoused by many theorists (Noddings, 1984; Orem, 1980; Paterson and Zderad, 1976; Peplau, 1952 and Watson, 1988 *for example*) then nursing ethics should focus on responsibilities and obligations. However, we need to take notice of Doyle's advice on relativity in relation to patient suffering for the sake of our own emotional comfort. Kant's interpretation of the categorical imperative can offer the nurse a way of limiting such emotional misplacement, exercise responsibility and prevent doing harm to others. Sullivan (1990) argues that the categorical imperative need only play a background role in our everyday moral life. We usually have substantive moral maxims already, or adequate policies to guide our decisions. We need only judge when and how to act on them in various situations. But we do need to use the categorical imperative when we are having difficulty deciding whether a problematic maxim *is* morally right and we wish to avoid rationalising our desires, or when, like Kant, we need to defend our maxims from the attacks of moral skepticism (Sullivan, 1990). Sullivan appears to be taking a similar position to Hare (1981) in relation to moral deliberation, with our 'substantive moral maxims' operating at the intuitive level and the categorical imperative acting as the baseline for critical decision making when there is conflict of moral values.

Conclusions

This chapter has highlighted the diversity and complexity of the literature pertaining to the concept of autonomy. It demonstrates the different meanings of the concept - from the individual's right to self-government on the one hand, to moral responsibility on the other. It highlights two opposing positions to autonomous decision-making - one based on universal principles and the other, a contextualised approach based on humanistic principles of attachment and responsibility. Both positions are often presented as an 'either/or' choice in moral deliberation. However, it has been suggested in this chapter that universal principles can be enriched through the acceptance of the significance of deliberative and contextualised moral reasoning in the context of individual relationships. Such contextualised decision-making is seen to occur in a relationship that holds the concept of 'partnership' as central. Through such a partnership, the significance of autonomy is established from an understanding of the situation - an understanding that is worked out within the relationship of nurse to patient. In order to understand the importance of autonomy in the relationship, it is suggested that an ability to see a person's life as a whole as identified through a life plan that highlights an individual's value history is important.

Universal moral principles (these are principles that can be applied to everyone) are not being rejected, but it is being suggested that the operationalisation of such principles needs to occur in the context of an individual relationship based on principles of partnership. The example of the right of all older people to have free access to continuing health care has been highlighted as a principle that can be applied universally. However, it has been further argued that such a principle can both empower and disempower older people if their individual life values and choices are not considered.

The positions presented represent a diversity of perspectives and therefore it is perhaps understandable why there is a paucity of nursing research that 'measures' the operationalisation of the concept of autonomy in practice. Many studies (Pankratz and Pankratz, 1974; Gortner and Zyzanski, 1988; Wood *et al*, 1986; Marchette *et al*, 1993; Bristow Ott and Nieswiadomy, 1991 *for example*) attempt to 'measure' the existence of autonomy in differing care settings and practices. This is clearly an impossible task without a clearer understanding of the gradations of meaning of the concept in nursing and a clear articulation of the definition of autonomy being used. A greater understanding of the patient's experience of different approaches to care and the nurse's response would add to our knowledge. Understanding more fully the aspects of patient interaction that nurses find problematic would help to redefine autonomy in a nursing context. Rather than taking the classic texts of (*for example*) Kant and applying them to practice, in order to understand practice, an approach that starts with practice may lead us to uncharted territory. It is this endeavour that the remainder of this book is dedicated.

4 'Seeing' Autonomy in Practice

Introduction

The previous chapter has analysed the concept of autonomy from a variety of perspectives. It is clear from the literature that while there is much philosophical conceptual clarification of autonomy, little attempt has been made to understand the concept from a 'practical' perspective; thence there is a lack of clarity about the practical discourse of autonomy. This chapter, outlines the approach adopted in the research presented in this book in order to determine a practical discourse of autonomy with nurses working with older people. It is set against the background of the philosophical and societal challenges identified in previous chapters.

The chapter will present the development of the theoretical position adopted in the research and how this shaped methodological decisions. It will finish with a description of the process of data analysis and a discussion concerning the way this data analysis has shaped the model of autonomy as authentic consciousness that will be described later.

The Research in Context

It could be argued that the concept of autonomy has little everyday meaning as it is not one that people are able to describe easily. Indeed some authors interpret work such as that of Gilligan (1982) with its emphasis on 'connectedness' instead of individualism, as evidence of the inappropriateness of the term for nursing (Johns, 1995 *for example*). How does one *see* autonomy? We usually recognise the concept through other concepts such as choice, self-determination and rights. Research so far into autonomy in professional practice has tended to yield little meaningful results because of the problems with defining the concept. Studies have tried to quantify the existence of the concept in practice (*for example* Pankratz and Pankratz, 1974), or describe the operationalisation of the concept in clinical decision making (*for example* Bristow-Ott and Nieswiadomy, 1991; Fried *et al*, 1993).

Each of these areas of research has proven problematic because of the differing meanings of the concept identified in practice and the researchers' assumptions about autonomy that are implicit in the research methodology. Additionally, few of these studies have started from practitioners' understandings of the concept, but instead have accepted existing theoretical positions as frameworks of analysis or do not explicitly identify which theoretical position is being adopted.

Studies exploring the extent to which autonomy exists in practice have tended to focus on the development of professional autonomy and the impact of the existence of professional autonomy on patient participation in decision-making. For example, Pankratz and Pankratz (1974) sought to establish the views of nurses regarding their dependence versus independence for themselves and patients. The degree of independence versus dependence experienced by both nurses and patients was seen as an indicator of the degree of autonomy of both groups. Indeed, while Pankratz and Pankratz (1974) do not attempt to define autonomy, they implicitly describe it as independence and without such a definition being made explicit, they developed a 'nursing autonomy and patients' rights scale'. The underpinning assumption of the tool is that the more autonomy (as independence) that nurses have in their role the more latitude patients will have or are allowed to have in knowing about or participating in their own care or treatment. While the research identified a high correlation between the level of education of the nurse, their attitude and patient participation in care decisions, no account of individual difference and perceptions about rights and independent decision-making is offered. In spite of these problems, the tool developed by Pankratz and Pankratz (1974) has been used in many other studies (Pinch, 1985; Wood *et al*, 1986, *for example*).

Pinch (1985) investigated decision making in ethical dilemmas and attitudes towards professional autonomy among a variety of nursing groups. The approach was based on Kohlberg's (1981) developmental theory and particularly focused on the role of the nurse as patient advocate in the nurse/patient relationship. Again, no working definition of autonomy is offered, although an individualistic concept is assumed because of the focus on the nurse as an independent decision-maker. The research demonstrates a positive correlation between graduate nurses and the degree of autonomy experienced, based on the extent of independent decision-making observed. However, only a cursory consideration of the impact of context on ethical decisions is made and no attempt is made to extrapolate the nurses' own understanding of the concept in relation to their role perception.

Wood *et al* (1986) make explicit their definition of autonomy as independence to make decisions, to take actions in accordance with self-determined plans and the amount of discretionary control over actions experienced. Like Pinch (1985), they see this achievement in Kohlbergian terms as 'the completely socialized professional'. Again, the research demonstrates a positive correlation between graduate nurses and the degree of autonomy experienced. But while there is a cursory acknowledgement of the impact of socialisation, clinical experience and the context of clinical practice, little attempt was made to account for these. In all of these studies an individualistic understanding of autonomy is assumed and underpins the research findings.

In exploring the operationalisation of the concept of autonomy in practice, studies have predominantly operated within an individualistic perspective of autonomy, but have used a variety of approaches to articulate this. For example, Bristow-Ott and Nieswiadomy (1991) examined critical care nurses' beliefs concerning the support for patient autonomy in 'Do Not Resuscitate' (DNR) decisions. Although they assume the importance of autonomy in clinical decision-making, they do little to define it and consistently equate autonomy with advocacy without explaining either term. A replication of this study by Marchette *et al* (1993) adopted a similar approach and conceptual framework. Others, such as Fried *et al* (1993) and Schwartz and Blank (1986) use characteristics of personal autonomy to measure its existence and subsequent operationalisation in practice - characteristics such as compliance with specific patient requests, provision of evidence to justify a decision, the extent to which patients make a specific request, and measures of competency to make rational decisions. A similar approach has been adopted in the measurement of the existence of nurses professional autonomy (Blegen *et al*, 1993; Singleton and Nail, 1984; Carlsen and Malley, 1981 *for example*).

All of these areas of study adopt an implicit individualistic understanding of autonomy that both underpin the theoretical approaches adopted and the conclusions drawn from the research evidence. A similar picture exists with research into the autonomy of older people. Given the dominant focus on an individualistic notion of autonomy in the literature (Ryden, 1985; Morganti *et al*, 1980; Powers, 1992; Saup, 1986), it is clearly evident why theorists such as Agich (1993) have argued for a conceptual understanding of autonomy that transcends notions of individualism and instead focuses on interdependence. While little attempt has been made to explicitly define autonomy in these studies, an individualistic conceptualisation is assumed from the existence of other defining characteristics such as independent choice, environmental control, functional ability and coping behaviours. Many studies focus on the older person's ability to make independent choices in their lives and in care/treatment plans (Heidrich, 1993; Hulicka *et al*, 1975; Jirovec and Maxwell, 1993; Pinch and Parsons, 1993). In these studies, 'choice' is identified as a central defining characteristic of autonomy. While attempts at measuring the existence of autonomy through structured approaches to data collection have been made, all of these studies fail to delineate the essential characteristics of autonomy other than viewing it as an ability to make independent choices.

Some studies have recognised the inherent problems of 'measuring' the existence of autonomy. Hertz (1991) undertook a concept analysis and measurement of the emerging defining attributes in practice. She identified voluntariness, individuality and self-direction as the defining attributes and from these, identified and outlined the antecedents and characteristics necessary to support these defining attributes. Hertz (1991) identified factors that could be observed to measure the existence of autonomy (empirical referents), such as absence of restraints, refusal to follow others' directives, use of the word 'I', communication of desires, preferences and goals and following one's own plan, which have been developed into 'the perceived enactment of autonomy scale'. However, these factors are dependent on a number of other variables such as the context of decision-making, individual competence and individual perception and socialisation. While Hertz acknowledges this, her account promotes an individualistic understanding of autonomy in a way that significantly reduces the impact of the identified empirical referents and the resulting scale.

Macmillan's (1986) study of autonomy shown in the life histories of older people identified three dimensions of autonomy - autonomy of action; autonomy of will; autonomy of thought. Macmillan viewed these dimensions as existing in a hierarchical fashion and in a functional relationship to each other. Autonomy of will was seen to be most vulnerable in older people and when this dimension was interfered with, there was the potential for synergistic interference with autonomy of action. Macmillan concluded that nurses appeared to be insensitive to patient autonomy and its implications in decision-making. She identified the significance of the individuality of persons and the differences in decision-making experienced in older age.

Mattiasson and Andersson (1995 [i]) utilised Collopy's (1988) dimensions of autonomy to elucidate nursing home staff attitudes regarding ethical conflicts. While the authors were able to measure the existence of each of Collopy's dimensions and staff attitudes within each dimension, their significant finding was that the dimension of 'authentic autonomy' required particular attention in the care of older people, that is, staffs' ability to infer consistency between past and present values in the determination of care needs and approaches to care delivery.

Research Aims

The majority of these studies fail to elucidate the meaning of autonomy in practice and its impact on the nurse-patient relationship. They also fail to distinguish between contextualised and universalist distinctions and how this can affect the nurse-patient relationship and the exercise of autonomy. The majority of these studies commence with a prior understanding of the concept that was used to guide the theoretical framework of the research or do not explicitly define the underpinning assumptions of the research approach. This occurred either overtly through the explicit definition/description of an individualistic concept of autonomy or covertly through the adoption of a particular research instrument/approach developed from an existing definition of the concept. As Macmillan (1986) identified, the problem with measuring autonomy, particularly with older people, is the individuality of the person and the impact of their life experiences. But, given the multi-dimensional nature of the concept as identified through philosophical, applied and empirical studies, attempts at measurement would always be futile unless individuals' concepts of autonomy can be accessed inductively through empirical evidence. Therefore, the intention of my research was to:

- Create greater conceptual clarity about the concept of autonomy in relation to the notions of professional and personal autonomy.
- Describe and explore the necessary and sufficient conditions for autonomy to exist in the relationship between nurses and older patients.

To do this, I considered two questions to be of particular importance to this research, for as Benner (1994 [ii]) suggests, the interpretive researcher's questions (like those of all researchers) inadvertently shape and foretell the possible answers to the question:

- What is the meaning of autonomy in a relationship between a nurse and an older patient?

- When working with older people, can the nurse promote the principle of patient autonomy while functioning as an autonomous practitioner?

Creating a Practical Discourse of Autonomy

The challenge in the design of the research methodology was to determine an appropriate approach to access practitioners' and patients' concepts of autonomy. There is a general dearth of research that attempts to elucidate the presentation of autonomy in practice or to inductively generate theories of autonomy from patients' and practitioners' own concepts. This approach to research is gaining prominence and holds much opportunity for the development of 'practical research' approaches and the generation of practice based theory that can be understood and used by practitioners (Fay, 1987; Carr and Kemmis, 1986; Schön, 1991; Benner, 1984; Savage, 1995; Johns, 1997; MacLeod, 1994 *for example*).

Wilson (1963) argues that in seeking to clarify the meaning of a concept, it is important not to behave as if there is one 'real' meaning of the word [autonomy] that would answer all questions relating to its use. The fact that autonomy adopts different guises and meanings in practice, demonstrates that it does not have a 'single meaning', but instead has different uses and different applications. According to Wilson (1963) the job of the researcher is to map out these uses and applications. However, Wilson raises the dichotomy inherent in the process of concept clarification. Usually the concepts we use are embedded in our subconscious and are taken for granted. For example, when a patient asks for privacy in their care, nurses will engage in a series of actions (the drawing of curtains, the closing of doors *for example*) which imply a particular set of meanings of the concept of privacy (the protection of personal space), that are used without thinking and are a part of usual everyday practice. However, if specifically asked about the concept and challenged about their understanding, nurses are being asked to become self-conscious about words that previously were used unconsciously. This process of consciousness raising and reflection, Wilson argues can very soon lead to the person becoming 'baffled' about the word and its use. Indeed Schön (1991) has demonstrated that this process can lead to dysfunctional practice if the practitioner is not helped to unravel such conceptual conflicts.

The fundamental problem of accessing practitioners' concepts provided the greatest obstacle to my achieving any more than a collection of rhetorical accounts of a concept as seen through individual practitioner's ideals. As already stated, one of the problems in attempting to gain an understanding of the concept of autonomy from practitioners' perspectives is the problem of recognising when the concept does and does not exist. How can we *see* autonomy? What does it look like to us when we confront it in practice? When I make decisions about action, on what grounds do I decide if they are autonomous or not? Given that autonomy is described in different ways, then social research methods that rely on retrospective reflection on action would not enable a real understanding of the meaning of the concept in practice to be gained. Processes of 'rational accounting', whereby the practitioner depicts their practice as reasonable and rational based on their practice 'ideals', would play a significant role in their verbal descriptions of the concept of autonomy (Scott and Lyman, 1968; Garfinkle, 1967; Goffman, 1959). That is, a disparity might exist between espoused practice ideals and the reality of practice. In nursing, communication studies between nurses and older people demonstrate this disparity (Macleod-Clark, 1991). When asked about the importance of effective communication with clients, nurses offer clear evidence of its importance to the individuality of the patient and the nurse-patient relationship. Subsequent observations of practice demonstrate that these same nurses spend little time communicating with patients (Macleod-Clark, 1991). Elliott (1987) suggests therefore, that while practitioners can make their practice ideals explicit and justify them, because of the separation of such accounts from the context of practice and their relationship with other elements within the practice context, critiques of such principles can only ever be partial critiques. For critiques to be 'complete', descriptions and principles from practice need to be derived. To be able to describe such practices, a methodological approach that captures the actual interactions of nurses and patients needed to be adopted in this research.

Theoretical Position

Previous studies of autonomy that have adopted a qualitative methodological approach have used biographical and narrative methods (Gilligan, 1982; Macmillan, 1986; Agich, 1993). There is a general dearth of research, however, that attempts to elucidate the presentation of autonomy in practice. Given the status of much of the research into the presentation and operationalisation of autonomy in practice, there is a need to inductively generate theories of autonomy from practitioners' own concepts. An interpretative methodology was considered appropriate to achieving the research aims. But even with the adoption of an interpretative methodology that focuses on creating 'a map' of the possible uses of the concept by practitioners and patients (*after* Wilson, 1963), the problem of interpreting a concept from individual practitioners' perspectives remained problematic. The problem remained of whether a contextualised or a universalist position should be pursued in determining an operational definition of autonomy.

The autonomy literature espouses the values of both philosophical positions with the merits of both applauded. However, Elliott (1987) argues for a synergistic relationship between contextualised and universalist principles, where practitioners' individual theories can be scrutinised in relation to the validity of the wider frameworks of beliefs and values they presuppose. Therefore an approach to this research that aimed to critique individual concept analyses within the broader philosophical theoretical frameworks available, offered a means of making visible the tacit ideals of practitioners. As Elliott (1987) asserts, research within a practice discipline must allow questions about the beliefs and values of the practice discipline to be answered. This means that research must be grounded in an awareness of the operational principles underlying practice and the contexts of beliefs and values in which they are embedded. A relationship therefore between the development and testing of operational principles and theoretical understandings is fostered. But how can such an interpretation be gained? How can the descriptions of practice gained through naturalistic inquiry methods be transformed into interpretations that preserve the underlying practice beliefs and have universal significance?

While Heidegger's existentialist phenomenology accounts for the importance of the researcher's values in the research process, I felt unclear about how my values could be articulated in the research design and their impact on the phenomena identified in the data, that is, the problem in interpretive social science of restricting an explanation of action to the actors' concepts. Therefore, it was to Gadamer's Hermeneutics that I turned.

Gadamer's Hermeneutics and Action as Text

Gadamer's hermeneutics (Gadamer, 1993) is a philosophical perspective that aims to offer solutions to the problems of moving beyond descriptive accounts of practitioners' concepts. Originally used by the Greeks as a method of interpreting texts, hermeneutics is concerned with 'bringing to understanding' the nature of the social world from both the subjective interpretation of the individual and the more general underlying abstracted meanings. Therefore, the hermeneutic process according to Gadamer is a dialogical process between the interpreter's understanding and the object being studied. Hermeneutic research does not attempt to interpret the data from an 'objective' position, but instead creates a dialogue where insiders' and observers' conceptions interact. Even when the interpreter feels constrained to reject the actor's view as totally off beam, it remains relevant that the actors have that view and that the interpreter be able to describe it accurately (Guba and Lincoln, 1994). Therefore, for Gadamer, understanding does not arise from a vigorous interrogation of a text or object under the gaze of an investigator, but instead the investigator allows himself to be 'questioned' by the subject matter. The investigator must be open to the concepts they wish to understand, be aware of pre-judgements (described by Gadamer as *prejudices*) that might be problematic and to critique them in the light of newly formulated meanings. The recognition, acceptance and management of 'prejudice' as an explicit part of the research process distinguishes Gadamer's approach from many other interpretative approaches (Husserl, 1964; Schutz, 1967 *for example*). Gadamer argues that the pursuit of objectivity as an ideal of the Enlightenment (that is, knowledge that is free from all particular perspectives), is at worse an illusion, and at best an unnecessary limitation.

Central to Gadamer's thesis is the notion of 'effective historical consciousness'. In saying that understanding is historical, Gadamer is arguing against the idea of creating the 'perfect' understanding. Understanding is always embedded in the prior assumptions that the interpreter brings to the interpretation. While other philosophical positions, such as that of Schutz (1967) recognise the influence of pre-understanding on the interpretative process, unlike Schutz, Gadamer does not suggest that such prejudices should be put in suspension (bracketing). Guba and Lincoln (1994) argue that bracketing represents the Cartesian dualism of disengaging the individual from their subjective (lived) experience in order to objectify it. Instead the awareness of these prejudices leads to the process of 'self-reflection' whereby the interpreter turns them into questions that challenge and clarify the interpretative scheme. However, Gadamer does guard against becoming too immersed in the data and self-reflection and he uses the analogy of the work of art in a gallery to indicate why it is important to 'distance' oneself from that being interpreted. Gadamer (1993; 149) argues that the worst judges of a portrait are the nearest relatives of the portraiture or the person themselves:

for a portrait never tries to reproduce the individual it represents as he appears in the eyes of people close to him.

In other words, being able to keep a distance lets the true meaning of the data emerge fully (Gadamer, 1993; 298). It not only lets local and limited prejudices die away, but allows those that bring about genuine understanding to emerge as such (Gadamer, 1993; 298). Understanding then, necessitates the desire to grasp the tradition (prejudices), of what is said in such a way that it 'fuses' with the interpreter's own traditions. Although Gadamer does not offer any direction about how this distance can be operationalised within a research design, his view of how the researcher engages with the data is important here.

In stating that the reader should allow himself to be 'questioned' by the data, Gadamer appears to be suggesting that the interpreter should not accept 'first impressions'. Instead the interpreter should raise questions about the data and first impressions, think laterally about alternative meanings and challenge his interpretations through application and referral to other sources. Research participants' active involvement in this interpretative process is also important so that a 'meeting of understanding' can be achieved.

Gadamer refers to this meeting of understandings as 'the fusion of horizons', where the prejudices of research participants and the interpreter meet in order to create a new understanding. Understanding then becomes a living event, that is, we enter the data through conversation with it and actively participate in the story that unfolds. Thus hermeneutics is concerned with:

- Gaining a comprehensive understanding of the world while helping to make it understandable to others;
- The identification and explanation of the structural and internal barriers to gaining a true understanding of a situation.

It aims to offer an account of the world as understood by those participating in it and the barriers that might prevent such an understanding from being achieved. For this research, this was particularly relevant as the barriers to understanding the nature of autonomy in a nurse-patient relationship are great; problems with the contexts of practice, the language used by practitioners, acceptance of cultural norms by patients, professional power and the prior conceptions of autonomy as held by the researcher, all influence the rigour and authenticity of the new understandings gained.

Understanding is always in constant movement, from the whole to the parts and from the parts to the whole. The approach to such practice is described as the 'hermeneutical circle of understanding' (Heidegger, 1990), that is, an understanding of the whole in terms of the detail and the detail in terms of the whole. When analysing data, therefore, the researcher undertakes analysis at two levels:

- interpreting individual data sets for particular meanings;
- integrating individual data sets into a whole picture and understanding the meaning of the picture created.

The 'hermeneutic circle' adopts three phases that interact and relate with each other and together encompass the notion of 'reflexivity':

- *Prior understanding* Every researcher starts the investigation with some knowledge or assumptions about the domain of inquiry. As a nurse and researcher, I have assumptions and understandings about autonomy and the socio-political context of nursing practice (as outlined in Chapter 1). I am aware of the theoretical domains of the field of inquiry and similar empirical work that has been undertaken. Unlike Husserlian phenomenology (Husserl, 1964), the investigator is not required to 'suspend' these assumptions, but instead make them explicit and open to critique - what Gadamer refers to as the testing of our prejudices in order to reach a valid understanding rather than a misunderstanding.
- *Interrogation of the social phenomenon* The data gathering and in-depth analysis.
- *Reflecting on presuppositions* During the analysis, the investigator reflects on prior assumptions in view of the data gathered and considers the effect on the data and the understandings gained.

Viewing social phenomena through the interpretive schema of Gadamerian hermeneutics thus allows the social sciences to side-step one of the main problems of interpretive social science, i.e. restricting the explanation of action to the actor's concepts. His position does not reject the basic principle of interpretive social science of starting with the actor's concepts. But Gadamer provides what is missing in the interpretive approach, i.e. a legitimising of the integration of research participants' concepts with the conceptual scheme of the interpreter. Thus, the purpose of inquiry is more than a re-creation of what already exists (what Gadamer refers to as 'a mirror image'), but instead what emerges is an interpretation that both captures the original context of the data and also identifies motives not present to the original participant (Hekman, 1983). For example, in analysing an individual practitioner's understanding of patient autonomy, the context in which that practitioner's understanding is created would be captured by me. However, further analysis would allow me to relate that understanding to more general philosophical understandings and thence expose 'hidden meanings' that are not in the practitioner's interpretive scheme, but which may influence the general understanding of the concept, that is, move between a contextual understanding and universal principles. The use of the hermeneutic circle creates a mirror image of practice for the particular practitioner, while at the same time applying something universal to the particular situation. Thus Gadamer draws on Aristotle's *practical philosophy* (Koch, 1995) and his notion of *phronesis* - reflection concerned with the translation of universal ethical values into practical forms of action in particular situations (Elliott, 1987). Knowledge is personalised by the practitioner through reasoning and experience and is always in a state of development, that is, knowledge is personal, subjective and never fully formed, but instead is always in a state of 'being formed' (Grundy, 1982). What is right cannot be determined independently of the context, and decision-making is therefore characterised by choice and deliberation (Gadamer, 1993) about what constitutes a 'good' action in the particular situation.

However, even within this ontological hermeneutic approach, the framework remains problematic. On what grounds do I base my interpretations of autonomy as presented through periods of data collection? As a nurse I have views about practices that constitute autonomous action and those that do not. My beliefs and values guide my practice towards a moral framework that is based on universal principles of autonomy set within a humanistic philosophical view of persons and the importance of the context of the situation. However, do these beliefs and values provide me with sufficient justification to critique another's practice as autonomous or not? That is, would I be able to reach an understanding through the fusion of horizons or a mere misunderstanding based on my own invalid prejudices?

Achieving a Valid Understanding

Ricoeur (1977) argues that a valid understanding will not be based on something 'hidden behind the text', but rather something disclosed in front of it. In other words an interpretation of autonomy should not just aim at a theoretical understanding of the concept, but should provide a sufficient map of the processes utilised in gaining the understanding and the context within which the understanding is gained. Ricoeur argues that structuralist analysis may be necessary as part of this process. Through systematic and structured analysis, an interpretation can move from a naive interpretation to a critical one and from a surface interpretation to an in-depth one. Therefore this hermeneutical arc of understanding places description and understanding at different ends of the interpretative scheme with the movement of analysis progressing from description to explanation to understanding.

In deciding that the research questions demanded an interpretive methodology informed by Gadamer's ontological hermeneutics, I needed to consider the most appropriate methods of collecting data. The problem of seeing autonomy through my own conceptual 'lens' concerned me, as I felt that there was a danger of achieving little other than a clarification/verification of my own understandings, or what Ricoeur (1977) describes as a 'partial understanding'. The importance of 'language as text' to Gadamer's hermeneutics began to offer directions for choosing research methods, i.e. the language of autonomy in the nurse/patient relationship provides a basis for understanding the rules of practice and the tacit concepts that underpin it. Therefore, the design of the methods needed to describe the linguistic features that characterised nurse-patient interactions and to develop hypotheses regarding the demonstration of power in nurse-patient interactions in different practice settings. The theoretical justification for this position lies in the theory of 'ceremonial order' in interaction (particularly doctor-patient interactions). Both of these approaches focus on the rules of discourse between the professional and client/patient. Strong and Davis (1977) and Strong (1979) use a Goffmanesque approach and describe 'situations' and 'frames' in doctor-client interactions. These are seen as ready made formats for social interaction that constrain all participants and make them vulnerable to being judged as to whether their performance accords with the moral regime associated with the situation. In relation to nursing in particular, May (1995) argues that it is through conversational practice that these rules are made explicit and the authentic person may be reinstated and revealed (or not).

But on what basis should autonomy-orientated data be chosen from recorded transcripts? Given that much of the focus of debates about autonomy concern issues of power and control and I had identified that language offered an appropriate medium for accessing practitioner's tacit concepts, then a conversation analytical approach, derived from ethnomethodology, could be adopted. In this research design, conversation analysis would be used as a 'structuralist' (Ricoeur, 1977) approach to describing the data and deriving interpretive themes - that is, as a 'tool' for the selection and description of data sets. By using an established framework derived from conversation analysis, then decisions about data choices for analysis would in the first instance be informed through the structure of the framework rather than my own subjective choices as a 'data interpreter'.

Conversation Analysis

Conversation Analysis (CA) originates from the work of Harvey Sacks and his two associates, Schegloff and Jefferson. They have produced no definitive text, but instead the methodology of CA has arisen from an analysis of a series of empirical studies of 'mundane conversation', that is *ordinary* everyday talk (*for example*, Sacks, Schegloff and Jefferson, 1974). The methodology of CA has been developed by researchers such as Jefferson (1984; 1988); Heritage (1984; 1988; 1991); Heath (1981; 1986) and more recently by Drew and Heritage (1992).

CA identifies a limited set of turn-taking rules within which discourse is constructed and within which participants perform particular acts within the constraints of this rule system. CA approaches discourse as action *in its own right* and not as a secondary route to understanding things beyond the text, like attitudes, particular events or cognitive processes (Drew and Heritage, 1992). Thus CA is compatible with Gadamer's view of language as action. The essential mode of data collection for CA is the recording of naturally occurring conversations.

However, in the context of professional-client interactions, Drew and Heritage (1992; 3) question the 'naturalness' of such conversation and argue that conversations always reflect or are at least influenced by the social context within which they are constructed:

> Talk-in-interaction is the principal means through which lay persons pursue various practical goals and the central medium through which the daily working activities of many professionals and organisational representatives are conducted.

They refer to talk of this kind as 'institutional interaction' or *talk at work*. Interaction is institutional insofar as participants' institutional or professional identities are somehow made relevant to the work activities to which they are engaged. Sentences and utterances are designed and shaped to occur in particular sequential and social contexts and that the sense of such sentences and utterances derives in part from the social context in which they are placed:

> ... utterances are interpreted in terms of whether or to what extent, they conform to or depart from the expectations that are attached to the 'slots' in which they occur (p 12).

CA combines a concern with the contextual sensitivity of language use with a focus on talk as a vehicle for social action. Its approach to the understanding of interaction and language is distinguished from other approaches through its *activity focus*. Therefore, the overriding concern of CA is on the particular actions that occur in some context, their underlying social organisation and the alternative means by which these actions and the activities they compose can be realised. Ordinary conversation is viewed as the predominant medium of action in the social world. It is also the primary form of interaction, to which, with whatever simplifications, the person is initially exposed and through which socialisation proceeds. Thus the basic forms of mundane talk constitute a kind of benchmark against which other more formal or 'institutional' types of interaction are recognised and experienced. The context of interaction cannot be taken for granted nor may it be treated as determined in advance and independent of the participants' own activities. Instead, context and identity have to be treated as inherently locally produced, incrementally developed and by extension, as transformable at any moment.

Drew and Heritage (1992) outline some differences between 'Institutional Talk' and ordinary conversation:

- Institutional interaction involves an orientation by at least one of the participants to some core goal, task or identity (or set of identities) conventionally associated with the institution in question. In short, institutional talk is normally informed by goal orientations of a relatively restricted conventional form.
- Institutional interaction may often involve special and particular constraints on what one or both of the participants will treat as allowable contributions to the business at hand.
- Institutional talk may be associated with inferential frameworks and procedures that are particular to specific institutional contexts.

These distinctions are particularly important to the methodology of this research. They represent the importance of understanding power relationships in the research because:

- Before the patient can instigate autonomous action the nature of the interaction process between the nurse and the patient determines the type of ensuing action (*for example* Heath, 1986; Baldcock and Prior, 1981).
- Immediate constraints may be imposed through conversation turns, thus limiting the extent of autonomy (*for example* Heritage, 1988; Brewer *et al*, 1991).
- Conversation 'rules' may only be known to either one of the parties involved and thus present a potential limitation on action (Drew and Heritage, 1992).

CA originates from an ethnomethodological perspective rooted in a rational philosophy. Ethnomethodology derives its origins from Schutzian phenomenology (Holstein and Gubrium (1994; 264). Holstein and Gubrium suggest that ethnomethodology combines a phenomenological sensibility of individual experience with a concern for the individual in society:

> From an ethnomethodological standpoint, the world of 'social facts' is accomplished through members' interpretive work-activity through which actors produce and organize the very circumstances of everyday life.

Given that the essence of this research was the relationship between individuals in a particular social world (*hospital wards*) then this focus on an individual's interpretation and the way that interpretation shapes the social world of the individual was particularly relevant. Garfinkel's (1967) ethnomethodology was based on the premise that people in society were more than what he referred to as 'social dopes', that is, responding to external forces and motivated by internalised directives and imperatives. Instead, for Garfinkel, ordinary individuals create society through their ongoing, embodied interpretive work. Persons possess the practical linguistic and interactional competencies through which the observable, accountable, orderly features of reality are produced (Holstein and Gubrium, 1994). Because of the embededness of the ethnomethodological concern in the nature of social order, then its central focus is the participation of the individual in the creation of that order. Other sociological theory (such as that of Parsons, 1968) understands social order through rules, norms and shared meanings as explanations for individual behaviour. Ethnomethodology also understands social order through rules, norms and shared meanings, but not as external creations that are responded to by an individual. Instead, rules, norms and shared meanings are seen through the actions of persons, that is, the appearance of an event is an instance of compliance or non-compliance with a rule. The aim is not to provide causal explanations of patterned behaviour, but to describe how members recognize, describe, explain, and account for the order of their everyday lives (Zimmerman and Wieder, 1970). The focus of ethnomethodology is that of understanding how a person practically produces a sense of reality. Social structures are locally produced and are produced through an individual's interpretive work. Therefore, meanings are context specific and the circumstances that provide the context are themselves self-generating, that is, interpretation is both *in* the setting and *about* the setting.

This rational philosophy of ethnomethodology is severely criticised by Gadamer (1993). However, Gadamer makes it clear throughout his hermeneutic philosophy, that the aim of his work is not to describe a methodological ideal for the social sciences, but is an ontological endeavour to discover the meaning of understanding. Indeed he makes it clear that while his work would have important implications for researchers, he did not intend to '... revive the ancient dispute between the natural and social sciences' (Gadamer, 1993; xxix). Although this stance is easy to demonstrate in his work, as Hekman (1983; 340) states '... it is no easy task to specify in concrete terms what methodological approach is dictated by his work'. However, elsewhere, Gadamer states that this lack of attention to a methodological debate does not '... prevent the methods of modern natural science from being applicable to the social world' (Gadamer, 1993; xxix).

Therefore, while it is recognised within the theoretical framework of this research that the structured approach being adopted for the analysis of discourse does not 'fit' within a subjective interpretative stance, the context within which it is being used is important. The central concern of CA is that of describing the power relationships that occur in discourse. It utilises a structured deconstructive approach to data analysis, from which general inferences and descriptions are drawn. The starting point of hermeneutic analysis is to understand the 'horizon' of action, that is, what the action means to participants (Hekman, 1983). The aim is not to 'get inside the actors' minds' but to discover the meaning of action that is detached from the actors' subjective intentions through the creation of layers of interpretation (Ricoeur, 1977). Hermeneutics does not reject an understanding of action in actors' terms (indeed this is fundamental to the process), but this is seen as only one stage in the dialectic of interpretation.

In this research, CA is being used to select data that reflects the subjective interpretation of the actors so that universal interpretations can be achieved. Without such an approach the danger of achieving 'misunderstanding' as warned against by Gadamer is great. By applying structure to the initial analysis of data, appropriate data sets that reflect the essences of the power relationships between the nurse and patient can be chosen. (Individual interviews with nurses using the initial transcribed data ensured that the meaning of actions to the participants was captured. This will be discussed later in this chapter.)

Reconciling Philosophical Conflicts

Wainwright (1997) argues that, the tendency towards triangulation of method in nursing research, represents a failure of such research to undertake methodological triangulation. In arguing for a realist paradigm in nursing research, Wainwright raises the issue of epistemological integrity in research design. He is critical of interpretive approaches because of their inability to capture and shape social order, but instead are introverted self-reflections of a reality. While Wainwright fails to recognise the *reflexive* underpinnings of interpretive approaches (Holstein and Gubrium, 1994), the issue he raises is an important one. In designing the research methodology, I was conscious of the need to make a statement that I was doing research in a particular paradigm - that is the need to say, 'I am doing a hermeneutic study'. However, I was also conscious of 'being trapped' by philosophy and restricting my choice of method to those that would be consistent with a particular philosophy in order to avoid what Guba and Lincoln (1994) have referred to as the 'paradigm wars'. While I did not want to enter a paradigm war, I was conscious that a 'purist' hermeneutic approach would not answer the research questions that I was in danger of achieving a partial understanding (Ricoeur, 1977) and of falling foul of 'rational accounting' (Scott and Lyman, 1968; Garfinkle, 1967; Goffman, 1959). Hammersley (1992; 203) argues that:

> Decisions should flow from particular research contexts rather than the commitment to general methodological principles.

In combining hermeneutic and ethnomethodological philosophies, I was entering methodological triangulation (Wainwright, 1997) in order to maximise the research context. Drawing on the philosophical writings of

Gadamer (1993) and Garfinkel (1967), common ontological and epistemological assumptions are shared between hermeneutic and ethnomethodological approaches:

- Human beings create meaning through their interpretive schema.
- The objectification of subjective experience through 'bracketing' is rejected.
- Reflexivity as interpretation both *in* and *about* the context of interpretations is emphasised.
- Analysis focuses on the properties of practical reasoning and the interpretive work that produces a stable reality, while avoiding the making of judgements about the correctness of interpretations.
- Ethnomethodology views language as action through its 'ordinariness' and hermeneutics treats language as action through 'text'.
- The structures of language (as ordinariness or as text) reveal and conceal.

A research approach was developed that captured the natural conversation between professionals and patients, combined with an opportunity for professionals and patients to reflect on their tacit concepts and practice ideals. I saw this as appropriate with the research aims of achieving clarity about the concept of autonomy in the relationship between nurses and older people and clarifying the necessary and sufficient conditions for autonomy to exist in such a relationship.

My aim was to create a 'dialogue' between various layers of data collection and analysis. For example, I had entered this research with prior assumptions and understandings (prejudices) about autonomy (as outlined in Chapter 1). I had subsequently read a diverse range of philosophical and applied literature that began to challenge, confirm or re-focus my central concern with autonomy and older people. I was aware that a dialogue between my reading and myself was occurring and that such a dialogue could inform the approach to data collection and analysis. Figure 1 outlines the subsequent theoretical framework developed to inform data collection.

**Figure 1: The Place of Structured Analysis within an Overall
Interpretive Approach**

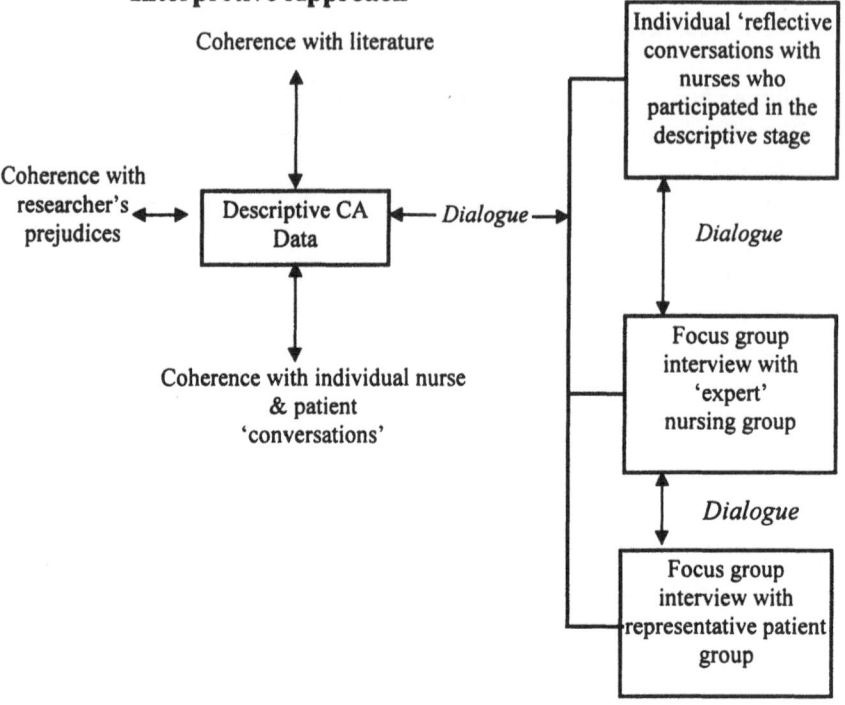

Data Collection Methods

As illustrated in figure 1, a two-stage approach to data collection was
identified:

- Stage 1: Description
- Stage 2: Interpretation and Understanding

Description Recording discussions and conversations between patients
and nurses; nurses and doctors; nurses and professionals allied to medicine
(PAM's). This was performed through two approaches:

1) The continuous recording of nurse-patient interactions through the use
   of a 'tie microphone' attached to a mini-cassette recorder (Philips
   Pocket Memo 696 with external microphone). Nurses were asked to
   wear the microphone during their shift. They had control of the
   microphone, that is, could turn it *on* and *off* as they wished. They were
   asked to wear the microphone for two-three shifts per week and were

asked to record conversations with patients that particularly pertained to discharge arrangements.

Although this was not a study about the quality of discharge arrangements, I was conscious of initial discussions with nurses who had difficulty deciding what conversations they would record and how they would do that with patients. I therefore decided to use the theme of 'discharge planning' as a focus, as this is a dominant care theme in the rehabilitation of older people in hospital (CSAG, 1998; Clark and Dyer, 1998; House of Commons Health Select Committee, 1996; Kadushin and Kulys, 1994). Nurses were asked to record all conversations with patients relating to discharge planning. This would include information gathering and educational conversations and would therefore include the initial assessment of care needs, skills teaching (self-medication for example), lifestyle information (to inform decisions about future care arrangements) and health status assessment. This focus would also involve the family in decision-making - a factor that is significant in the decision-making of older people in hospital (Jecker, 1991; High, 1991; Barker, 1991). It was intended that eight nurse/patient relationships would be recorded in each practice setting.

2) Audio recording of multi disciplinary meetings, discharge planning meetings and case conferences. The aim of this approach was to understand if and how the nurse represented the patient's perspective. Other opportunistic interactions between the nurse and other health care professionals would be recorded by virtue of the nurse wearing the 'tie microphone'. Again, during these interactions, the aim was to understand how the nurse represented the patient's wishes, desires, needs etcetera.

Interpretation and Understanding Follow up 'reflective conversations' with nurses who wore the 'tie microphones'. They were provided with transcripts of the recorded data and my initial interpretations and asked to participate in a short individual interview (30 minutes). This interview occurred within six months of the final audio recording of conversations they had made. The participants were not being asked to validate the accuracy of the transcript, but instead to reflect on the interactions outlined in the transcripts. Therefore the time between recording the data and engaging in the interview was not so crucial. The purpose of this interview was to clarify emerging issues in the recorded transcripts, to offer their interpretations of events and to offer an opportunity to describe the contextual issues that would be important to the recorded conversations.

The term 'conversation' rather than 'interview' was chosen, as it more fully describes the actual process that was used (Bergum, 1991). The word 'interview' implies one person asking questions of another (Polit and Hungler, 1987), the word 'conversation' implies a discussion (Bergum, 1991) and more accurately reflects the approach adopted. Bergum (1991) stresses the similarity between an interview and a conversation, in that both have a central focus, but in the conversation it is not one-sided. This was an important principle to establish, as the aim was to enable participants to reflect on the data collected and my initial interpretations of it.

Each participant was given a full copy of the coded transcript for each of the patient case studies that they had participated in. In addition, two weeks prior to the reflective conversation, participants were provided with a transcript of the interpreted data of each of the patients with whom they recorded data. A cover letter with suggested reflective questions was also provided. I was mindful of the problems of raising to people's consciousness issues that had previously been unconscious (Elliott, 1987). Each participant was therefore offered the opportunity to have more than one reflective conversation as a means of support and to assist them with identifying solutions and practice changes. Only one participant availed of the opportunity for ongoing support. The conversations were undertaken in the participating nurses' own homes at a time convenient to them. A schedule based on issues emerging from my initial interpretations was devised and shared with participants. The conversations were audio-recorded and transcribed verbatim. Participants were supplied with a written transcript of the conversation for their own reflections.

A focus-group discussion with a group of expert nurses following my initial interpretation of the data was then undertaken. The aim here was to use the data collected during the recording period to explore autonomy issues further in order to 'map out' the concept of autonomy and to verify or falsify my initial interpretations. Five gerontological nurse experts who have a national profile were asked to participate in a focus group interview of three hours. Each of the nurse experts fulfilled criteria for expert practice as described by Benner (1984), Benner *et al* (1996), Jasper (1994) and Greenwood and King (1995).

- acknowledged expertise in the speciality;
- 4-8 years experience in the speciality and in a variety of settings;
- possessed a specialised body of knowledge and skill;

- graduate level educational preparation;
- demonstrated leadership skills in the speciality.

Two weeks before the focus group discussion, each member of the expert group was supplied with four data sets that had undergone initial interpretation. Data sets were chosen to represent the different clinical settings, a mix of male and female patients and differing care foci. Members of the expert group were provided with key questions to consider when reading the interpretations prior to the focus group. The same 'conversation' style used in individual reflective conversations (Bergum, 1991) was adopted.

A focus-group discussion with a group of patients was held following my initial interpretation of the data. A group of six patients (representative of the population) were asked to participate. The aim here was to offer the patients the opportunity to clarify their perspectives on autonomy issues and to compare this to nurses' perceptions. 'Vignettes' based on the conversations recorded with patients by the participating nurses and considered to be 'significant' by the expert group, were audio recorded and played back to the patient group. A written version of the vignettes was also provided. The group was asked to tell their story of being a patient and to compare that to the recorded vignettes.

Ever conscious of my own prejudices, I recorded in the form of a reflective diary, my own reflections on the data as I listened to tapes and developed transcripts. I recorded my initial 'feelings' about the data and any issues arising that seemed important to me. 'Importance' was defined as:

> segments of interactions that caused me to reflect on the particular interaction; invoked feelings of surprise, anger, satisfaction etcetera; or those that challenged my prejudices.

The approach outlined established 'trustworthiness' (Ely *et al*, 1991; 93) in the data collection process:

> Being trustworthy as a qualitative researcher means at the least that the processes of the research are carried out fairly, that the products represent as closely as possible the experiences of the people who are studied. The entire endeavour must be grounded in ethical principles about how data are collected and analyzed, how one's own assumptions and conclusions are checked, how participants are involved, and how results are communicated.

No specific time frame for completing the collection of data was provided to the participating nurses. They knew, that the recording of data would begin when a patient was admitted to the ward and to each of them as Primary Nurses. It would end when a decision about the patient's discharge arrangements had been made and agreed with the patient and team members. They also knew that they were being asked to record conversations with up to four patients. The length of time it would take the nurses to collect data with up to four patients would vary according to a number of factors, including:

- the willingness of patients to participate;
- the patient's presenting health status and multiple pathology;
- reason for admission;
- long term care arrangements;
- nurses workloads.

In all the participating settings, the average length of stay for patients was three weeks, but obviously some patients were admitted for much shorter or longer periods than this. In all, the data collected in all sites occurred over an eighteen-month period.

Choosing Patients Many of the participating nurses had difficulty with 'getting started' with data collection and needed much encouragement to do so. The nurses made decisions about choosing patients based on criteria of their overall workload and the patient's mental state and care needs. Difficulty with commencing data collection predominantly related to the nurses' perceptions of their overall workload. It was evident that if they felt pressurised by their workloads, then they were unwilling to initiate data collection when new patients were admitted. It was also evident that the nurses chose patients to participate whom they perceived to have complex care needs and would be in hospital for a long enough period of time to enable them to establish a relationship. The majority of the patients were approached the day after they had been admitted, as the nurses felt that they needed to 'see them for a shift' before deciding if they were appropriate participants.

Choosing Conversations Although the nurses wore the microphones and audio-recorders throughout their working day, they only turned them on for specific conversations. These conversations predominantly related to care assessments, discussions about care options, discharge planning, patient education and case reviews with members of the multidisciplinary team. While there were multiple individual conversations recorded, the average amount of conversation recorded with each patient was three hours. While few research studies have identified the actual number of hours nurses spend in verbal communication with patients, several research studies have reported that nurses only spend a small proportion of their time communicating with older patients (Stockwell, 1972; Norton *et al*, 1975; Wells, 1980; Macleod-Clark, 1982). The majority of conversations recorded were deliberate, intentional or planned.

This can be considered to be a weakness of the data collection approach, as it could be argued that the deliberateness of switching on the audio-recorder affected how genuine the communication approach adopted was and the authenticity of the data recorded. Robinson (1986) addresses this problem (described by her as 'distortion') in her study of Health Visiting. She argues that because of the interest shown in interactions between Health Visitors and their clients, then any distortion may be a positive one and would in fact make the interaction 'more typical'. Robinson's argument is based on the premise that observation of work (or in this case interactions) can result in the person being observed paying more attention to the work being undertaken and therefore making it more typical of all similar work. Even though the nurses were aware that the focus of the study was patient autonomy, they did not know from what perspective it was being explored, nor indeed if it was being viewed as a positive or negative concept in patient care. In order to overcome the potential problem of distortion, participating nurses were asked to treat their first attempt at recording as a 'trial run'. There is little evidence in the data of it being staged. Cross comparison of conversations suggest that the conversations were indeed authentic and that the recording of these conversations had little effect on the overall data collected.

In addition, the patients themselves acted as a 'control' in two significant ways. Firstly, they were unaware of the audio-recorder being switched on, as the nurses had been asked to do so prior to approaching the patient. This occurred in most cases. Two conversations suggested that the recorder was switched on at the patient's bedside (identified by the patients comments). This data was not rejected, but its structure was compared with other conversations before it was included in the data set and prior to any interpretation of it being made. Secondly, the patients were unaware of the focus of the data being collected. Patients were told that the research was focusing on elements of the nurse-patient relationship rather than on patient autonomy. The patients who would not be participating in this performance would have counteracted any distortion to conversations pursued by the nursing staff. Further, in this study, as identified by Robinson (1986) there were ample opportunities for the nurse participants to destroy data that they thought to be unrepresentative of their work. From the tape recordings returned for analysis, I was not aware of this being done. In addition, during follow-up reflective conversations, while nurse participants considered much of the data analysed to be less than ideal practice or indeed poor practice, they did not consider it to be 'abnormal' practice arising from their focus on the tape recorder.

Typically, data collection occurred in the following way:

- The patient would be approached by the primary nurse participating in the research, on their second day of admission to hospital.
- The patient (and family where appropriate) would be provided with a consent form and background information about the study and given up to 24 hours before asked to make a decision to participate.
- Throughout the data collection period the nurse would wear the microphone and audio-recorder (usually hidden in a pocket or 'bum-bag').
- Data collection would begin when the nurse approached the patient to undertake their initial assessment and planning for care needs.
- Further conversations would be recorded periodically throughout the patient's stay, relating to discharge planning or associated activities.
- Discussions about participating patients' progress were recorded at weekly multidisciplinary review meetings throughout the patients' hospital stay.
- The final conversation to confirm discharge plans and arrangements made, usually ended the data collection period (although some nurses continued to record data up to and including the patient leaving the ward).

Ethical Issues Patients who were approached to participate were provided with a letter of explanation and consent form which explained the study aims and what their participation would entail. In addition, they were provided with an information sheet (which included my name and place of contact) for their family and friends. Throughout the study, only two patients refused to participate and one withdrew from the study. This degree of compliance is consistent with other research evidence and represents the compliant behaviour of older people in hospital (Ebersole and Hess, 1990).

The issue of 'indirect participation' was a significant one in this study. Because of the data collection method adopted (audio-recording of naturally occurring conversations), there existed the potential for patients who had not been asked to participate, having their voices recorded. The approach agreed with the ethics committee to overcome this, consisted of gaining consent from all patients on the ward during the data collection period. A letter for patients 'indirectly participating' in the research was prepared. However, in practice this proved very problematic. As participating patients would be located in various parts of ward areas, all patients on the ward would need to provide their consent. This would need to be done for all patients being admitted over a long period of time (up to one year in some cases). The time involved in doing this would be considerable and none of the managers were prepared to support this approach. Instead, agreement was reached that a poster and information sheets would be prepared. Posters would be displayed in various parts of the ward area and information sheets would be included with the admission packs for all patients and their families. A number of patients and their family members inquired about the research from ward nurses, but none objected to it.

Participating nurses were provided with a letter and consent form which explained the study aims and what their participation would entail. In addition, they were provided with a supply of patient letters, consent forms, information sheets and letters for members of the multidisciplinary team. The nurses participating discussed the research with other nurses in their team and I was available to answer any further questions that they were unable to answer. In no case was this necessary and the nursing teams in all the participating settings supported the research.

Members of the multidisciplinary team were also provided with information about the research and asked to consent to having their voices recorded during 'naturally occurring' conversations and during multidisciplinary team meetings. The research was discussed in detail with managers of occupational and physiotherapy services (the dominant therapists in ward teams) and these managers in turn discussed the research with members of their teams. Managers of other 'visiting' therapists were sent information about the research.

In the community hospital settings, medical support is provided by General Practitioners (GPs). A letter was sent to the senior partner of each practice informing them of the research in progress, the possibility of their 'indirect participation', the need to record multidisciplinary team meetings and patient participation. GPs' consent for patients to participate in the research was assumed, unless they objected to specific patients participating. While some GPs inquired further about the research design, none objected to patient participation or to their conversations being recorded.

Although the Consultant Geriatrician in the specialist department had initially agreed to the research proceeding, he subsequently withdrew support for *his* patients to participate in the research. This limited the number of patients available to participate and delayed the overall data collection period. The other consultant in the unit did not object in this way and supported the research.

The Nurse and Patient Sample The final sample consisted of 4 hospital based primary nurses, one community based specialist nurse and an expert practitioner (hospital based) (figure 2). These participating nurses were asked to complete a 'profile' of their biographies as a means of demonstrating their typicality to the reader (Ely *et al*, 1991).

Figure 2: The Nurse Participants

HOSPITAL	NUMBER OF NURSES
Community Hospital A	1 Primary Nurse
Community Hospital C	2 Primary Nurses
Specialist Department	1 Primary Nurse
Specialist Nurse	1
Expert Nurse	1

The nurses were asked to record the conversations with up to four of their patients from admission to the time that a decision about discharge arrangements had been agreed (Figure 3). Only one nurse (Laura) managed to achieve this for a variety of reasons, including workload pressures, duty rotas, sickness and annual leave. All of the nurses recorded conversations with two or three patients. The clinical nurse specialist only recorded conversations with one patient. However, this was acceptable given the nature of her work. She carried a large caseload of patients over a large geographical area. When a new patient was entered onto her caseload, her visits to their homes were for long periods (usually one hour). In this research, she recorded four such conversations (i.e. four home visits) over 6 months. A gap of at least one month exists between each conversation/visit and therefore in this research, these visits are treated as separate cases, although undertaken with the same patient. The expert nurse did not have a set caseload of patients and therefore, the conversations she recorded are not so 'deliberate, intentional or planned' as other participating nurses. Her work role was predominantly supervisory, supportive and advisory and therefore, the conversations recorded are not located with particular patients or spread out from admission to discharge.

Figure 3: Participating Nurses and the Patients they Worked with

SETTING	NURSE [Pseudonyms]	PATIENTS [Pseudonyms]
Community Hospital A	Ann	Shirley; Jim; Mabel
Community Hospital C	Laura	Mrs. Burke; Mrs. Day; Sid; Jack
Community Hospital C	Nicola	Mrs. Archer; Reg; Molly
Specialist Unit	Leslie	Aidan; Len
Specialist Nurse	Pat	Neil
Expert Nurse	Barbara	Various patients

Note: The differing patients' titles reflect individual patient choices offered by participating nurses.

The Settings In order to maintain anonymity of participants, detailed descriptions of the settings are not provided. Munhall (1991; 269) raises the problems of confidentiality and anonymity in qualitative research:

> In qualitative research, can we promise confidentiality when we include precise quotations from transcripts in our publications? The answer is 'no', but we can provide anonymity by protecting the identity of the participant.

While in this research, actual names have been removed from data sets, the provision of details about the care settings could potentially result in identification of participants. Therefore, common characteristics of the settings are offered, rather than detailed descriptions:

- All settings operate a primary nursing system of care set within a team structure.
- The ratio of primary nurses: patients is approximately 1:6.
- The percentage ratio of registered: unregistered nurses is 60:40.

- All settings are managed by a G Grade ward manager (except for community hospital C which is managed within a team structure).
- The community hospital wards are of a 'race track' style, i.e. a long central corridor with four bedded bays, double rooms and single rooms off it.
- The ward in the specialist unit is a converted 'Nightingale Style' ward, i.e. a large open room with partitions erected in order to create private spaces.
- Both community hospitals cater for a similar client group - rehabilitation, respite care and sub-acute care.
- The specialist unit's client groups are those who need rehabilitation, but with acute care needs that require regular medical intervention.
- Patients who are on the 'list' of local General Practitioners are admitted from local District General Hospitals and directly from home to the community hospitals.
- Each setting has weekly multidisciplinary review meetings.

Regular contact by telephone and periodic visits to the participants was maintained throughout the period when they were collecting data. While I was not continuously present with the participants, I needed to create a relationship with them that was quietly encouraging, yet gave them the freedom to make decisions for themselves about what data to collect. I remained conscious of the need to balance being supportive with not appearing coercive. As Ely *et al* (1991; 51) suggest:

> there really is no short cut and no magic ... Qualitative researchers have to be there with all our senses, with much of our time, and with a quiet stubborn streak that says, 'There is a way. Maybe we haven't found it yet but with patience and skill, maybe tomorrow'.

The approach was successful in assisting the participants to maintain their momentum in data collection. In all, the data was collected over an eighteen-month period.

Establishing an Analytical Framework

The analysis of data was guided by the philosophical principles underpinning conversation analysis and hermeneutics, as earlier identified in this chapter. However, as Ely *et al* (1991) identify, it is important at the beginning of the analytical process to establish 'the rudder' of analysis, that is, the framework that will guide the decision-making process. The framework adopted is drawn from the work of Drew and Heritage (1992) and Field and Morse (1985). This framework will be unfolded in the next sections, by making explicit the decisions made in:

- organising,
- describing and
- interpreting the data.

Organising the Data

By the end of the data collection I had accumulated fourteen case studies (NB: the interactions of the nurse expert are counted as one case study, because of the approach to data collection adopted and earlier described in this chapter) accumulating approximately thirty-three hours of tape-recorded data. The process of analysing data began with the organisation of the data collected. With reference to the preparation of transcripts for analysis, Silverman (1993) argues that the preparation of transcripts is not simply a technical detail prior to the main business of analysis. For conversation analysis, this is not only an important consideration in relation to transcript preparation, but in the preparation of the recorded data. The technology used to record data forms an essential consideration in conversation analysis prior to data collection. In this study, this was particularly difficult, as the conversations were not occurring in a formal setting, that is, nurses were often engaged in other work while recording the data - for example, doing treatments, assisting with patients' hygiene needs. Therefore it was essential that the technology used would capture the voices of all those involved in the conversation without the need for the establishment of a deliberate 'interview type' setting. The tie-microphones fulfilled this purpose. However, some data was lost due to background noise.

Each tape had a backup copy made prior to their transcription. Once the initial transcription was made, each conversation was listened to at least twice before any further work was undertaken. This was useful for a number of reasons, including:

- achieving an overall sense of the conversation flow and its focus;
- gaining a sense of the accuracy of the transcription made by the secretary;
- planning time for data analysis.

Each conversation was then listened to for a third time, with missing words inserted, data omissions and inaccurate interpretation of words altered. In addition, conventional grammatical structures needed to be removed from the data. As will be discussed later, the use of these structures is limited in conversation analysis and their use have different meanings to those in conventional sentence construction. Although the secretary had been asked not to insert these constructions in the initial transcription, she found this difficult to achieve.

A coding frame was then established based on the work of Jefferson (1984, cited in Heritage, 1984). The aim of the frame is to establish a very detailed transcript, translating onto the page, three facets of speech:

- what was said - words, sounds;
- when it was said - timing, silences;
- how it was said - intonation, emphasis.

The details of the coding used in this research are outlined in Figure 4.

Figure 4: Conversation Analysis Coding Conventions

1.	Text A ⌈more text A ⌊Text B	Overlap.
2.	⌈Beginning of text A ⌊Beginning of text B	Talk starts simultaneously
3.	⌈Beginning of text A* more text A ⌊Beginning of text B	The point at which two overlapping or simultaneously started utterances end
4.	Text A=more text A= =text B	"Latching", i.e. no interval between the end of a prior and start of a next piece of talk.
5.	Text A= =⌈Beginning of text B ⌊Beginning of text A	'Latching' and simultaneous talk
6.	⌈Beginning of text A ⊨ ⌊Beginning of text B ⊨ =text A	two utterances end simultaneously and are latched onto by a next.
7.	Text A(**number, e.g. 0.3**)more text A *or* Text A (**number**) Text B	elapsed time in tenths of seconds
8.	Text A, *or* Text A. *or* Text A?	question (symbol used to indicate intonation rather than grammar.
9.	Te:xt A	the prior syllable is prolonged
10	Te:::::xt A	a more prolonged syllable.
11	<u>Text</u> A *or* <u>Text</u> A	indicates various forms of stressing and may involve *pitch* and/or *volume*.
12	Te(**h**)xt A	explosive aspiration (e.g. laughter)
13	°Text A	the talk it precedes is low in volume.
14	**TEXT A**	increased volume.
15	(text A)	not sure about the accuracy of words contained in parentheses.
16	( )	no hearing was achieved.
17	((e.g. cough))	indicates features of the audio materials other than actual utterances, or utterances that are not transcribed.

Describing the Data

Atkinson and Drew (1979) highlight six characteristics of descriptions that acted as important considerations in this research:

- any description is potentially infinite;
- any description can be as small as a single word, yet be sufficient;
- anything can be described in more than one way. A choice of description is always a choice between viable alternatives;
- the choice of description depends on the context. The same event in a different context may invoke a different description;
- the recognition of a description as appropriate is independent of knowledge of the subject described. The description is validated without specific reference to the subject;
- descriptions are part of the subjects they purport to describe independently.

Analysis in qualitative research relies heavily on the quality of the transcript of data (Ely *et al*, 1991). Burnard (1992) raises the issue of the differences between a particular reality and the way that reality is captured in a transcript. Burnard argues that a transcript can never represent a true reality and that indeed, transcripts present a different reality to that observed in context. The collection of naturally occurring data and its detailed coding that captures the conventions of everyday talk enables the conservation of the reality of the talk rather than descriptions of it. The inter-relationship between the transcription of talk and the recorded talk itself enables the reader of such talk to have access to the original data and not just a description of it. Atkinson and Drew (1979) suggest that given direct access to the data, a reader can follow the logic of interpretations made as well as decisions about the process of interpretation. If, for example, I have interpreted interruptions by a nurse as a form of power and control, then the reader can read the originally recorded data to review the utterances in question and, secondly, to check the validity of the interpretation of the utterance.

The objective is to describe how particular institutions are enacted and lived through as accountable patterns of meaning, inference and action. Descriptions of data combine a concern with the contextual sensitivity of language use with a focus on talk as a vehicle for social action. The initial and overriding focus is on the particular actions that occur in some context, their underlying social organization, and the alternative means by which these actions and the activities they compose can be realised. Following the initial coding of transcripts, a framework for describing the data was developed from the work of Drew and Heritage (1992). The framework has three foci:

1) Goal orientation;
2) Special and particular constraints;
3) Inferential frameworks.

and five dimensions of analysis:

1) Lexical choice;
2) Turn design;
3) Sequence organisation;
4) Overall structural organisation;
5) Social epistemology and social relations.   (see Figure 5)

Figure 5: Data Analysis Framework

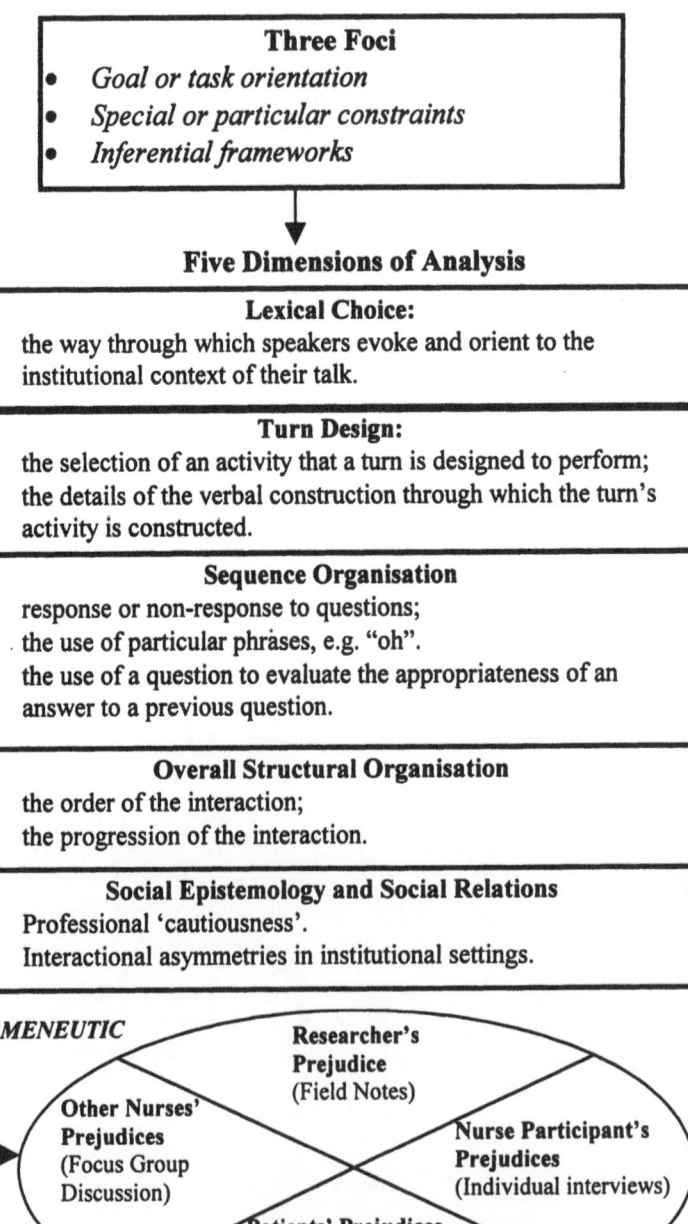

CONVERSATION ANALYSIS

Three Foci
- *Goal or task orientation*
- *Special or particular constraints*
- *Inferential frameworks*

Five Dimensions of Analysis

Lexical Choice:
- the way through which speakers evoke and orient to the institutional context of their talk.

Turn Design:
- the selection of an activity that a turn is designed to perform;
- the details of the verbal construction through which the turn's activity is constructed.

Sequence Organisation
- response or non-response to questions;
- the use of particular phrases, e.g. "oh".
- the use of a question to evaluate the appropriateness of an answer to a previous question.

Overall Structural Organisation
- the order of the interaction;
- the progression of the interaction.

Social Epistemology and Social Relations
- Professional 'cautiousness'.
- Interactional asymmetries in institutional settings.

HERMENEUTIC

Researcher's Prejudice (Field Notes)

Other Nurses' Prejudices (Focus Group Discussion)

Nurse Participant's Prejudices (Individual interviews)

Patients' Prejudices (Focus Group Discussion)

Using this framework and through comparative data analysis, research aims to demonstrate the way that particular features of talk in institutional contexts embody systematic asymmetries that are not ordinarily found in mundane conversation. By highlighting the particular emphases on words, particular interruptions, etcetera, the meaning of these linguistic structures can then be understood using the framework described. Each conversation was analysed in this way.

Following the application of the analytical framework to the data, each transcript was then 'segmented' and a descriptive account of the data made, including my initial interpretations of the descriptions. Each case study was analysed in this way. This approach enabled the selection of relevant data to be chosen to take to the next stage of analysis, that is, the interpretation of the data for themes and meanings. Throughout this period of analysis, reflective notes (reflective diary) were maintained by me. These notes served the same function as those of a qualitative researcher 'in the field'. Listening and re-listening to tape recordings invoked feelings, ideas, hunches and views that I needed to capture because:

- they minimised the impact of my feelings etc. on the approach to data analysis. Each time I responded to a particular interaction, I recorded my response in reflective notes as a means of minimising its impact on the way the data was analysed;
- they acted as a means of checking out emerging issues from the data that I may wish to discuss with participants in the 'reflective conversations';
- they maintained the hermeneutic focus of the research approach, that is, the making explicit of my 'prejudices'.

Interpreting the Data

The second stage of data collection (reflective conversations and focus group discussions) formed the basis for achieving 'layers of interpretation' (Morse, 1991). The relationship between the conversation data and the second stage of data collection is illustrated in figure 4. It demonstrates how the 'hermeneutic circle of understanding' is being utilised as more than a methodological framework, but as an approach to framing the relationship between researcher and participants; as a means of achieving shared interpretations through situational understandings; and as an approach to achieving 'fusion of horizons' through the different layers of interpretation. The aim was to create a 'dialogue' between naturally occurring data and interpretations offered by participants, patients and expert nurses.

The data were analysed using principles of thematic analysis developed from the work of Ely *et al* (1991). My aim was to develop understandings based on the way participants in the research understood the language of autonomy and their justification for these understandings. The continued focus on language was also consistent with the overall focus of the work. My overall intention was to move from descriptive understandings achieved through conversation analysis to an interpretation of these descriptions through the development of themes and categories. Members of the 'expert' focus group were asked to identify themes from the interpreted transcripts provided to them prior to the focus group interview and following discussion in the focus group itself. These themes were used as the 'rudder' to develop other themes and as a basis for comparing themes generated by the researcher and nurse participants. Ely (1991; 150) defines a theme as:

> ... a statement of meaning that (1) runs through all or most of the pertinent data, or (2) one in the minority that carries heavy emotional or factual impact. It can be thought of as the researcher's inferred statement that highlights explicit or implied attitudes toward life, behaviour, or understandings of a person, persons or culture.

This definition was used to guide decision-making in the thematic analysis of data. In addition, while qualitative research texts (Field and Morse, 1985; Leininger, 1985 *for example*) advocate the use of categories as elements of overall themes, thereby forming a matrix of categories and themes, I made the decision to use Ely's definition of themes and develop 'Themes' and 'sub-themes'. A sub-theme being:

> a label applied to particular data characteristics that highlight explicit or implied attitudes, behaviour, or understandings. The amalgamation of the common characteristics of sub-themes leads to the generation of data themes.

For example, the sub-theme 'lack of skill in dealing with emotion' was seen to have similar characteristics as the sub-theme 'deference to professional opinion'. From these, and a number of other sub-themes, the theme of 'Socialisation and Enculturation' was developed. To achieve this thematic analysis, an adapted version of Ely *et al's* (1991) structured approach to the generation of themes was utilised (based on the work of Bussis *et al*, 1978). This process involved:

- Study and re-study the raw data to develop detailed, intimate knowledge.
- Note initial impressions.
- List tentative sub-themes.
- Refine sub-themes by examining the results of steps 2 and 3 and returning to the entire database of step 1.
- Group data under the still tentative sub-themes and revise sub-themes if needed.
- Select verbatim narrative to link the raw data to the sub-themes.
- Study results of step 6 and revise if needed.
- Write theme statements based on the common characteristics of sub-themes, and by linking data in and across sub-themes.
- Integrate findings of each case study.
- Compare findings for commonalities or patterns, differences, and unique happenings.

Five themes that characterise the concept of autonomy as exercised by older people in hospital and facilitated by nurses were identified through the data analysis (figure 6).

Figure 6: Research Themes

THEME	FOCUS
1. **Communicative Style**	The use of language to enhance or limit individual action.
2. **Power and Control**	The power relationship between participants and its impact on individual action.
3. **Constraints on Autonomous Action**	Interactions and contextual factors that enhance or inhibit individual action.
4. **Socialization and Enculturation**	Socialization processes and cultural norms that enhance or inhibit individual action.
5. **The Professionalisation of Relatives**	Interactions that enable a patient's family to make decisions on his/her behalf without explicit authority from the patient and which are corroborated by the nurse.

The theme of 'Communicative Style' is a consistent theme throughout the data. Through the methodological focus on 'language as action', the communicative style of nurses and other health care professionals was identified as a central focus of much of the data, as a means of either facilitating or inhibiting autonomous action. It is through the focus on the structure of language and the style of communication used by nurses and other members of the health care team that other themes were identified in the data. The relationship between the themes and sub-themes is illustrated in figure 7.

Figure 7: Relationship Between Themes and Sub-Themes

THEME 1: COMMUNICATIVE STYLE **(Chapter 5)**	**SUB-THEMES** • The Conversation Agenda • The Conversation Focus • Signposting • Sensitivity to Cues & Appropriate Response • The Control of Conversations.

THEME 2: POWER and CONTROL (Chapter 6)
 	
SUB-THEMES
• Professional Power and Control
• Hopes, Dreams and Desires
	THEME 3: CONSTRAINT on AUTONOMOUS ACTION (Chapter 7)
	
	SUB-THEMES
	  • Organisational Constraint
	  • Routinised Practices
	  • Emotional Constraint
	  • Lack of Synchronicity

THEME 4: SOCIALISATION and ENCULTURATION (Chapter 7) **SUB-THEMES** • Deference to Professional Opinion • Lack of Skill in Dealing with Emotion	**THEME 5: THE PROFESSIONALISATION OF RELATIVES (Chapter 7)** **(NO SUB-THEMES)**

As each theme was developed, 'Principles for Action' were identified. These are factors/issues that would need to be considered if a patient-centred approach to practice that was built on contemporary issues of partnership and empowerment was to be realised.

All principles for action identified in each theme were then listed and grouped according to their common focus. Five new themes were identified that represented all of the individual principles for action contained in the data. The five themes identified were:

- Informed Flexibility;
- Sympathetic Presence;

- Negotiation;
- Mutuality;
- Transparency.

The data from the practice of an expert nurse and a clinical nurse specialist in the community were compared with the themes derived from the principles for action, to see if the removal of some of the contextual inhibiting factors and greater expertise would make a difference to the way a patient-centred approach to involvement in care and decision-making happened, that is, would these five themes be present in their positive form, rather than as constraining factors. Two 'types' of data were identified:

- data that illustrated a 'different approach', that is, a is patient-centred approach;
- data that demonstrated no difference in approach.

By doing this it was possible to identify factors that could be altered through a change in approach to practice while no change in approach would illustrate the structural constraints that exist in organisations/institutions irrespective of the philosophical approach to practice.

Presentation of Data

Chapters five, six and seven that follow will discuss in depth, each of the themes and sub-themes derived from the analysis of the data. Chapter five will address the theme of 'communicative style' and focuses on the impact of communication on the nurses' facilitation of patient autonomy. Chapter six will discuss the theme of 'power and control' and the way inwhich power in the nurse-patient relationship and between members of the multidisciplinary team is manifested. Chapter seven incorporates the three themes of 'constraint on autonomous action', 'socialisation and enculturation' and 'the professionalisation of relatives'. These themes have been amalgamated in this chapter because of the way they collectively represent the continuous interplay that appeared to exist between nurses, other professionals, patients, their families and the culture of the care environments. The phrase 'Speaking for you or Speaking for me' consistently re-emerged in my reflections as I worked with the data and therefore has been used as a metaphor to represent these three themes.

Each chapter integrates conversation data, with reflective conversation and focus group interview data. It should be noted that the data from the 'older people focus group' is predominantly included in chapter seven, as the majority of the issues identified in the analysis of this data were located within these themes. Each of these chapters ends with an identification of the 'principles for action' from the data analysis presented. As outlined in chapter four, these principles for action were developed into five themes. Chapter eight then, presents data collected from the expert nurse and community nurse specialist that illustrates the articulation of these themes with the removal of contextual inhibiting factors and evidence of increased practice expertise.

5 Communicative Style

Introduction

Through the methodological focus on 'language as action' (Drew and Heritage, 1992), the communicative style of nurses and other health care professionals is the central focus of the data in this chapter. The style of communication used by professionals with patients serves as a means of either facilitating or inhibiting autonomous action. As outlined in chapter 4, it is through the focus on the structure of language and the style of communication used by nurses and other members of the health care team that initial themes were identified from the data. The participants' orientation to social institutions (professional groupings), as either representatives or clients of the institution (Drew and Heritage, 1992), as demonstrated through the style of interactions, is the focus of this chapter. Participants in the 'expert nurses focus group' and 'the patients focus group' validated the initial themes and provided them with 'labels'.

By focusing on the structures of language and the linguistic styles of nurses, patients and other health care workers, issues concerning older patients' abilities to participate in their care and nurses/health care workers' abilities to facilitate such decision-making are raised as critical factors in understanding the nature of autonomy in the nurse-patient relationship. The aim is to describe how the structures of a social institution such as a hospital, are enacted and lived through as patterns of meaning, inference and action. Five sub-themes describe the structures of language and communicative styles:

- The Conversation Agenda.
- The Conversation Focus.
- Signposting.
- Sensitivity to Cues and Appropriate Response.
- The Control of Conversations.

The data examples used are illustrative of the themes in the data analysis. They are chosen because they are representative of all the data in that theme rather than for their particular unique attributes.

The Conversation Agenda

While there were some examples in the data of conversations following the patient's agenda, the majority of conversations followed a pre-determined agenda set by the professional:

Case Study 5/Interaction 1/Molly

```
28 P:   just ordinary bits and pieces around the flat-there's
29      nothing strenuous
30 N:   (0.1) do you see your self (      )=
31 P:   =she always carries it she carries it (     ) coffee
32      please not too strong.
33 N:   (0.2) would you like it made with milk or water=
34 P:   =oh no water's fine thank you=
35 N:   =would you like sugar?=
36 P:   =no thank you (0.1) em oh yes she does that yes
37      and there's a little (0.3) it's not really a laundrette
38      it's a washing machine dryer and that down on the
39      site so that's handy there's no washing to do only
40 N          ⌊right
41      smalls and things like that
42 N:   (0.1) and you can do that?=
43 P:   =yes that's alright but most of it will go in the
44      washing machine-have an extra load if I have to=
45 N:   =what about em (0.4) cooking?
46 P:   thank you (0.1) thank you very much I don't see
47      that will be any problem because if it's difficult
48      (   ) you know all you do is (        ) oh and it
49      shot up lost the lot ((can't hear this something
50      about a microwave)).  I can use the top of my
51      other oven but I'm (      ) as you might say
52      (   ) waist level as you might say  there's no
53      (   ) problem you see it's getting up the stairs
54 N:   (0.4) and how many stairs do you have to go up?=
55 P:   =inside ones and concrete ones to the front door
56      (   ) count stairs when they go up one (0.1) two=
57 N:   =(        ) (about thirteen)
58 P:                        ⌊it could be ten I really don't
59      know (0.3) we do have a rail like (     )
```

In the above conversation, the nurse followed up her responsibilities agreed at the discharge planning meeting regarding discussing discharge issues with the patient. The conversation followed an orderly question and answer sequence organisation. The nurse worked through a 'tacit' list of issues that needed to be discussed with the patient about her discharge arrangements. There were differences in perception between the nurse and patient concerning the goal of the conversation that arose from a conversation 'asymmetry' (Schegloff, 1992). This asymmetry appeared to arise from the tension that existed between the nurse's perspective of collecting routine social information and the patient, for whom these questions were unique and personal to her situation. While the goal of the interaction for the nurse was the collection of this information in order to plan further action (for example, a home visit) the patient treated the conversation as an opportunity to tell the nurse about the details of the problems she experienced. The information gathering focus of the conversation was indicated through the lengthy and detailed answers to questions given by the patient and the limited responses by the nurse or the moving onto another question without acknowledgement of the previous response. What was not made explicit throughout this section of the conversation was an already established plan for the patient to stay in hospital for two weeks.

The dominant theme throughout many of the case studies is the agenda of patients' families and the nurses' ability to respect patients wishes while trying to balance these against the wishes of the family. It is this tension that forms the agenda of many conversations in the case studies and will be addressed further in Chapters 6 and 7.

The overall structure of interactions was dictated by the agenda of the nurses. Because of the focus of much of the settings where the research was undertaken (i.e. rehabilitation with an emphasis on enabling older people to return home or to a suitable residential alternative), how best to proceed with patients' discharge arrangements formed the basis of many of the interactions between nurses, patients and other health care workers. A health care climate with a dominant managerial focus (Traynor, 1996), an emphasis on rapid throughput (CSAG, 1998) and a prevailing view that older people are a burden on hospital resources (House of Commons Health Select Committee, 1996) places pressure on nurses and other health care workers to achieve early discharge. Others (*for example* Bogoch, 1994) have found that the linguistic style of professionals often is focused on the convenience of the organisation rather than the expressly stated wishes of the client:

Case Study 11/Interaction 1/Mabel

48 P: I haven't been out for years not out on me own (0.1) just

```
49 N:                                        ⌊right
50      come from my door and get in the car (0.07) (   ) to my
51 N:                                      ⌊right
52      daughter's (0.1) no I haven't been out in the village they
53 N:              ⌊right
54      come and pick me up you see in the day centre so I don't
55 N:                                  ⌊right
56      have to walk=
57 D:   =she can't=
58 N:          ⌊right
59 P:   =I get up and walk in there and that but em not a lot=
60 N:   =so what do you hope from this admission just to get your
61      chest better and then you go back home

65 N:   =right °right your daughter was just saying that she didn't
66      feel that you'd be able to go back to your own home
67 P:                                                  ⌊no
68 N:   (0.3) Do you think you would be able to go back home to
69      yo::ur house if we put in some help? (0.2) What do you
70      think
71 P:   (0.3) Eh not on me own=
72 N:   =yeah but if I spoke to Kathy Sugden to see if we could
73      get someone to pop in each morning (0.2) to help you get
74      up=
```

This control of the conversational agenda is further illustrated in case study 11. Between lines 48 and 59 the patient told her story to the nurse about her ability to mobilise. Throughout this story the nurse reinforced its validity by the use of supportive interjections - 'right'. The nurse did not use the story told by Mabel as an opportunity to understand how she 'coped' with her disabilities or to ask further questions to gain a greater understanding of her coping abilities. Instead, in line 60 the nurse latched a question onto Mabel's previous statement in order to initiate a topic shift and return to her agenda.

The question is both asked and answered by the nurse in lines 60-61. Mabel predictably agreed with the nurse's assumption, because it conferred with her expressed wish. However, in line 65 the nurse latched a supportive 'right' to Mabel's previous assertion, before introducing the daughter's view. The nurse, however, overcame the constraining nature of this assertion by following it up with a question that sought Mabel's views. Mabel qualified that she would not be able to cope on her own. This remark was understood by the nurse as a request for help at home rather than a suggestion that she did not want to return home at all.

The organisation of further conversations in this case study are dominated by professional agendas. For example, throughout the various interactions with professionals, Mabel described her usual weekly routine. While Mabel was provided with opportunities to input into the conversation and control the agenda, a major asymmetry (caused by a hidden agenda) existed, i.e. the views of the patient's daughter. Although the patient was provided with the opportunity to make choices and suggestions, and plan for her care needs, she was continually unaware of the views of her daughter and these were not made explicit to her. Each suggestion she made about her care needs was responded to by the professional with a suggestion of the daughter's views and her desire for Mabel to have morning and evening carers. This agenda was not however made explicit to Mabel and she did not link the significance of the care manager's utterances with the suggested care plan.

At no time was Mabel's explicit agreement sought about the care planned. The sequence organisation of the conversation disadvantaged her as she was unable to assert what she really wanted because of the many agendas being played out through the professionals' perceptions of her 'best interest'.

Although, on some occasions, the professionals did not appear to explicitly aim to hide the real conversation agenda from patients, their skill in introducing the agenda was generally limited. Rarely was the agenda for the conversation clearly set out by the professional, but instead the agenda appeared to unfold as the conversation progressed. Baldock and Prior (1981) found a similar lack of clarity in their study of social worker interactions with clients. Social workers were seen to avoid the main reason for meeting with their clients and spent considerable time talking about 'unimportant' issues. While the importance of setting the scene for a conversation is recognised, the social workers, like the nurses in this study, appeared to lack an ability to switch from 'general chat' to a focused agenda. Case Study 12 illustrates the lengthy route that many of the nurses adopted in order to reach the 'real' conversation agenda:

Case Study 12/Interaction 1/Shirley

```
374 N:  (0.1) Shirley what would you say are one of your problems
375     whilst you are here you know we have these care plans
376     what would you say is your ma::in problem whilst you are
377     here in hospital do you think (0.3) is there anything that
378     really troubles you at the moment?
379 P:  E::h no no because (0.1) em (0.08) you know Don and
380     Anita my next door neighbours =
```

381 N: Yes I do=
382 P: =Don (0.05) he's done you eh know looked after the
383   turning up and turning down or whatever of the gas (0.3)
384 N: ⌊Right
385   and eh (0.1) no I think it's all been looked after at home
386   alright=
387 N: =ri:::ght em from a nursing point of view whilst you're
388   here what would you say would be one of your difficulties
389   while you are here (0.2) do you think it's more trying to
390   learn (0.1) well not learn but become more mobile do you
391   think or do you think its the fact that you've got no interest
392   in food
393 P: (0.1) Well yes at the moment I haven't and I think (I've got a
394   freezer full of food) (I go out and) look and see and
395   sometimes its ever so nice but I don't want it but I have to=
396 N: =push yourself?=
397 P: =yes
398 N: (0.1) Are you sleeping at night?
399 P: Yes not too badly really I suppose you could say=
400 N: =right
401 P: (0.3) Yes and ( ) unless these pains in my back and legs if
402   they start aching I can't go to sleep ( )=
403 N: =right right
404 P: °Yes I feel more dry now=
405 N: =do you want to have a drink?
406 P: Yes yes
407 N: (0.5) No keep on ( ) have a glass (10.0) Shirley how would
408   you say your mood was would you say your moods ( )
409   fresh this afternoon
410 P: (0.3) The only thing is I haven't got anybody at home to do
411   the laundry I dunno I shall have to get somebody to do it
412   ( )=
413 N: =well that's alright we can sort that out whilst your here
414   (0.07) no I meant from the point of view (0.1) Jim died last
415   June wasn't it=
416 P: =yes yes (0.06) yes
417 N: (0.2) I should imagine it's still very (0.1)
418 P: Oh yes I ( ) (0.1) comes over you sometimes=
419 N: =yes=
420 P: =but as I say I'm not afraid of being at home on my own=
421 N: =right
422 P: (0.1) But just sometimes you wake up in the morning and
423   think 'well, what's to get up for' (0.2) I do get up of course
424   I do but I could almost do without getting up so I get up
425   and go back to bed and eh something that sort of feeling

426   (0.3) but anyway I'm still here to tell the tale=
427 N: =m:::::m you are aren't you (0.08)do you chat to Reg about
428   Jim much
429 P: (0.05) O:h yes yes I do
430 N: (0.1) Do you find that helps?=
431 P: =yes I do yes and my friend her husband went down to the
432   village to get his pension on the Thursday before Christmas
433   and he came back home and he went upstairs to put the
434   money away and dropped down dead=
435 N: =o:::::h Shirley that's a shock isn't it=

In this interaction, the nurse sought Shirley's perception of her main problems. The nurse, in line 375 referred to this question being related to 'these care plans' that are used. The way that the nurse expressed this question resulted in Shirley misinterpreting the aim of the question, i.e. the nurse begins by asking the patient what she thinks her main problems are while she is in hospital, then links this to 'we have these care plans' and then rephrases the question to 'is there anything that really troubles you at the moment'.

Shirley's response related to her support at home, i.e. she was not worrying about her home whilst in hospital. The nurse recognised the misinterpretation and responded supportively (line 387 - =ri:::ght ...). She then attempted to rephrase the question and narrowed it to a choice between her mobility or her loss of appetite. Shirley's response confirmed a loss in appetite. The nurse then asked the patient about her sleeping pattern (line 398) and in line 407 asked Shirley about her 'mood'. Following a three second pause, Shirley did not answer the question, but instead talked about needing help with her laundry. Eventually in line 414 the nurse directly asked the patient about the death of her husband and her grief response to this. In line 422, Shirley provides a full explanation of how she felt.

It is clear that the nurse's agenda was to discuss the patient's 'low mood' and that she attempted to do this by seeing what Shirley's perception of her problems were. Shirley did not raise the issue of her grief and therefore the nurse eventually picked up on this and raised the issue explicitly. To some extent, the nurse appeared to be avoiding making explicit her perception of the problem and indeed, the nurse did not make any reference to her perception of it. Even when she raised the issue of Shirley's grief reaction and mood she still did not explain to Shirley that this was her agenda. Baldock and Prior (1981) describe 'client-centred' interactions as those that are determined by what the client wants rather than what the professional wants. Although the style of interaction may encourage participation (broad questions, encouragement, using client ideas, using silence and exploring) it does not mean that the patient's agenda formed the focus of interactions (Baldock and Prior, 1981).

In only one case study (case study 13) is there evidence of the patient's agenda being acknowledged. Even on this occasion when the patient's agenda was made explicit, this was for short periods only and the acceptance of the patient's issues as an explicit agenda was controlled by the professional:

Case Study 13/Interaction 2/Jim

```
6 N:    Hello Jim
7 P:    (   )
8 N:    em:: after yesterday's conversation about you
9       wearing the conveen all day and all night  is that
10      working better?
11 P:   (   ) as I (   ) working very well=
12 N:   =it is=
13 P:   =because I'm at ease=
14 N:   =right  are you drinking plenty?
15 P:   I'm drinking a lot more than what I used to=
16 N:   =yes  now I see from your prescription chart Doctor
17      Haigh came in yesterday and has put you on some
18      antibiotics=
19 P:   =for the water infection yes=
20 N:   =that better? do you feel a bit better from that?
21 P:   Well in what way can I feel better from that=
22 N:   =well  have you got any stinging when you pass
23      water?
24 P:   No (   ) it went away very quickly=
25 N:   =right (the) urgency=
26 P:   =yes (   ) like an urgency yes (   ) got this on I just
27      go and not worry about it=
28 N:   =right okay=
29 P:   =so it's a big relief
```

In this conversation, although the nurse has set the agenda, she was focused on the patient and facilitating feedback from him about his condition. In line 8 the nurse asked an open question to begin the conversation and to enable Jim to express his views. Jim's response (line 13) highlighted his continued focus on his emotional state. In line 13 he stated that he was at ease. The nurse's response was to ask if he was drinking plenty and changed the focus of the conversation to that of the infection and his hydration. Although the nurse was focused on physical treatments, Jim's responses indicated his continued focus on aesthetics and his concerns about being incontinent.   In line 26, he continued this focus by his response to the previous utterance. He stated that he didn't have to worry about it (incontinence) now because he had a sheath on and in line 29 described this as a big relief. This difference in focus suggests the differing goals of conversation that the nurse and patient have in the conversational agenda. The nurse was concerned with the physical treatments that Jim was receiving and the outcomes from these treatments, while Jim's focus was that of reducing his worry about being incontinent and its emotional effects. This also illustrates how autonomy can be enhanced. In this scenario the patient's autonomy is promoted by actions that reduce the emotional impact of incontinence. While the actions that have been undertaken do this, the goal of those actions does not appear to be the same as the patient, i.e. they are physically orientated. Generally, however there is little explicit recognition of the dual outcomes of such actions.

Control over the conversational agenda was instigated through a number of linguistic processes implemented by professionals, including their response or non-response to previous utterances, which suggested an ability to identify salient features of conversations and introduce topic changes in order to control the agenda. This resulted in a conversational asymmetry between the professional and patient and the placing of the patient in a powerless position to initiate decisions. Other studies (Bogoch, 1994; Crawford *et al*, 1995; May, 1995 and Brewer *et al*, 1991) also identified the professionals' control over interactions and this has been referred to by Dingwall (1980) as 'orchestrated encounters'.

The professionals achieved control over the conversational agenda through their ability to control the flow of the conversation and the introduction of topics (Smits, 1984). One method of achieving such control, that appeared to be predominantly open to professionals only, was that of not responding to previous utterances (Heritage, 1988; Jefferson and Lee, 1981).

Case Study 3/Interaction 1: Mrs. Archer

In this example a focus on the patient's discomfort and the use of medications to minimise this is maintained through most of the interaction.

```
65 N:    (  ) what about the em swelling (2.0) well that one's
66       (  ) then if it's down all the day ( ) do you think
67 P:    ⌊well it would be
68       it's because this is too low (7.0) and that's not
69       comfortable for you?=
70 P:    =it's all right for a little while
```

71 N: (0.5) Now the other thing I've got to talk to you about
72   is the medication that you're taking at the moment do
73   you know what you're taking? (0.1) have those
75   medications changed very much? ( ) So the aspirins are
76   new and the paracetamol (0.2) is new (   )=
76 P: ⌊yes

84 N: they do use the aspirin when ( )
85 P: yes after an op yeah=
86 N: =very often they have to make a decision about whether
87   you want to go home on it and quite often they do   .
88   like you to stay on it to be able to ( )
89 P: yes *((both nurse and patient laugh))* but I don't often=
90 N: =oh we would actually (0.2) as part of- she could come
90   to you then couldn't she-when you get back on your
91   feet (0.2) but what about the feeling of going home and
92   being grounded.

In line 65, the nurse inquired about 'the swelling' and offered Mrs. Archer a reason why the swelling might be as it was and also that the position she maintained might cause discomfort, i.e. Mrs. Archer was not raising her leg high enough. She did not directly take on board what the nurse had said and instead focused on the degree of comfort, suggesting 'it's all right for a little while'. The nurse did not use this opportunity to reinforce what she meant, but instead her reply changed the focus of the conversation to that of general issues about Mrs. Archer's medication.

Such changes in the orientation of the conversation style are directed by the nurse and do not always naturally flow from the preceding conversation. For example, lines 70-71 (the nurse changed the conversation focus from pain and discomfort to general issues about medication), lines 90-91 (the nurse changed from establishing the patient's knowledge about a particular drug to the patient's feelings about 'being grounded' when she went home).

Such control over the organisation of the interaction illustrates the power of the professional over lay participants to dictate the agenda of the conversation (Smits, 1984). It further highlights the limited opportunities there are for lay participants to take the initiative during conversation and retain or change topics (Heath, 1986).

Throughout nurse-patient interactions, it was the nurse who directed the flow of the conversation and its progression. The nurses chose to keep the conversation open by the way they responded to questions. They appeared to be able to do this because of their access to wider information and knowledge that enabled them to decide how the interaction would progress and the topic areas that would be discussed.

This access to wider information and knowledge enables the professional to identify salient features of the conversation and initiate topic shifts where he/she feels it appropriate to do so. Rarely however are topics changed by the patient, thus reinforcing the powerlessness of the patient and their reliance on the professional to control the care processes. Heath (1986) identified that patients' interactions with general practitioners displayed an extraordinary 'passivity' when they received news or information about their illness. Heath suggests that the demonstration of such passivity enabled the doctor to progress from diagnosis to management of the condition and as such reinforces the asymmetry that exists between the status of the patient and professional.

The ability of the nurse to identify salient features of prior answers in order to select 'next questions' and thus prevent particular issues becoming topics in their own right, was evident throughout their interactions with patients:

Case Study 7/Interaction1/Mrs. Day

```
42 N:   (0.09) right (0.05) is she worried about you going
43      home?
44 P:   · (0.2) no=
45 N:   =no?=
46 P:   =no she thinks I'm quite sensible=
47 N:   =does she=
48 P:   =yeah=
49 N:   =because I expect you have been told there are certain
50      things that you mustn't do (0.2) for six weeks=
51 P:                       ⌊yes I have yeah  =( ) told
52      me=
53 N:   =oh right yeah what did she tell you?=
54 P:   =she promised that I would do no lifting (0.1) and I'd
55      just lift a cuppa tea (    ) just make a cup of tea and
56      not do a lot at all (0.09)⌈ °not yet anyway*
57 N:                             ⌊what will you do about meals*
58 P:   (0.1)Well my daughter's getting me a lot in from
59      Iceland=
60 N:   =right=
61 P:   =I just have to put it in the oven=
62 N:   yeah (0.07) that sounds good doesn't it?=
63 P:   =yeah they do nice meals there=
64 N:   =do they?=
```

65 P: =yes yeah and reasonable too*
66 N: =and breakfast and tea *are quite light things aren't
67   they so you can manage-=
68 P: =I can manage that yes my Daughter will be coming in
69   at quarter past four
70 N: (0.1) °yeah (0.05) it's no vacuuming or carrying the
71   vacuum cleaner upstairs=
72 P: =N::O I don't go upstairs I have all what I need
73   downstairs (0.1) my °bedroom the lot=
74 N: ⌊yes fine =because you were self-sufficient
75   for your kidney for your dialysis weren't you?
76 P: ye::s I had a bedroom downstairs for that
77 N: im yes so you could ⌈(   )
78 P: ⌊(   ) °I'm very sensible=
79 N: =what are you going to do about the shopping?

In this case study, the emphatic statement made by the nurse in line 47, was connected to the explanation offered by her, regarding her concern about Mrs. Day being aware of what she could and couldn't do. The response made by Mrs. Day suggested that she did understand because she had been told. The nurse's response to this utterance was in the form of a question, whereby she asked the patient to explain what she had been told. The nurse controlled the order of the conversation and initiated topic changes as she felt appropriate. She had an advantage over the patient in doing this. Because of her previous experiences, she was able to make decisions about the responses offered by Mrs. Day and evaluate their appropriateness. In line 78, Mrs. Day reiterated her feeling that she was sensible. The nurse did not respond to this statement but instead continued to ask questions regarding the patient's home arrangements.

What is significant about all of this is the asymmetry between the ability of the nurse and patient to control the agenda. While the nurse appeared to follow a particular routine assessment, the patient did not know why the nurse was asking these questions in particular. She may just have been following a routine, i.e. institutionalised/routinised practice, based on her previous experience of undertaking similar assessments many times before (this theme will be discussed further in chapter 6). Alternatively, the nurse may have made decisions about issues that she needed to discuss with the patient based on previous assessments. The significant issue is that the conversation agenda is not made explicit to the patient and therefore her ability to create symmetry in the conversation is prohibited.

It can be concluded from these data that the setting of the conversation agenda is an important factor for the facilitation of patient participation in decision-making. Nurses appeared to take control of the agenda and determine appropriate topics for conversation. Thus, topics that were not seen by the nurse as being important to the patient's care were avoided or controlled by them.

The Conversation Focus

With the conversation agenda established, the success of the interactions between professionals and patients was dependent on the way the focus of the conversation was maintained. Although it could be argued from a linguistic perspective that 'conversation agenda' and 'conversation focus' have the same meaning, in this study, they are identified as being different. The conversation focus is understood as:

> the process of maintaining the conversation agenda within an overall interaction.

Maintaining a focus on the agenda of the conversation would appear to be an important factor in enabling patients to exercise their decision-making potential and thence their autonomy. This is particularly so for older hospitalised patients, where the combined effect of illness and unfamiliar surroundings can affect the person's decision-making abilities (Haug and Ory, 1987). Baldock and Prior (1981) identified that the lack of provision of any clear indication of 'what is relevant to the discussion' provides a limitless array of potential interactional foci and conversational agendas.

Expert group participants felt strongly that in the data generally, there was an inability among nursing staff to maintain the conversation focus while at the same time facilitating a 'natural' conversation:

Expert Group Interview (lines 231-234)

EX1:   One of the things I picked up from most of the data was the idea of either a lack of focus or multiple foci that kind of came and went and yes this grappling with continuity of an issue. But I couldn't work out whether or not that was because the nurse wasn't controlling it or because the patient wasn't able to control it. I sort of made comments - does this nurse know what she is trying to achieve?

This was referred to as the 'conversational competence' of the nurse, i.e. the nurse's ability to maintain an overall intention while facilitating a free-flowing conversation:

Expert Group Interview (lines 488-893)

EX1:   But if that's what they were intending to do, have this social sort of conversation, what made me cross was that the patter that they used was so appalling. You know, let's have a natter or let's you know, and the sort of language, I mean you said that in some cases it was quite patronising and I think it was.

Some participating nurses suggested that it was their responsibility to maintain the focus of the conversation, but also recognised the problems they had in doing this:

Nicola (Lines 74-86)

N: The actual agenda when, when you were heading off down to that particular patient you would have an agenda in your mind. Whether it was just to update them or whatever.
BMC: Mmm, and I just want to get clear. Are you saying that sort of inhibits the way you talk or you become more conscious of it?
N: ... I think you are very conscious of it. Um, in conversation I would on the whole, I would think carefully about what I said and how I said it ...

This nurse was clear that it was her responsibility to ensure that her conversations with patients had been thought out and planned before she approached them. Later, she offered a reason why this was an important consideration in interactions:

Nicola (Lines 173-179)

N: Well, I suppose if I passed my self in the role of patient going to the doctors ... you go in and you talk to the doctor and then you come out and you think, ah I didn't ask this, I didn't ask that and I didn't feel I could and as soon as I got in there I felt as if I'd forgotten everything.

This nurse's particular style was based on how she felt as a patient herself. Because of this particular experience, clarity and focus in communication was an important issue to her. This nurse's account of her approach raises the issue *of* 'repertoire versus stylisation'. One factor that appeared significant in maintaining the focus of the conversation was the repertoire of conversational approaches available to the nurse. Expert group participants acknowledged that it is not easy to maintain the focus of conversations and that there would be a danger of nurses becoming too 'stylised' in their approach as described by Nicola:

Expert Group Interview (lines 569-577)

EX2:   Yes, but that's about tackling opportunities as they arise and (failing) in those opportunities rather than falling into it. It sounds like she (a particular nurse) fell into it but then went into assessment mode. I worry about encouraging nurses to do focused discrete assessments because I don't think the majority have the capacity to work in that focused way.... I worry that it goes into the robotics of 'Right yeah I've come to assess you' (*as described by Nicola*) ...

Members of the expert group also felt, that although Nicola was explicit in her stylised approach, stylisation also occurred among the other participating nurses because they had a limited repertoire of communication approaches. Smits (1984) has suggested that while nurses have acquired plenty of communication skills, their use tends to be unconscious and routine. Crawford *et al* (1995) in concurring with this assertion assert the importance of nurses paying attention to their language use and the linguistic symbolism articulated:

Expert Group Interview (Lines 453-459)

EX2:   It seems to me that rather than having a repertoire that these nurses are very stylised, that they have a 'This is my approach' and how can that approach be adapted with different people. It doesn't change though (*in other case studies*).

Nurses having a repertoire of responses appeared to enable patients to tell their 'stories' and thence provide important information to the conversation agenda. In some interactions, nurses used patients' responses to previous questions to determine appropriate 'next utterances'. For example, nurses used the word 'right' as a means of reinforcing what had been said. It was only when the nurses found themselves having to go against the patient's wishes that they changed these responses, as illustrated in the following example:

Case Study 1/Interaction1/Jack

436 N: I don't want you getting on the bus into ((City)) and then
437   it all being too much=
438 P: =no no no I just get off the bus it's not very far to walk
439   ⌊°im
440   down (0.1) well it stops just outside the Post Office the
441 N: ⌊°im

442   bus does

The nurse's conversation became more hesitant as demonstrated through the use of such phrases as 'I mean' and 'em'. The importance of these monosyllabic utterances in demonstrating engagement with the patient is highlighted through the following data example:

Case Study 6/Interaction 1/Mrs. Burke

469 P: and he said to me 'I think I'll get that for you' well I said I
470   got a card get on the 'phone (0.1) so he got on the 'phone
471   and it was at our house the next day=
472 N: =really!=
473 P: =and the people I've had stop asking me what the name is
474 N: ⌊stop yes
475   the people is and (   ) there's the telephone number and I
476   give them that the number of people .....course it's
477 N: ⌊ yeah
478   like a pram=
479 N: = yes yeah it's dead good
480 P: ⌊you know and* it's no trouble whatsoever
481   (0.07) you put it in the ((*paused*))
482 N: no sorry I'm meditating
483 P: °oh I put it in the shed at night and - eh no I love my-
484 N: ⌊im   ⌊ yeah=do
485   you manage to use your bath at home yourself?

In previous conversations, Mrs. Burke expressed satisfaction with the use of her trolley that she used to mobilise. In this section of the conversation, she continues her story about her trolley and its merits. The nurse offered supportive utterances that encouraged the patient to continue with her story. The importance of these supportive utterances to the patient's story telling is evidenced in line 482. Mrs. Burke noticed that the nurse was not paying her full attention and paused her story. The nurse interpreted the pause as the patient checking on her and apologised for not paying attention. Mrs. Burke (line 483) responded with a quietly spoken 'oh' and picks up the story from where she had left off. However, the nurse who wished to introduce another topic area stopped the story through an interruption.

In some interactions, nurses used responses to previous utterances to establish more detail about the patient's condition and to decide on the most appropriate action. Throughout these interactions, patients played an active role in providing appropriate information for nurses to work with. Further, the nurses used questions to evaluate the previous response and to build up a picture of events. In these interactions, while the nurses were undertaking an assessment of patients, they didn't appear to follow a predetermined agenda, but instead determined 'next questions' from previous utterances. Empathetic utterances by nurses appeared to enable patients to 'tell their stories' and facilitate emotional expression:

Case Study 13/Interaction 1/Jim

```
106 P:   (  ) yeah a little bit of headache but (  ) ((crying))
107 N:   ri::ght ri::ght  (0.2) °it's alright=
108 P:   =all I was thinking about was (  )
109 N:   all you were thinking about?=
110 P:   =was what was going to happen (0.2) I was
111      ((crying)) I wish I had died=
112 N:   =°o::::h
113 P:   (0.3) that would have solved everything thing
114      wouldn't it
115 N:   (0.9) I can appreciate that's how you think (0.08)
116      and how you feel when you're feeling really down
117      do you feel that when things are going well for you
118      at the minute?=
119 P:   =(  ) not really well (  ) again (0.1) all last year in
120      nineteen ninety five I was in and out of hospital all
121      the time (and it feels like this) year's starting the same
122 N:            ⌊im                              ⌊im
123      (0.1) wha' would you think?=
124 N:   =I'd think the same Jim=
125 P:   =I mean I can't get about like I (used to years ago)=
126 N:   =I mean you were very unfortunate with the
127      dislocation of your hip weren't you (0.1) I mean
128      how do
129 P: ⁻      ⌊(how could I) cope with that (  )=
```

Between lines 106-126, the nurse changed her conversation style and worked with Jim's conversational agenda. During this time, he became distressed about what was happening to him. He cried when he described his symptoms and fears. The nurse's utterances were empathetic and supportive of him. She used repetition of Jim's incomplete utterances to assist his expressions of how he felt (see for example lines 108-109). In line 110/111 Jim expressed that he wished he had died. The nurse used an open and supportive response (°o::::h) which enabled Jim to describe his feelings. In line 115, the nurse continued to express support for Jim. She was empathetic and used her supportive utterances to question further his feelings and if he was actually depressed. Jim explained that his feelings related to his continuous admissions to hospital that made him fear for the future. In line 123 he asks the nurse what she would think and the nurse freely responded that she would think the same and in line 126 she expressed further empathy with Jim's situation.

In contrast to this approach, the nurse in Case Study 15 did not demonstrate such sensitivity, but instead concentrated on maintaining her established agenda of discharging the patient to a residential care unit:

Case Study 15/ Interaction 3/ Aidan

```
 3 N:   That's Prof. ((name)) (0.06) the consultant that you
 4      saw at the ((Hospital)) (0.05) he has beds down here in
 5 P:                    ⌊yea::h
 6      the rehabilitation unit of which you've come down to
 7      (0.04) e::m and he's obviously followed you down to
 8      (continue) your 8 care under him=
 9 P:   (oh yes)
10 N:   (0.08) e:m did you understand what he what he said
11      (0.06) did you understand what he said?
12 P:   (0.1) well sort of yes=
13 N:   =sort of what he does he does a ward round every week
14      and finds out what's gone on on the previous week (0.1)
15      and the::n tries to:: organise with the multidisciplinary
16      team what the right plan of action would be with your
17      approval (and make sure you know about what's) going
18      on (0.07) so the   next stage now will be to continue with
19      your physio and occupational therapy (0.1) get you
20      stronger it can still go on
21 P:           ⌊( )
22      in here (0.1) get you back on your feet and then Stella
23 P:           ⌊(I suppose it can do yes)
24      will come and have a chat with you to see if you still
25      thinking about residential care okay=
```

The nurse's intention was to establish Aidan's understanding of events following a previous ward round. In lines 10 and 11 she asked Aidan directly if he understood what had been said. He suggested a partial understanding and this was followed by an explanation that was an interpretation of events set within her overall agenda of discharging Aidan to a residential care home (somewhere he is unsure about going). In line 23, Aidan's response to the nurse's explanation about his rehabilitation was uncommitted, but the nurse did not react to this. Instead she continued to focus on her established agenda.

From this data, it would appear that professionals need to be able to maintain the overall focus of the interaction while at the same time facilitating a free-flowing conversation. Maintaining the focus enables the agenda to be reinforced with the patient and the integration of new knowledge into the conversation.

Signposting

Another means of maintaining the focus of the conversation agenda and the patient's involvement was through 'Signposting', i.e. creating opportunities in the conversation to direct the patient through the conversation agenda. Such approaches as regular reinforcement of the conversation agenda; reinforcement of the patient's goals and the steps taken to achieve these; the clear articulation of questions and explicitly stating the reason for questions, were seen by the expert group as being essential to effective patient participation:

Expert Group Interview (Line 495)

EX1:   they didn't sign post in their language

Expert Group Interview (Lines 488-515)

EX5:   Yes, they didn't actually offer an approach of partnership. If one particular patient needs a gentle introduction to their (interaction, such as) 'it would help us to be able to sort out' or 'if you could tell us such and such'. It was lacking in sort of assisting the patient in becoming more knowledgeable about what the purpose of the conversation was ... so then making them more informed about the information they might give back

Expert Group Interview (Lines 517-563)

EX1:   I think that it was Sid, who a nurse was asking him a lot about his drugs and to me it appeared she wanted that information for the case conference for the discharge planning. She needed to know that. Now, she to me kind of fumbled through it, and you know 'do you know what your Frusemide's for?' and 'your ameloride' ((laughter)). But she was testing that patient and she had set the questions in advance and depending on what that patient said, she would evaluate it and take that information to the case conference and that would affect this patients discharge. And he didn't have a clue about it... it wasn't fair because he was being assessed he had no idea that he was taking an exam.

However, signposting approaches were not very evident in the data. Examples of where some attempts at signposting or failure to signpost effectively are seen in the following data extracts:

Case Study 1/Interaction 2/Jack

```
 5 N:   right then (0.1) °so:: so were you on tablets before you
 6      went into the ((Hospital))? were you on tablets for your
 7      heart then? (0.06) before you had the opera:::tion?
 8 P:   (0.05) e::::h yes I had tablets=
 9 N:   =did you? and did you just used to get them from the
10      chemist yourself?=
11 P:   =when I was in the (Hospital)) they gave me some the
12      ((Hospital))=
13 N:   =yeah::: I mean befo::re that when you were at ho::me=
14 P:   =OH no no I never had no tablets=sorry I got mixed up
15      love
16 N:   (0.07) you weren't taking any tablets then at a:::ll=
17 P:   =⌈no no
18 N:    ⌊no no (0.2) you're going to be going home on tablets
19      obviously (0.1) so::
20 P:                       ⌊don't worry about it (if leads to) (   )
21      you know=
22 N:   =yeah so we need to::: (0.08) you we need to make sure
23      that you are able to take them okay and that you
24      understand how to take them
```

In this interaction, the conversation focus changed to that of assessing Jack's competence with self-management of his medicines and teaching him about their safe administration. The nurse began the conversation by determining Jack's previous experience with medicines. However, he interprets 'before you had your operation' as meaning immediately prior to his surgery. It was only when the nurse asked if he got them from the chemist himself that she established that he wasn't on tablets previously. Jack interprets this misunderstanding as a 'mistake' and apologised to the nurse. The nurse did not acknowledge the apology, but instead the response was used to confirm that the patient had not been previously taking medicines. The nurse repaired the situation by explaining to Jack that he would be going home with tablets this time and that therefore he would need to know how to administer them safely. This interaction highlights the importance of questions being specific in order for the patient to effectively participate in care planning. Misunderstandings because of lack of specificity in the asking of questions could also be seen in Case Study 12, as illustrated by the following example:

Case Study 12/Interaction 3/Shirley

```
23 N:    (0.2) Now what would you like to do this morning?
24 P:    Well tell me what=
25 N:    =well obviously have a cup of tea that's the first in the
26       morning isn't it and then breakfast=
27 P:              ⌊yes              =I thought you was
28       going to say go out somewhere or other when* you said
29 N:                              ⌊we::ll
30       what would you like to do=
31 N:    =well
32 OTHER VOICE: It's Friday today (   ) go up the markets=
33 N:    =would you like to go up the market today?
34 P:    °No no=
35 N:    =well I mean there's enough bodies around we could (em
36       take you in) a wheel chair if you wanted to (0.3) have a
37       think about it have I sprung it on you I have haven't I=
38 P:    =°yes::
```

The goal of this interaction was that of facilitating Shirley's choice about her plans for the day. The nurse's initial approach was 'open' and not set within any limits (line 23). Shirley did not wish to make the choice and suggested to the nurse that she told her what to do (line 24). The nurse began to paint a picture of a routine and Shirley interrupted this utterance with an interjection that suggested she misinterpreted the nurse's initial question. She interpreted the initial question as 'going out somewhere'.

This raises issues about the way choices are presented to patients and their ability to respond to such presentations. The question 'what would you like to do today?' can be interpreted in numerous ways and the answer would depend on the particular perspective that is being adopted by the respondent. The nurse was asking the question in her capacity as a nurse planning care with a patient, to which there is an established (informal) routine (line 25 and 26). The patient however, was not responding as a 'patient' with a knowledge of that routine, but instead responded from the context of 'person', where doing something related to those things other than the usual routines of the day. This is an important issue and confirms some of my own feelings as a practitioner:

> *Reflective Diary Extract* We all have a morning routine for washing and dressing that we usually adhere to. Everybody caring for the particular patient should know this and care should 'just happen' in that way. While as practitioners we need to be mindful of the effect that a 'strange' environment has on an individual's routines (Haug and Ory, 1987) it may be disconcerting for patients to be asked everyday how they would like the morning routine performed as it raises issues of lacking security in the care givers. Real choices are those that concern the rest of the person's day and their rehabilitation focus.

In Shirley's case, as this interaction progressed, she became increasingly anxious about her misunderstanding and the more choices offered to her the more anxious she became.

Creating opportunities for 'signposting' interactions would appear to be an important consideration when facilitating decision-making with older people. In doing this, professionals demonstrate an awareness of ageing processes that affect the older person's ability to assimilate new information with previous understandings (Slater, 1995).

Sensitivity to Cues and Appropriate Response

The professionals' focus on a particular agenda often resulted in an inappropriate response to 'cues' that patients offered in conversations. Cues are defined in this study as:

> *A non-response to a previous utterance or a response that does not directly relate to the previous utterance, but which provides the professional with evidence of the patient's emotional status or health and social care concerns.*

In general, professionals in this study, demonstrated a lack of sensitivity to the patients' cues:

Expert Group Interview (Lines 312-325)

EX5:   Yes I felt quite cross at times because I felt that the nurses had gone in to do something and in fact they'd got a task to do. They'd got to find out something and they'd got to check up on something or got to achieve something and there was lots of messages and suggestions being given by patients about what they wanted to talk about and what the problems were or how they perceived things but these things were just missed or brushed aside. They weren't given the opportunity to explore or even given the option for someone to go back later to talk to them and I felt quite angry at times that these things were just being completely ignored...

Members of the expert group agreed that in general, nurses in the study failed to respond appropriately to 'cues' that emerged in their interactions with patients. This was seen to occur because nurses treated their communication with patients as another 'task'. In their study of general practitioners' interactions with their clients, Byrne and Long (1976) were critical of the unsophisticated way that doctors used language. Zimmerman and West (1975) highlight the importance of responding to cues in interaction, because they act as 'positive reinforcement for continued talk'. In addition, Anderson (1979) argues that even if the professional is not interested in the patient's story, these stories are imbued with meaning for the patient and therefore demand respect. In relation to the interactions of professionals, Anderson (1979: 192) suggests that:

> the (professional) who interrupts or shuts off such a story, risks appearing cold and uninterested, so reducing the patient's further communicability: she risks losing access to the domain of home, family, work and friends in which actual health decisions are made: and she risks missing the end of the story, an end that might be of diagnostic relevance.

The extent to which cues were not recognised or were inappropriately responded to was concerning:

Case Study 13/Interaction 3/Jim

```
7 N:    Jim how was last night you know we talked about
8       (0.08) Jim  you know we talked about you having a
9       conveen on?=
10 P:   =°ye::s=
11 N:   =with a long leg bag=
12P:    =yes I felt a lot better it really was (nice) and I felt
13      top of the world=
14 N:   =did you and there was no accidents or anything in
15      the bed last
16 P:              ⌊no no no
17 N:   And a good nights sleep?=
18 P:   =I had a wonderful night sleep yes but (I wish there
19      weren't) things thats been worrying me (0.2) (   )=
20 N:   =yea::h would you like to pursue the same routine
21      this evening?  you know have the conveen*=
22 P:              ⌊I most certainly would
```

23 N: =and theres no Kylie on the bed is there?=
24 P: =no I most certainly would
25 N: OKAY then well that's something positive isn't it?
26 P: (0.07) yes ( ) this all started at home wetting the
27   bed (0.3) no now I've been told tha' when I go
28 N: ⌊yeah
29   home I'll get one of these things put on so ( ) I'll
30   wake up in the morning the same as I went to bed=
31 N: =yeah
32 P: ( )
33 N: No I think that will cut all the problems down a bit
34   won't it now with respect to the diarrhoea the stool
35   specimen you know we took a sample and it went
36   off to be scree::ned? its come back as negative
37 P: ⌊yeah   ⌊yeah
38 N: so what I might do I might get a sample again
39   tomorrow and we'll just check it
40P: (0.2) ( ) as I said I went down to the Day Hospital
41   (today) and I was absolutely I was absolutely no
42   interested and I met lot of people down there I
43   known for a long long time (0.1) but I just didn't
44 N: ⌊yeah
45   want to know=
46 N: =no that's fine Jim you get days like that=
47 P: =yes (0.4) ( ) I sat on the toilet there and I cried me
48   bloomin' eyes out I shouldn't be doing that should
49 N: ⌊o::h Jim
50   I?
51 N: (0.2) we:::ll (0.2) if it's going to make you feel
52   better sometimes a cry helps you know=

This interaction began with the nurse inquiring of the patient's satisfaction about the care overnight in relation to the management of his incontinence. Jim expressed his satisfaction with the arrangements, but in line 18 continued to explain that although the management of his incontinence was all right he was still worried about 'things'. The nurse was still focused on the physical aspects of care and in line 20 highlights this overriding concern and the continuing lack of acknowledgement of Jim's worries. The nurse tried to get him to see that this progress was positive (line 25) thus acknowledging the patient's worries, but only in the context of the physical care that was organised. Jim used the opportunity to explain his feelings. In line 33, the nurse initiated a topic shift and returned the conversation to her agenda of sorting out the physical aspects of his care. Jim did not respond to the nurse's previous utterance (line 40) but instead tried to return the conversation to his worries and concerns and explained how he felt when he went to the day hospital. Again, the nurse did not offer to help him explore these feelings, but instead suggested that it was okay for him to feel like this because he would have days like that, i.e. part of the course! Jim went on to explain in line 47 just how depressed he felt and explained how he sat on the toilet and cried. In line 51 the nurse suggested that it was all right to cry but again did not respond in a way that facilitated Jim's understanding of what was going on.

It is evident in this data that Jim was asking for help in all of these emotional expressions and that the nurse was not identifying or acknowledging such expressions. In an earlier section of the case study during a multidisciplinary meeting, Jim had been identified as 'emotionally labile'. It could be suggested therefore that this failure to respond appropriately to Jim's emotional expressions was because of the label that had already been applied (Slater, 1995). This approach to Jim's emotional expression continued throughout his stay in hospital. He continued to express fear for his future and an inability to cope. It is important to recognise that Jim was readmitted because of a 'failed care package' soon after his discharge from hospital. How much of this 'failure' was due to Jim's lack of emotional resources to cope with his state of dependency is difficult to elicit from the data. However, it is clear that Jim's emotional resources were low and that the restoration of these resources was not a recognised goal in his care plan.

Patient embarrassment at discussions about aspects of their physical functioning (particularly regarding incontinence), without the nurse recognising this embarrassment, was also evident in the data:

Case Study 15/Interaction 1/Aidan

```
32 N:   =right so you were using a commode at home?=
33 P:   =yeah a mate of mine was coming round to empty it for
34      me
35 N:   (0.1) how did you get access to your mate to come in to
36      help you (0.07) was it just a one off:::?=
37 P:   =on the phone=
38 N:   =on the ⌈phone
39 P:          ⌊yeah (    ) too late=
40 N:   =ri:::ght=
41 P:   =he wasn't very quick=
42 N:   =so were you having accidents then=
43 P:   =°yeah °I °was °yeah
44 N:   (0.2) were you able to help yourself then to get yourself
```

45   clean again or:::
46 P: (0.1) up to a fashion=
47 N: =were you (0.1) if you have a commode at home (0.08)
48   then obviously somebody's assessed your need for one
49   (0.2) did you have a carer coming in to help you at any
50   time during the day?=

In line 32 Aidan described the way he managed his toileting needs - how he received help from a friend and that he experienced periods of incontinence. The discussion that followed suggested a practice that was seen as unsafe. Aidan's response in line 43, in which he lowered the volume of the response, suggested that he was embarrassed by his situation. The nurse did not respond to this embarrassment (line 44) but instead asked a further question about his ability to cope. This suggested a focus by the nurse on her agenda and not responding to the particular concerns of the patient. Although the nurse structured her discursive style according to Aidan's previous utterances, because of the way the conversation was structured and managed by the nurse, there was little deviation from the overall goal of the conversation.

Other forms of lack of sensitivity to cues and failure to respond appropriately occurred between professionals when discussing care arrangements. Throughout the case studies, it was commonplace during case conferences, multidisciplinary meetings and discussions between health care professionals to override or ignore previous choices made by patients, as illustrated by the example below. Indeed throughout this case study, non-response to the patient's cues manifested itself in the form of power and control and will be discussed in Chapter 6.

Case Study 11/Interaction 5/Mabel

6 N: Right you've spoken to the daughter
7 CM: Right yes what do you want to know=
8 N: =you spoke to her daughter and:::=
9 CM: =em she thinks she's going to need help mornings and
10   evenings=
11 N: =right
12 CM: And eh:: I've got to talk to her and see what she thinks=
13 N: =right is that going to be a problem do you think setting it
14   up?=
15 CM: =I shouldn't thinks so no I haven't asked yet but I don't
16   think it will be=
17 N: =⌈right
18 CM: ⌊(do you want to know)

19 N: ⌊well she doesn't want to stay in 20 more than
    another day or so because she thinks she is
21   quite fit and there's some sick people around her=
22 CM: =(huh huh)=
23 N: =e:::m (0.1) and she actually keeps telling me she is a
24   hundred and she doesn't think we need to test her urine
25   because she lived 'till she was a hundred so what's the
26   point in testing it etcetera etcetera etcetera

In this interaction the nurse and the care manager discuss ongoing care
arrangements for Mabel. In line 9, the care manager informed the nurse
that Mabel's daughter wanted her to have morning and evening care (in an
earlier conversation Mabel had already refused evening care). The nurse
did not raise the issue of Mabel not wanting evening care arrangements and
it was the care manager who suggested that she needed to see what Mabel
thought about it. The nurse's concern was with the availability of the care
needed. In line 13, the nurse asked the care manager if it was going to be a
problem getting care morning and evening and the care manager replied
that it should not be - again accepting that morning and evening care would
be provided. The nurse used her turn to provide an explanation that wasn't
asked for by telling the care manager about the patient's views and wishes.
It is unclear what the nurse aimed to achieve from this utterance. While it
summarised Mabel's views, the tone of the conversation was one of
amusement (as interpreted by the care manager, line 22) rather than a
genuine representation of her perception.

Being sensitive to cues in interactions with patients, would appear
to offer opportunities for the professional to discover patient concerns that
are indirectly communicated. Such sensitivity illustrates an engagement
with the patient that is focused on seeking to understand their perspective
as expressed through their emotions and feelings. May (1995) argues that
such sensitivity requires the suspension of an elaborate set of moral
pressures on the nurse to adopt a proactive role in information seeking (e.g.
pressure of time resulting in the following of a predetermined set of
questions). It requires the nurse to create a 'sympathetic presence' and to
construct 'spaces' for patient participation.

Control of the Conversation

The conversations recorded by nurses in this study were predominantly
information seeking as part of an assessment process on which to base
decisions, or actual decision making conversations in themselves.

Although these conversations occurred with patients and were therefore part of a shared decision making process, the control over the conversation, including the conversation agenda and the maintenance of its focus, predominantly remained with the professionals (Baldock and Prior, 1981; Byrne and Long, 1976; Crawford *et al*, 1995). Professionals were able to do this because of their ability to identify salient features from previous utterances and integrate those features into their already established 'picture' of the patient (Drew and Heritage, 1992). Such a picture arose from their access to a broader knowledge base than the patient, including discussions with other health and social care professionals that were not directly reported to the patient and as a result were able to initiate topic shifts in the conversation where they felt appropriate to do so:

Case Study 5/Interaction 3/Molly

```
79 N:   I'll just em (0.05) no I'll just do that and then it's
80 P:                Lis that an easy top?
81      just em
82 P:              LTHEY DON'T CONSIDER people with
83      arthritic joints do they?=
84 N:   =well=
85 P:   =or do they?
86 N:   I think what they tend to do is they routinely put
87      click lock lids on for everybody (0.3) but if
88      you've got a problem then we just go back and
89      explain that=
90 P:   =well you can see I have yeah yeah=
91 N:   =it's no problem to change it.
92 P:   (0.1) I stand here and I wrestle with the blooming
93      thing you know (  ) that's eh (0.1) that's the same
94      (0.1) one to be taken twice a day and I take those
95      with the others (0.2) you know (0.7) break those up
96      'till they get small and then swallow them down
97 N:   (0.2) and then the other one
```

In line 82, Molly expressed anger and frustration with the bottle lids 'THEY DON'T CONSIDER people with arthritic joints do they?'. She was clearly frustrated with this constraint on her actions. The nurse's response however, diffused Molly's anger and frustration (line 84) and she became less emphatic in her view. The power of the single word response 'well' with its cautious and questioning tone, resulted in Molly choosing not to continue to express her emotion and question the accuracy of her original expression. The nurse's explanation that followed (lines 86-89) illustrated how routine/ritualised practice prevents individual autonomy and acts as a constraint to autonomous action. Such routine practice relies on the action of the professional to prevent the constraint and facilitate more autonomy for the patient. In line 90 Molly continued to express irritation with the practice, but the nurse's response (line 91) was controlled and set within her perception of her role. In line 92, Molly's irritation was still evident, but was not being overtly acknowledged by the nurse.

However, even when patients' emotional responses were acknowledged, this was done within the overall control of the nurse as directed by his/her agenda:

Case Study 11/Interaction 4/Mabel

146 N: When do you normally go to bed at home what time?
147 P: All times
148 N: All times
149 P: Half past nine
150 N: Right
151 P: Very seldom after that ( )
152 N: Well it's only quarter to eight in the evening
153 P: O::H is it?
154 N: Yes there'll be a hot drink coming round shortly=
155 P: =( ) if I got to bed too early I=
156 N: ⌊wake up too early=
157 P: =no it's not a matter I can get up any time=
158 N: =right=
159 P: =yes=
160 N: =°ok=
161 P: =in fact I'm very seldom in bed well nearly always half
162   past seven my son - when I'm up my daughter's you see
163 N: ⌊right OK
164   the weekend he brings a cup of tea in well I don't go off
165   to sleep no more see and by the time I'm dressed it takes
166   me a long while to dress because I have to sit down and
167   take my breath like=
168 N: =right ok well look Mabel I'll em I'll sort out the sheet
169   and everything (0.8) em I'll just see where your hot cup
170   of tea's coming or hot drink should I say
171 P: ( ) because I mean my daughter does my washing you
172 N: ⌊yeah
173   see and sheets and that (0.1) ((tearful)) and I don't like to
174   be moaned at me too much=
175 N: °right do you think you've settled down today in
176   hospital?=

177 P: =EH=
178 N: =do you think you've settled down today in hospital
179 P: (   ) really since I've been taking them biotics not feel so
180   bad *((tearful))*
181 N: You're feeling better
182 P: Ye::s
183 N: Good
184 P: I mean
185 N: ⌊but do you think since you came into hospital this
186   afternoo::n do you think you've settled down here now=
187 P: ⌊ye::s
188 P: =eh?
189 N: Do you think you've settled down here now?
190 P: =well I think so *((laughs))*
191 N: Yes?=
192 P: =it's a case of having to isn't it yes=
193 N: =well there's nothing that's troubling you at the minute?
194 P: No:: I don't think there is (0.1) I mean everybody's been
195   as they should you know like kind to (0.2) I don't try to
196   make much trouble regarding helping (   ) and I'm always
197   grateful for what anybody does (0.1) and I mean when
198   anybody does anything for me working or anything like
199   that (   ) I always pay (are we having a hot drink) tonight=
200 N: =there's one just coming no::w
201 P: O:h is it oh

This conversation began with a discussion about the time Mabel normally went to bed, as part of an ongoing assessment by the nurse of Mabel's continence. In lines 161-167 Mabel uses the opportunity to tell the nurse more about her routine and includes information about her physical problems (breathlessness) (line 167). The nurse did not see the significance of this story as indicated by the latching of her input to the previous utterance and the urgency of the 'right ok' in line 168. The nurse used this response as a means of initiating a topic shift and a means of beginning to close the conversation. Mabel responds with more information about her routine and the support from her family. She became tearful in the conversation as she expressed her value of not liking being 'moaned'· at too much. The nurse acknowledged Mabel's emotions (line 175) and wondered if she had settled down in hospital. This question by the nurse, which was not overtly related to the previous utterance, was misinterpreted by Mabel as a question about her general physical state. The nurse realises that and asked the question in a different way (line 185). However, given Mabel's tearfulness, the nurse follows this up with an apparent inappropriate and closed question in line 193. The response by Mabel provides a further indication of her values and passiveness.

This conversation highlights the way nurses can control their interaction with patients by having a particular agenda to follow. While it is necessary for nurses to follow an assessment agenda with regard to issues like continence, it is also necessary for them to be open to taking on board other information that patients input (May, 1995). As earlier identified, utilising a repertoire of approaches in interaction enables the maintenance of the overall focus of the interaction (e.g. continence assessment) while simultaneously being sensitive to other information provided by patients.

An asymmetry occurs in these situations, whereby the nurse follows an established proforma that is not known to the patient. Patients are expected to follow this proforma by responding to the questions that the nurse asks. However, an alternative approach would be to ask patients to tell their 'story' about, for example urinary and bowel habits with questions asked that seek to elaborate, clarify or complement information given. In this way a 'sympathetic presence' (May, 1995) is maintained, while the power relationship shifts with the control of the structural organisation of the conversation shifting from the nurse to the patient and a reversal of the order of the interaction (Baldock and Prior, 1981).

Conclusions

Through exploring the communicative style of professional-patient interactions, it can be seen that the power to control interactions is located with the professional rather than the patient. Achieving control over interactions with patients is maintained through professionals determining the conversational agenda and controlling inputs into the conversation. The communication skills of professional staff, particularly in managing the focus of the interaction and signposting the conversation appear to be particularly important in enabling older patient's participation in their care. How the agenda and focus are determined appears to have a significant impact on the professional's ability to deviate from the agenda in order to respond appropriately to issues that emerge through implicit cues offered by the patient. Because it is the professional who establishes the database of information that is used in the planning of care, then it is necessary for the professional to be sensitive to such cues and integrate them into already established knowledge. A number of principles for action have been identified from this data.

Principles for Action

- Make explicit the care agenda.
- Recognise that the questioning style adopted affects the ability of the older patient to contribute to the setting of the care agenda and their contribution to a conversation.
- Be aware that actions to achieve one outcome may have an effect on a previously unrecognised need.
- Have a repertoire of interactional approaches that would enable patient decision-making and participation in the planning of care plans.
- Pose specific and clearly formulated questions that have a clear aim.
- Respect individuals' important routines in daily life and negotiate new components of the care agenda each day.
- Be aware that older patients depend on professionals to minimise/prevent constraints on their autonomy.

6 Power and Control

A consistent theme throughout the case studies was 'power and control'. Power and control were manifested in terms of the power relationship between participants and their impact on an individual's potential for action. Within the theme of power and control, two sub-themes were identified:

- Professional Power and Control.
- Hopes, Dreams and Desires.

Professional Power and Control

Expert Group Interview (Lines 817-829)

EX4:   I felt there was a very fundamental feeling that came out for me and it was one of ownership. It seemed to me to relate very much to autonomy and it was almost like the patients' sort of power and control had been removed by the relatives before they got into hospital... and it seemed to me that in a lot of the language it was like the staff not only owned the solution to the problem but also seemed to own the person's permission as well in that they, they didn't seem to leave the ownership with the person...

Power and control over patients' health states and their resolution appeared to be 'owned' by the professionals. While in some cases, patients were encouraged to participate in decision-making, it is difficult to see how patients could take responsibility for decision-making, given that the ownership of their health state and potential resolutions were taken away from them. Professional power and control over the patient's decision making capacity was exerted in a number of ways, including:

- Orchestration of the Conversation.
- Knowledge as Power and Control.

Orchestration of the Conversation

- Control of Discharge Arrangements.
- Medical Control.

As already identified in Chapter 5, the communicative style of nurses and other health care professionals either enabled or inhibited decision-making by patients. Fairclough (1989) identified that, in their 'practice', professionals express their power over users in discourse. Three factors enable this to happen - the content of the conversation, the relationship between participants and the roles that they perform. Fairclough's (1989) work concurs with the work of other conversation analysts, in that it highlights how the professional controls the content of professional-client conversation and that an implicit structure (this has been discussed as 'the conversation agenda' in chapter 5) exists that highlights the social roles of each of the participants. The control of the conversations exerted by professionals in their interactions with patients manifested itself as power and control over the patient's decision-making capacity. The power that professionals exert is often characterised by the way their utterances are framed (Fairclough, 1989). Utterances were often framed as a suggestion/statement and because of this it would therefore be unlikely that the patient would disagree with the suggestion because of their deference to professional opinion. As Hugman (1991; 37) suggests:

> language is a central aspect of discourse through which power is reproduced and communicated.

Strong's (1979) notion of 'an orchestrated encounter' has been used to describe the interactional relationship between nurses and patients in this research. Strong's research into the relationship between medical consultants and families in children's out-patient departments highlighted a series of rules that together maintained the 'bureaucratic format' of the professional-client interaction. In this study, conversations often had a 'fait accompli' feeling about them, which appeared to exist because of a lack of overt planning in the conversation to present a range of alternatives that patients could choose from. This appeared to be a feature of much conversation between older patients and professional carers in this study. Although the language of conversation may have often been aimed at offering choice, the reality of the patient making choice was limited by their lack of understanding of the range of alternatives available to them.

The controlled and limiting response to questions by the hospital professionals was probably one of the most common formats in professional-client interactions in the data and acted as the main reason for patient powerlessness. Fairclough (1989) highlighted the way the conversation agenda is used to control the dimensions of conversation, i.e. acceptable and unacceptable communication. The uncooperative client is one who does not conform to the rules of the conversation and cooperation exists when the client's actions conform to the professional's expectations. In this study, the patient was at the control of the doctor/nurse to decide on the most appropriate treatment/care plan. As a result, there was little opportunity for the patient to control the agenda and have the decisions made based on his/her agenda. Although there appeared to be the 'trappings' of partnership, in reality, this was based on the professional's agenda. The patient's input into the agenda was only that which fitted into the parameters dictated by the professional. Decisions outside of that parameter were the remit of the professionals with the patient having little formal opportunity to influence that agenda. It appeared that such influence was determined by the skill of the individual practitioner and the extent of their focus on the patient's views rather than the views of the professional team.

The orchestration of interaction with patients could be seen as a positive approach to maintain the focus of the conversation and the patient's involvement in it (as already discussed in Chapter 5). However, in this study, professionals used orchestration as a technique to maintain power and control over conversations and thence the interactional agenda. Instead of working towards addressing the imbalance of power that existed in the conversational agendas, this research has highlighted ways inwhich nurses exploit this imbalance as a means of encouraging compliance with care plans.

Knowledge as Power and Control

It was evident in the data that the autonomy of the patient was enhanced or limited according to their access to relevant and appropriate knowledge. Differences in the relationship could be seen to occur in the case studies according to the amount of knowledge that the patient possessed. The patient's ability to engage as a partner in the conversation was primarily dictated by their level of understanding of the conversation agenda. In ordinary conversation, the participants generally assume that while they may not always be equally knowledgeable and informed about every topic, such imbalances will be short lived and will shift among the speakers from topic to topic (Drew and Heritage, 1992). This data demonstrated that even in professional-client interactions where partnership in the relationship was emphasised, that assumption could not be made. In most cases assumptions were made by nurses about the amount and type of knowledge possessed by patients. They rarely sought information from nurses about the way their care would progress. Even when they did so, the information provided was limited and controlled:

Case Study 13/Interaction 7/Jim [with District Nurse (DN) Clare]

```
95  Wife: =(I'll just get ya) to explain some of these ta::blets
96        (as well) (   )=
97  N:   =yea::h a:::ll the medicines have changed as well
98        Clare he's gone on to Phenytoin a hundred BD
99  DN:  (0.2) yea:h
100 N:   (0.1) now the Phenytoin (0.1) tha:t's one of these
101      capsules twice a day and what we've been doing is
102      one in the morning and one when he goes to bed=
103 P:   =⌈that's right
104 Wife:⌊(    ) whatever they're called=
105 N:   =now the Tagamet a:::h (0.1) they're the
106      Carbamazepi:::ne one to be taken twice a day so
107      they
108 Wife:    ⌊what with those=
109 N:   =yeah: same time (0.2) so that's to stop him having
110 Wife:              ⌊that's right
111      any fits or anything  (0.2) he's got the combination::
112 DN:                ⌊he's got the combination?
113      (0.07) because he was on a very high dose of the
114      Carbamazepine and we probably thought that that
115      was one of the reasons for the diarrhoea (0.1) so
116      we're reducing that okay? so that's  yeah mo:rnin'
117 Wife:                         ⌊(   )
118      and night this is the Perimide needs to be taken each
119      morning oh hang on where are we Lofepramine
120      one to be taken twice a da:::y so you can have one
121      in the morning and one in the evening
122 Wife:                    ⌊what's that for?=
123 N:   =that's to buck Jim's spirit up a little bit=
124 P:   =oh the 'a::ppy pill as he calls it yeah=
125 N:   =yeah that's your anti-depressant  alright=
126 Wife: =it's not doing any good at the mo::ment but we
```

```
127      ⌈hope it will
128 N:   ⌊well:: I think I think once Jim gets ho::::me=
129 Wife: =yeah yeah::
130 N:   (0.1) then the Loperimide eh two to be taken with
131      each very very loose bowel action so if he gets an
132      accident in the ni:::ght (0.1) take two alright? (0.2)
133      and then thats his inhaler=
134 Wife: =yeah I could have done with a blue one not the
135      brown one (0.2) because he's got two or three
136 N:                 ⌊the °blue °one °right°okay::
137      brown ones because then you see they always seem
138      to la:::st longer than the blue:: one=
139 N:   =yeah well he's alway-
140 P:                         ⌊(   )=
141 Wife:        =ye:::s  he has got one at ho:::me so it doesn't
142      (really make much difference)˙
143 P:   (    ) (got this wrong)
144 N:   (0.3) right okey dokey then did you do a continence
145      assessment form when he was home last Clare?=
```

This conversation begins with Jim's wife asking the nurse to explain his tablets to her. The nurse 'latches' a response that directly answers the wife's request. However, she directs her answer at the District Nurse. The nurse begins to explain the tablets in line 98. However, it is clearly not an educative approach that is being taken. Instead the nurse works her way through a 'list' and provides brief explanations of each drug. Jim's wife initiates interruptions in order to ask questions and seek further clarification. In line 122, she asks what a particular drug is for (Lofepramine). The nurse chooses a response that does not directly explain this (line 123). Jim 'latches' a response, suggesting that it is the 'happy pill'. This utterance leads the nurse to state clearly what the drug is for. She ends her utterance with a question 'alright?', thus highlighting her insecurity with suggesting that Jim is depressed. The nurse asserts that the drug is not doing any good. Her response is chosen to affirm the rationale behind her determination for Jim to go home (line 128) and is cautious. She does not provide Jim's wife with the opportunity to clarify any issues or ask any questions. There is also no attempt made to check out the wife's understanding.

While this data example is being used to illustrate the limited and controlled nature of information giving in this study, the subject area (medication teaching) is in direct contrast to some of the other case studies (from one particular clinical area) that were focused on lengthy education sessions with patients about their medicines and initiating self-medication regimes.

When detailed information was provided, this often appeared to be 'coercive', i.e. it was provided in a way that encouraged patients to follow a particular decision:

Case Study 15/ Interaction 1/Aidan [with daughter-in-law (DL)]

178 P: I think I (feared) I'd be cared better for if the eh::: (0.3) if I
179 was living away from the flat=
180 N: =if you were away from the ⌈flat? (0.2) so are you thinking
181 P: ⌊yes
182 along the lines of residential ca::re (0.2) where::: you could
183 be::: staying in an area where there is people around twenty
184 four hours a day
185 P: (0.1) (was it em:::) (0.1) res(0.07)idential care what is it
186 then-what?=
187 N: =a residential ca::re area is: (0.1) a unit or u:::::m flats within
188 a contained area where people are on duty it's not hospital
189 P: (   ) like you know where e:::m Westside in Forest Way
190 there that's one that's a residential care unit=
191 DL: =no:: that's warden controlled flats
192 P: ⌊warden controlled <u>flats</u>?=
193 N: =that's slightly different=
194 P: o::h is it oh?
195 DL: ⌊residential ca::re is where they've got a number of
196 like bed sits and they have a kitchen (°I work in a residential
197 home) (0.1) e:::m they have social workers who are <u>resident</u>
198 the:::re to make sure that you get the attention you need*
206 N: =yes yes (0.08) basically they have people working twenty
207 four hours a day within the complex (0.1) you have your
208 own a::rea you are able to do what you want when you want
209 but there's somebody there on duty that if you need it they
210 can help you
211 DL: (0.1) you can go out if you want to:::=
212 N: =you're not <u>confi:::ned</u> to the area (0.1) you can::: have
213 P: ⌊no
214 people to visit you (0.1) you can have friends in you can go
215 away there's no there's limited restrictions but there are
216 people on duty twenty four hours a day so that if you need it
217 they can help you (0.1) as opposed to a <u>fla:::t</u> or a house
218 where you're on your own and you're dependent on <u>yourself</u>
219 (0.1) or carers coming in tha:t perhaps

220 P: ⌊they eh::: they install
221   the pho::ne things like that?=
222 N: =⌈YEAH* it's no problem you can have one installed=
223 DL: ⌊yea:::h
224 P: =°and eh (0.1) television=
225 N: =⌈YEAH
226 DL: ⌊you have your me::als you can have communal in a like a
227   dining room (0.08) where all the residents will go at a certain
228   time when the meals are available breakfast dinner and tea
229   or you CA::N have them in your room (0.06) I mean that
230   must depend I suppose on the individual unit I don't know
231   (0.1) it depends if you were ill and you couldn't get out to
232   the dining room they would bring your meal to you that day
233   or (0.1) it's sort of like being in a ho::tel but you-in a way
234 N: ⌊yeah
235   isn't it=

This conversation occurred during the first assessment discussion with Aidan. Members of his family were present and the nurse had already identified that she had a prior conversation with them. The interaction appeared to have been established in order to convince Aidan to accept residential care rather than go back to his flat. It is what his family wanted.

Although Aidan was meant to have thought about going to residential care, he did not know what it was. The input/explanations provided (lines 188- 219) are all designed to paint a positive image of residential care and one that Aidan would accept. What is interesting is the factual way both the nurse and the daughter-in-law speak without knowing the particular care home that he may go to. In this way they paint an 'ideal' picture of residential care and one that would be acceptable to him. This is further highlighted in line 220, when Aidan asks if he can have a telephone and a television installed. The nurse gives an emphatic response in line 222 and 225. The daughter-in-law offers a simultaneous utterance to the nurse (line 226) and describes the food and organisation of meals, an issue that was debated earlier. In this way the daughter-in-law chooses an area of previous concern to present in a positive way. The nurse speaks knowledgeably about what meals Aidan can have and where these would be served. However, in line 229, she recognises that individual practice is done according to the 'rules' of the particular home, but goes on to support the daughter-in-law's description of residential care as 'sort of like being in a hotel' (line 233). This is an interesting metaphor to use, given that a hotel (usually) has guests and not residents, and guests' choices in a hotel are paramount.

It could be asserted that the goal of this input by the nurse and daughter-in-law was to coerce Aidan into choosing residential care. Later conversations continue to paint an ideal picture of residential care compared to a less than ideal picture of his flat. Studies in social gerontology highlight the importance of the meaning of 'home' to most older people. 'Home' is more than a physical environment. It has metaphysical value over and above a shelter to conduct everyday living (Willcocks *et al*, 1987). In such a situation, even though many social networks may have been eroded through disability and illness, there remains an expressive value of having links or connections with a wider society through traditional social networks (Willcocks *et al*, 1987). Howell (1983) suggests that home is a personal power base and a source of self-identity. Research by Willcocks *et al* (1987) highlighted the limited choice that older people have about moving to residential care. Few were given a choice and professional carers played a significant role in the older person's decision.

Throughout the nurse-patient interactions there was evidence of knowledge by the nurse being used as a means of controlling patient decision making. Four types of control appeared to be in use:

The nurses' understanding of the health and social care system This enabled the nurses to make decisions about patient care that would not always be obvious to patients. While the nurses in the study regularly emphasised the importance of patients making decisions about their care and encouraged them to do so, the fact that they possessed so much more knowledge about the relationships between different parts of the health and social care systems, enabled them to move into making decisions on their behalf. It was evident in the content of the conversations that the nurses desired to work with patients in decision-making. However the structure of the conversations suggested the need for decisions to be made quickly and because of a lack of knowledge by patients, then they were unable to participate as equal partners in this process. This knowledge was particularly evidenced during multidisciplinary meetings, where discussions about patients would occur, the detail of which was rarely reported back to them.

An important example of this, is demonstrated in Case Study 13 - Jim. The dominant feature of this case study was Jim's anxiety and his concern for his future. Throughout his interactions with the nurse and others, no attempt was made to help Jim deal with his anxiety and his emotional responses. However, during a multidisciplinary meeting, a detailed discussion about his anxiety occurred but none of this was used in subsequent interactions with Jim or his wife:

Case Study 13/ MDT meeting/Jim

```
77 N:    =I think he's very het up he gets very het up about
78       his incontinence that preoccupies his mind he forgets
79       how he's got to walk he's frightened because he's
80       had a hip replacement in the past that had to have an
81       open reduction because he dislocated and I just think
82       its a vicious circle
83 ?:    ⌈I think (   )*
84 P:    ⌊(   ) time generally het up
85 DHN: (   ) are so:::: hard (   ) I feel that it's something
86       that should be addressed and maybe he does need
87       medication I kno::w that its not always the answer to
88       (   ) medication to old people but he is particularly
89       anxious personality and it is has deeply affected his
90       wife with his wife she's anxious and she's not well
91       herself is she=
92 ?:    (                    )
93 DHN: =Well ever since I met them
94 ?:    He's always been an anxious person  not just (   )
95       making him anxious
96       ((multiple voices))
97 ?:    He's always been (    ) recently he seemed OK
98 ?:    He's always got fed up and nervous
99 N:    He's very nervous of hospitals and medical staff
100      e:::m
101 ?:   (   ) such a big problem (   )=
102 GP:  =The incontinence is making him more anxious than
103      ever  if you cure the incontinence the anxiety will go
104      away
```

In a later multidisciplinary team meeting, the nurse acknowledged the connection between Jim's incontinence, his overall health state and his anxiety. However, even with this understanding, these insights were not explicitly made known to Jim. In many interactions with him, the nurse demonstrated an understanding because of her focus on physical aspects of his care, but she never made her rationale known to Jim.

Prior Knowledge This theme overlaps with a later category of 'The Professionalisation of Relatives' which will be discussed in detail in chapter 7. For those patients who had family involved in their care, it was commonplace for the nurse to have a discussion with the family prior to her first interaction with the patient. This was never made known to patients themselves and it was obvious during their interactions that the nurse had prior knowledge and that this was being used to structure the interaction and the agenda. Because of this prior knowledge, nurses asked direct, specific and focused questions of patients, thus limiting their opportunity to tell their story from their perspective. Teasdale and Kent (1995) warn against the use of 'deception' in nursing, because of its effects on trust and the creation of an 'emotional distance' in the nurse-patient relationship.

Some patients in the case studies demonstrated prior knowledge of technical aspects of their care. In these cases, a greater partnership was seen to occur with the nurse. One patient in particular clearly possessed a lot of technical knowledge about his medicines. In this case the nurse was seen to take great effort to reinforce his understanding and regularly offered further information in order to expand technical knowledge:

Case Study 4/ Interaction 1/ Reg

116 P: except the Thyroxine-
117 N: ⌊except the Thyroxine which is
118 where (0.1) oh yes I've found it so I'll give you all
119 your medication for now (0.2) em and you'll need to
120 become more familiar (0.1) I'll tell you what they are
121 all for now (and explain them to you) (0.2) that's your
122 water tablet (0.1) the Frusemide=
123 P: =yes
124 N: (11.0) So that's the water tablet (0.1) that's the one
125 that actually makes you em-
126 P: ⌊( )
127 N: *((laughs))* yes it tends to keep you busy in the morning
128 doesn't it=
129 P: =yes definitely it does ( )
130 N: there's that one that's the (Ameloride)
131 P: ( )
132 N: Now Thyroxine that's the <u>one</u> that you're familiar
133 with=
134 P: =that's it I have my own eh::-
135 N: (0.1) these are the ones that have been dispensed by
136 the ((Hospital)) pharmacy

137 P: =oh I see (0.1)
138 N: So you shoul-
139 P: ⌊you should have got-there's a couple of
140   bottles of my own as well there some where (0.1)
141 N: Dispensed in the pharmacy is two bottles and then to
142   make up the dose to a hundred and fifty (0.2) they've
143   dispensed a fifty microgram strength as well (0.1) So
144   that's the Thyroxin a hundred and fifty how long have
145   you been taking <u>that one</u>?
146 P: (   )
147 N: <u>Oh:</u> right e::m and yet they're no (calling) back?
148 P: these are they these are my own Thyroxi::n
149 N: (0.1) oh right this is yours
150 P: (0.1) One hundred=
151 N: =oh good well we can use tho:se=
152 P: =yeah?=
153 N: =yeah they are in date they were dispensed on the
154   fifteenth (0.1) when we run out of these we can go on
155   to these=

In lines 117-122 the nurse uses a combination of professional and technical terms. Reg demonstrates that he has some understanding of what is being said by his ability to actively engage in the conversation without the need for many of the terms (particularly names of medicines) to be explained further. The nurse provides explanations about the actions of some medicines (line 124). Reg suggests that he has some knowledge of this by his interruption (inaudible). The response of the nurse (line 127) indicates that he knew of the effect of the medicine. In lines 141-145, the nurse uses a collection of technical terms in the conversation in order to provide an explanation for the presentation of the medicines. Again the lack of a need for a further explanation indicates that Reg has an established level of understanding and knowledge and this allows him to participate as a partner in the planning of his care.

Routine Case Many kinds of institutional encounter are characteristically organised into a standard 'shape' or order of phases (Drew and Heritage, 1992). Naturally occurring conversations by contrast are not. This order occurs because of the professional orientation of the practitioner and the fact that the practitioner may engage in many such encounters in any one day, whereas for the patient the particular encounter may be unique. Professional control manifests itself as a pattern of sequences through which clients may find themselves being led (Drew and Heritage, 1992):

- the order tends to be primarily shaped by the professional;
- the order may be prescribed, e.g. an assessment structure;
- the order may be the product of locally managed routines, i.e. institutionalised practices.

This research concurs with the manifestation of professionally ordered conversation as described by Drew and Heritage (1992), with little evidence of patients themselves setting the order of the conversation. While the nurses in this study emphasised the importance of the individuality of the patient, there was clear evidence of institutional routine. Koch and Webb (1996) have demonstrated how individual needs are ignored as they become the objects of inflexible routines in health care practices. How much of the routine in this research could be described as ritualistic is difficult to tell. However, one example of this routine in which patients were clearly disenfranchised was the collection of information on admission to hospital:

Case Study 1/ Interaction1/ Jack

```
16 N:   Yeah:: (0.1) I mean some of this you may have been asked
17      befo::re but we'll just check it briefly o::kay? so you live at
18      Yardley House

72 N:   I'm going to ask some questions which perhaps seem a bit
73      irrelevant but we just have to write them down=do you have
74      any allergies as far as you kno:::w=
75 P:   =°no::=
76 N:   =no:: right that's °good (0.1) right so I'm Laura and I'll be the
77      nurse that's looking after you while you are here oka::y?=
78 P:   =°thank °you °very °much °indeed=
79 N:   =when I am off duty it will be one of the others but I'll be
80      your na::med nurse oka::y? so (0.3) so you don't have any
81      help at home usually, you manage do you?=
82 P:   =I manage quite well
83 N:                      ⌊so you haven't got a ca::re manager as far as
84      you know
85 P:   (0.1) no no=
86 N:   =you don't have any home help (0.05) services
87 P:                                          ⌊no no
88      at all=
89 P:   =no
90 N:   (0.1) right (0.1) so you are Mister Thompson and you are aged
```

```
91        seventy one yes?=
92 P:     =I'll be seventy two next birthday next April=
93 N:     =right=
94 P:     =I'm seventy one now=
95 N:     =oka:::y (0.2) and you live alo:::ne=
96 P:     =yes=
97 N:     (0.1) e::m you came to us fro::m (0.08) hospital and you live
98        in flat number eight Yardley House right °okay (0.1) and
99        you've come to us
100 P:                        ⌊°correct.
101       following heart surgery you've had a double by-pass I think
102 P:                        ⌊°yeahs
103       haven't you? is that what they called i::t?=
104 P:    =I'm not su::re I wouldn't know they might*
105 N:                                ⌊no °right
106       (0.1) they haven't told me like but eh:: but I feel a lot better
107       since (then)=
108 N:    =do::: you? (0.1) yeahs (0.08) have you had any e:::m what
109       other medical problems have you had in the past illnesses or::.
```

In the example from the data, the nurse apologised to Jack for needing to ask the questions that then followed. Indeed she clearly stated that she knew he had already been asked these questions elsewhere and that the purpose of doing so was 'just to write them down'. However, although Jack may have been asked these questions before, this was his first time in this particular care setting and therefore it was a unique experience. However, the structure of the interaction indicates the 'routineness' of the action by the nurse.

Use of the Term 'WE' A further example of the exertion of professional power and control is through the use of the term 'WE'. Professionals were seen to change from a self- orientated ('I') form of discourse to a collective one ('WE') when they were trying to emphasise a particular course of action or a particular decision:

Case Study 1/ Interaction 1/ Jack

```
50 P:     I hope when I can come out this weekend (0.1) to be honest
51 N:     (0.1) Goodness that's a bit soo:::n isn't it=
52 P:     =yes I don't mind you know=
53 N:     =I know::: (0.05) I think we:: might mi(h)nd (0.08) let me just
54        have a chat with you fir::st and just see::: e:::::m (0.07) 'cause
```

```
55 P:                                    ⌐°okay:::
56      we would have to check with your doctor about that you know
57      and I e::h he might feel it was a bit soon for you to go yet (0.1)
58      who is your doctor::?
```

This interaction occurred on the day of Jack's admission to hospital. Even at this early stage, the nurse has made a decision that Jack would not be ready for discharge at the weekend. The nurse's response to his stated wish is one of surprise. Jack interprets this response as concern for him and replies that he doesn't mind. In order to give her response greater authority, the nurse invokes the term 'we', thereby suggesting that it is not she in particular who would disagree with this decision, but the organisation as a whole. Suggesting that the doctor may have the final say in the decision further reinforces this claim of authority.

This issue emerged throughout the data and appeared to be a particular approach used by nurses when patients were not conforming to desired outcomes. The approach further reinforces Fairclough's (1989) understanding of the need for patients to conform to the rules of the conversation agenda in order to be seen as a cooperative patient. Non-conformity is seen as uncooperativeness. In this study, professionals not only controlled the interactional agenda, but also the knowledge available to patients about their care. This limited knowledge by patients further contributed to their inability to fully engage in care decisions and subsequent actions and concurs with other research in this area (*for example* McWilliam *et al* 1994; Clark and Dyer 1998).

The idea of the older person as a consumer of health and social care (as discussed in Chapter 2) is challenged through this data. There is little evidence of these patients' choices and preferences being held central to care decisions. Limited knowledge of the health and social care context, a lack of understanding of professional decision-making frameworks and the need for health care decisions to be made 'quickly' because of competing pressures all act as barriers to effective consumer choice. Patients have access to large amounts of information and knowledge. Indeed one of the surprising aspects of the data is the extent of information giving and teaching that takes place between the nurses and patients. However, it is also suggested from the data that an increase in patient knowledge does not necessarily deliver greater autonomy. Bhaskar (1989) notes that knowledge is only one component of freedom; also required are the disposition and the power to act in one's own interests. Research into older people in hospital has clearly demonstrated that many of them lack the disposition to exercise autonomous action and are indeed powerless (*for example*, Raps *et al*, 1982; Clark *et al*, 1996; Clark and Dyer, 1998).

Control of Discharge Arrangements

Few of the patients in this study exerted authority over decisions about their ongoing care arrangements and the findings are consistent with other studies (*for example*, Clark *et al*, 1996; Macmillan, 1994; Dill, 1995; Abramson, 1990; Coulton *et al*, 1989). However, as has already been identified through the previous sections of this chapter, patients required a lot of physical and mental energy in order to sustain their determination to have their decisions implemented or pursued on their behalf. This was particularly the case for 'Aidan' as illustrated through such interactions as that on page 186 (interaction 1; lines 178-235). Issues already discussed regarding the nurses' communicative style, their approach to information giving and their perceived 'ownership' of the patient's health state further exacerbated this. Control of discharge arrangements appeared to act as another form of power and control exerted by professionals in this study and the findings concur with similar studies by Clark *et al* (1996):

Case Study 9/ Interaction 4/ Sid

```
17 N:   (0.1) they tell me that you are thinking about home
18 P:   (0.2) well I shall have to go home (0.2) I'm going to tell you
19 N:                                      ⌊getting itchy feet
20      like I told Ted I'm not taking my own discharge (0.1) if you
21 N:                                                        ⌊no
22      send me all's well and good I'll go (0.2) if you think I'm fit
23      enough I'll go 'amorra but no not=
24 N:    =Heidi was saying em that Heidi was saying the
25 P:                    ⌊eh
26      Occupational Therapist that em they'd arranged a home visit
27      for Thursday but you were saying ⌈that's a long way* and she
28 P:                                     ⌊yes °it's a long way
29      =the way she put it excuse me interrupting the way she put it
30      to me (0.07) I can't come before so and so when she told me
31      that's like a week Thursday yesterday 'ain it and she said (  )
32      make arrangements to go home after (that of course)=
33 N:   =yeah (0.1) if you're saying now that they could do it on
34      Wednesday but even that's not soon enough is it?
35 P:   (0.1) nothing's soon enough is it dear=
36 N:   =no I'll have a talk with I'll have a talk with* you and Meg
```

37 P: ⌊(I don't want no bother)
38   Later <u>OK</u>=
39 P: =(yes ok yes) it depends on you=
40 N: =because you are obviously much better than you were aren't you=
41 P: =c::o yes! ⌈(it doesn't make sense)
42 N: ⌊I think Heidi's main worry was (0.1) was the
43   stairs managing the stairs we just need to feel confident about
44   you doing the stairs but I'll talk to Megan later=
45 P: =I been up and down these stairs two or three times (   )=
46 N: = yeah yeah I'm on now all the week end so we'll see how
47   you get on over the week end alright and then we will talk
48   with Heidi on Monday and if we feel that you are going to be
49   able to manage the stairs you know perhaps you won't have to
50   wait until Wednesday eh?
51 P: (0.09)yeah
52 N: (0.1) we'll see how we go ⌈yeah ok then*=
53 P: ⌊yeah ok that's Meg's brother*

In line 17 the nurse informs Sid that she has been told that he is thinking about home. The nurse does not state who has told her this information and implies that it has been more than one person, thereby making it seem a more powerful response. Sid proceeds to provide an explanation that suggests that he wants to go home but that he will not take the initiative to do so without being told so by the nurse. It is the nurse's perception of his ability that will count and not his own. In line 24, the nurse initiates an interruption to the patient's story by telling him more specifically what she has been told and by whom. The nurse also included Sid's perception of that (line 27). He challenges the organisational constraints being put in place. He wishes to go home sooner. It is the organisation of the services that places an unnecessary restriction on his action. The nurse's response is challenging to Sid. She challenges his persistence to go home soon and suggests that even the earlier date would not be soon enough for him. The nurse is cautious in her response (line 36) and does not offer any possible solution. While Sid has some idea of what he wants to happen, he interprets the 'efforts' being made on his behalf as causing 'bother', something that he does not want (line 37) and again places the ultimate authority for decisions made in the hands of the nurse (line 39).

In line 43, the nurse offers an explanation about the perceptions of the staff, in that their concern is Sid's ability to manage the stairs. Again this perception differs from his. While the staff are concerned about his ability to manage, Sid feels that he has practised on the stairs and that he can manage. The nurse's response (line 47) does not serve to elaborate on his input ('yeah yeah'), but instead is cautious in that she suggests that she would be working all weekend and could see how he gets on. She would then consult her colleague on the Monday and make a decision. She still does not give Sid a definite answer, but instead suggests that if they feel he can manage the stairs then he may be able to go home sooner. This control by professional staff is evident throughout this conversation and is further highlighted in line 53.

This interaction provides evidence of the way nurses can control decisions with patients. Throughout this interaction, it was the nurse who directed the flow of the conversation and its progression. The nurse chose to keep the conversation 'open' by the way she responded to questions. She had access to wider information and knowledge that enabled her to decide how the interaction would progress and the topic areas that would be discussed. The power of the professional to manipulate the care agenda is also particularly evident. While Sid had a perception about his ability to cope at home, the nurse and Occupational Therapist appeared to have a different perception. His ability to have control over the planning of his care was limited by the lack of information giving by the nurse. The nurse did not encourage active participation, by not overtly considering Sid's wishes in planning care. The nurse exercised professional cautiousness in her responses, by continually referring to other members of the team and their input. In this way the nurse was not just limiting Sid's autonomy, but also suggesting limitations to her own autonomy.

Sid's lack of control was made further problematic by the lack of engagement by the nurse with his agenda. Although he made suggestions and offered his interpretations, the nurse did not overtly use this information. She evaded responding to his utterances and did not actively seek his opinion or views. The nurse was mainly concerned with considering the impressions of professional colleagues rather than assisting the patient with decision-making and informing him directly if his interpretations were accurate.

The 'we'll see how you go' approach is one that was used frequently in interactions between nurses and patients in this study. Sometimes a time frame was added to it, but most often not. While this approach can be appropriate in the rehabilitation of older people (Ebersole and Hess, 1990), it would be most appropriately used in the context of an overall plan of care that is communicated to the patient. In the context of this study however, this non-committed approach suggested professional control over decisions and further rendered the patient powerless, as no clear indication was given as to what had to be decided and how the decision would be made. Clark and Dyer (1998) identified that while there exists the trappings of involvement of older people in discharge planning, there is a dominant focus on professional interpretations of ADLs (Activities of Daily Living) based on an assessment of functional deficit, rather than by a recognition of the complexity of the meaning of independence to older people.

Medical Control

The control of discharge arrangements was also either directly or indirectly affected by the power of doctors over decision making. This power was seen in all care settings, even those that were nurse-led and utilised the medical services of General Practitioners. Doctors effected discharge decisions directly through their communications with patients (Interaction 2 below) or indirectly through their interactions with other staff (Interaction 3 below):

Case Study 11/ Interaction 2/ Mabel

```
7  P:    (   ) Mornings really=
8  Dr:   morning's the worst time is it?
9  P:    (   )
10 Dr:   Yes well I don't think we'll have you for long Mabel but we'll
11       just we won't have you in for very long just a few days to
12 P:        ⌊eh?
13       get you back on your feet again=
14 P:    =ye::s
15 Dr:   OK::=
16 P:    ⌊go home Saturday (    )=
17 Dr:   =well we'll work it out as we go along ok so I think two or
18       three days here to see how you get on
```

Case Study 11/ Interaction 3/ Mabel

```
40 DR:   Ha I know she's fitter than a lot of people half her age=
41 N:    =right right ok we know she is very proud of being 100 but
42       well look I'll ring
43 DR:                    ⌊well I think it would do everyone a lot of
44       good just to give them a break have her in get her back on
45       her feet get her moving give her a bit more confidence and
46       then
```

```
47 N:        ⌈get her home*
48 DR:       ⌊get her home* as soon as we can=
49 N:    =with a care package how about a respite bed? do you think
50       that would
51 DR:               ⌊I don't think so well we'll have to keep that in
52       mind she's so independent=
53 N:    =yeah=
54 DR:   =so that's the score=
55 N:    =fine fine ok then (0.2) the daughter's going to come in
56 DR:                     ⌊e::h
57       again o:::n (0.1) Thursday so I'll chat to her on Thursday
58       (0.1) and we'll have a better idea thank you
```

The sequence organisation of the conversation, demonstrates the power of the doctor in the relationship and the passive role of the nurse. The dominant inputs into the conversation are made by the doctor, with the nurse's input either being supportive or confirming. In line 41, the nurse begins to suggest a way forward with Mabel's care, but this is interrupted by the doctor (line 43) as a way of asserting his personal view. Again the nurse accepts this. In line 49 the nurse asks the doctor's view about a suggestion she has for care. Before the nurse has finished the question, the doctor interrupts with his view. The doctor is the dominant player and dictates the order of the conversation. The nurse does not assert her views other than those that support the views of the doctor. Finally the nurse asks the doctor's permission regarding organising respite care. Because of the overall structural organisation, it is clear why this has happened. The doctor is presented as the powerful player in the interaction. He interrupted the nurse when she made suggestions and asserted his view confidently. The nurse found herself in a position whereby she supported these views and therefore became more powerless as the conversation progressed. Therefore by the end of the conversation, the nurse felt unable to make a decision without seeking the doctor's permission to do so. However, the imbalance of power was maintained as the doctor did support the nurse's suggestion, thus maintaining his powerful position.

This data illustrates the interplay that exists between nurses, doctors and patients (Svensson, 1996). It highlights the power of the doctor in the patient interactions and the compliance of the nurse with the doctor's decision-making agenda. Instead of working with the patient to achieve the best outcome for her, the nurse is seen to comply with the decisions of the doctor and as such acts as an 'agent' of the doctor in facilitating patient decision-making.

Hopes, Dreams and Desires

There was evidence in the data of nurses and other health and social care professionals being non-specific about their goals of care and not specifying goals with patients. From the professionals' perspective, it appeared to allow flexibility in their decision-making and in the progression of the care plan. Being specific would necessitate an explicit discussion with the patient about goals and opportunities and a need to be specific in interventions. Being specific would also necessitate an acceptance of the patient's goal(s) and a need for frankness and honesty in discussing the feasibility of achieving such goals:

Expert Group Interview (Lines 1104-1116)

EX1: ... it's this idea that I think sometimes you know its alright ... to accept conflicting goals in people or conflicting hopes and that people can have dreams and wishes and desires ... and they may know or not know that they are never going to fulfill them but somehow we the professionals we don't allow people to have that ... and they have to know, we have to be objective and we have to be realistic and well I don't lead my life like that.

These expert nurses expressed concern at what they saw as nurses' need to 'objectify' their relationship with patients and their decision-making. In considering ongoing care arrangements, patients were expected to have an objective view of their lives and suspend any hopes, dreams or aspirations they might have had. In adopting such a position, nurses appeared to spend a considerable amount of time avoiding or trying to account for potential 'risky decisions'. In doing this, they appeared to have a need to ensure that every possible 'risky' situation was accounted for. This was particularly manifested through the assessment of patients' competence to 'do the stairs'. Therefore two issues emerge through the data in this sub-theme:

- Risk Taking.
- Doing the Stairs.

Risk Taking

Throughout this study, professionals demonstrated significant problems with the facilitation of what they perceived to be 'risky' decisions by patients. In general, patients' hopes, dreams and desires were controlled by the nurse and were only considered important if they fitted in with the discharge plan being arranged. Given that professionals tended to control the arrangement of discharge plans, then the individual aspirations of patients played a minor role in their consideration of the appropriateness of discharge plans.

Reflective Conversation - Ann (Lines 786-798)

A: ... I think at the moment in my practice what I do is I set the ball rolling about discharge and then say it's over to you to the Care Manager or whatever. Fait accompli. I can go off and nurse someone else ... Um and then I think well what have they said? You know, what choices have they got. Um, and again from this, there is someone that we discharged home that we all thought would have been wonderful at home and she fell down three times and she's come in with horrendous bruises and it was a failed discharge.

While they recognised the importance of respecting a patient's individual wishes, trying to go along with these wishes was more difficult. This suggested a conflict between acknowledging the importance of individual choice and the practitioner's ability to facilitate it:

Reflective Conversation - Laura (Lines 972-992)

L: ...I suppose you know feeling that you do know them and that knowing their capabilities and knowing the whole picture does certainly influence the amount of autonomy you give them. ... Um, but it shouldn't do should it? I mean I feel it probably shouldn't do... if you know that someone's going home to a safe patch with family around or somebody popping in ever five minutes and you know its warm and that risks are low, if you had all that information I suppose you would accept that and go along with it...

Laura illustrates the kind of implicit decision-making that can occur when a patient makes a choice that appears 'risky'. She identifies a number of criteria that need to be considered including the individual's capabilities; family and friends involvement; the safety of the environment and that 'risks are low'. For Laura, she clearly saw her responsibilities for effective discharge going beyond the parameters of her immediate responsibility and for ensuring that all considerations had been made before agreeing to the patient's expressed choice.

Nurses' understanding of their authority and accountability in the context of supporting individual choice and decision making, emerged as an important issue, and is supported by Macmillan (1994), Dill (1995) and Hennessy (1989). The degree to which nurses have a right to affect lifestyle post-discharge appeared to be an issue. In their reflective conversations, participating nurses expressed concern and confusion about their understanding of their responsibility for patient care following discharge and the extent to which they would be held accountable for 'failed discharges'. Nurses interpreted a failed discharge as a failing in their discharge planning process rather than the taking of a risk that was unsuccessful.

The objectification of patient's lives by professionals was a persistent theme throughout the data. As the expert group suggested, few people adopt such an objective view of their life in general, yet older hospitalised people are prevented from returning to a previous way of life because such a way of life is deemed 'too risky'. The case of Aidan was a particular example of this. Aidan was understood to have a problem with the amount of alcohol he consumed. His family expressed their dissatisfaction with his lifestyle and their unwillingness to support him. Throughout the case study, Aidan expressed conflict with competing desires - on the one hand he recognised his difficulties in caring for himself, while on the other he valued his freedom highly and did not want to lose this. The approach taken to his care planning was to confront him with the reality of his situation from the nurse and family's perspective, without consideration for how a compromise situation could be established, i.e. for Aidan to live in his own home with more support. Aidan was expected to have an 'objective' view of his situation and to suspend his hopes, dreams and desires. The conflict of understanding the objective view continuously expressed by family members and professional staff and his personal desire for his freedoms, prevented him from fully engaging in decision making about his care:

Case Study 15/ Interaction 1/ Aidan

```
166    about (0.1) now I'm here to help you decide (0.1) what you
167    want to do and I can guide you (0.1) but you have to
168    make up your own mind at the end of the day it's your
169    decision (0.2) but what I'd like you to do is listen to
170    everybody and just take in what the::y (0.1) what their
171    concerns are showing and what they think might be su::itable
172    (0.2) okay now I had a message form the ((Hosp. Name))
```

173   before you came down to say that you might be considering
174   residential care but when I asked you the day after you came
175   in you were saying no you wanted to go back to your flat
176   (0.3) now is there any reason why you either I got the
177   wrong message or why you changed your mind?
178 P: I think I (feared) I'd be cared better for if the eh::: (0.3) if I
179   was living away from the flat=
180 N: =if you were away from the ⌈flat? (0.2) so are you thinking
181 P: ⌊yes
182   along the lines of residential ca::re (0.2) where::: you could
183   be::: staying in an area where there is people around twenty
184   four hours a day

Later however, Aidan changes his mind about going to residential care and decided that he wished to stay at his own flat - a decision that the family disagreed with:

319 N: Have you tho:::ught about what we've been talking about
320   now?=
321 P: =yeah I have yeah
322 N: (0.2) why::: do you think ho:::me would work (0.2) in
323   opposed to:: going somewhere else? (0.1) what's the
324   po::sitive thing about home? (0.1) about the flat?
325 P: (0.3) too free and easy too-I can come and go as I please
326   virtually=
327 N: =okay (0.1) u:::m do you regard your indepen::dence
328   highly? (0.1) do you like being able to control (0.08) what
329   you want
330 P: ⌊°yeahs
331   to do?=
332 P: =°yeah but I don't want to be curtailed altogether you know
333   if I want a drink (then I want t'be able to) get one
334   (0.2) which I know a lot of people in ((Place)) won't get
335   me one=
336 S: =no because you don't just take one=
337 D: =you kno::w why though don't you?=
338 S: =you have a bottle bottle bottle bottles it's one after another
339   (0.1) it's not just one is it?=
340 DL: =it's seven or eight bottles a wee:::k not just one a week=

The nurse's response to Aidan's expression of his desires is a challenging one and because of the presence of the family, sets him up to be criticised by them. In a reflective conversation with this nurse, she expressed her concern about what had happened and offered a rationale for it:

Reflective Conversation - Leslie (Lines 10-21)

L: There are so many different um people, there are so many different influences towards this chap and I think the main problem I had or one of the main factors that really got me thinking along a certain pathway was because I had um knowledge from the ((other hosp.)) first before this chap came down. And they had actually talked to the family before he even came on to the ward ...so I had in my mind a picture of what this person was before I saw him.

Reflective Conversation - Leslie (Lines 70-78)

L: ... there were lots of them *[family]*. Even though I was in effect controlling the situation. They were a very dominant family when they were together and you could obviously see which way it was going. ... So it was a case of trying to do, trying to structure it in such a way that I could try and control it but trying to get out of Aidan (*patient's son*) why they wanted him to go to ((residential care home)).

Leslie highlights the problems she experienced in trying to work with Aidan, given her previous knowledge and the influence of the family. The family responded angrily to Aidan's explanation of his values and reasons for wanting to go home. He was placed in a powerless position as each family member painted a negative life picture to him. This 'mirror imaging' of his weaknesses in life further served to place him in a powerless position. If the overall aim (as earlier expressed by the nurse) was for Aidan to make the final choice about where he lived, then this was clearly not the view of the family nor was it facilitated by the nurse, because of the reasons she offered. As this interaction continued, each contribution by Aidan served as another example for the nurse and family to demonstrate his failure to cope. The complex relationship between patients and families will be further explored in Chapter 7.

'Doing the Stairs'

The issue of 'doing the stairs' was a significant one for older people and their control over discharge plans. 'Doing the stairs' is seen as a metaphor for professional control over risk taking.

Excerpt from Field Notes: May 28, 1996

'Doing the Stairs': for all of the participants in this research, being proficient at going up and down stairs appears to be a significant issue in controlling patient's ability to determine their own discharge plan. I am aware from my own practice that for older people, stairs become a major obstacle to their lives once they experience some kinds of handicap through illness. I can't help wondering however, how much this orientation on the stairs by professional staff acts as a metaphor for the degree of control that professionals exert over patients. It seems that the stairs issue acts as a control mechanism to dictate when patients can be transferred home and that it is professionals who determine achievement of proficiency. Is this always necessary? My feeling is that it is an issue of professional control. Except for two patients, doing the stairs was a significant focus in care plans. Doing the stairs acted as another process in the objectification of patient's lives:

Case Study 9/ Interaction 5/ Sid

122 P: Like going up stairs there (and walk along, when all) I'm
123   being told is slow down=
124 N: =that's right yeah ⌈and I mean* these areas are - you won't
125 P: ⌊they keep-
126 N: walk these long areas at home because your house isn't as big
127   as this is it so in fact people always go home quite a lot fitter
128   than- and very often I have to say to people you know well
129   they won't be expected to go that far at home you know
130   because the loo's next to the front room and the front room is
131   next to the bedroom isn't it so its a lot less the stairs are the
132   main problem well in my mind I was thinking well if you only
133   have to come down in the morning and go up at night then
134   somebody could go up behind you at night (0.1) and come
135   down with you in the morning and you just need to go
136   carefully=
137 P: =my son's always there and goes up behind-=

In this interaction, the nurse adopts a realistic view of Sid's coping abilities and how he could manage the stairs. However, in a later interaction, she demonstrates a more cautious position and wants to delay his discharge until a 'home visit' is performed:

Case Study 9/ Interaction 7/ Sid

8 P: =I'm going home lovely=

```
 9 N:   =beautiful listen would you really would it be really awful to
10       ask you if we can make it Wednesday
11 P:    (0.1) what!=
12 N:    =to go home
13 P:    (0.2) well if you say so I (    )=
14 N:    =because if we leave it Wednesday the Occupational
15       Therapist and Physio can come home with you to do a home
16       visit discharge all at once where they can just have a look at
17       how you
18 P:            Lyes
19       manage and I think they would really like to see you on the
20       stairs (0.2) and it's only one extra day and I think Meg would
21 P:         Lyeah                         Lyes
22       be happy (0.1) if they came with you=
```

Even when patients themselves were clear about their ability, this was not accepted until it was objectified through an assessment:

Case Study 11/ Interaction 1/ Mabel

```
106 P:   No I don't need anybody to get up the stairs*=
107 D:                          Lthere you are you see
108 P:   =Coming down the stairs yes=
109 N:   =you need help down right=
110 P:   =yes (0.1) not so bad going up I mean=
111 N:   =right (0.08) I think I think what's happening here is that
112      I'm (0.05) we have various people that can help you now
113      that you're in hospital besides Dr Jackson and us looking
114      after you the nurses there's people called physiotherapists
115      and occupational therapists and I think it=whilst you are
116      here (0.1) and you are at this great age of over a hundred I
117      think we ought to do like an MOT on you=
118 P:   =yes I would=
```

The home visit appeared to act as the 'gold standard' in deciding on patients' level of proficiency and in validating their participation:

Case Study 11/ Interaction 1/ Mabel

```
145 N:   =No I think what we'll do you know Kathy Sugden your
146      care manager I will ring her hopefully by about half past
147      four today to say that you are here and that I would like her
148      to pop in and visit possibly Thursday Friday so we can
```

```
149      discuss things and we've got your 'phone number (0.1) in
150 D:                                              ⌊that's
151      right
152      the meantime I'll ask the physiotherapist to put you through
153      your paces once your chest is feeling a bit easier with your
154 P:                                         ⌊h::m
155      walking (0.2) and we'll get the occupational therapist to
156      have a look over and see if there's anything we can help you
157      with because an occupational therapist can go home and do
158      a home visit and look at the house and it may be that you
159      just need another rail up the banisters
160 D:                                   ⌊no she doesn't I've
161      had two (already fitted)=
162 N:   =you've got two rails right well it may be that there's a few
163      things that they can add and then you can go home but it
164      will take a few days but we need you'll be meeting all these
165      new people so it might be a bit confusing (0.1) but I'll be
166      your nurse for your stay in hospital all right and I've noticed
167      you've got a little dressing on your left leg=
```

In this interaction, the nurse explains about the occupational therapist doing a 'home visit' to assess the need for alterations to the house and in particular to fit 'two rails' on the stairs. The daughter suggests that such a visit would be unnecessary, as these alterations have already been undertaken. The nurse persists with her suggestion by indicating that there may be other needs, thus implying that discharge cannot occur until a therapist confirms the daughter's views. Later, even though Mabel demonstrated on a number of occasions her ability to get up the stairs, a carer was organised to assist her with this activity. Clark and Dyer (1998) found similar practices in their discharge planning study.

Conclusions

In this study, professionals' ability to freely exert power and control over older patients was illustrated throughout the data. Such power and control manifested itself in the form of control of the interaction agenda and the structure of interactions, the control of information, the control of discharge arrangements and professional control by a dominant medical hierarchy. Professionals' abilities to make decisions about the degree of risk to take in decisions about care needs appeared problematic. There appeared to be an emphasis on objectivity at the expense of attention to patients' hopes, dreams and desires. The inability to make such decisions effectively in a way that respected and acknowledged the hopes, dreams and desires of the patient manifested itself in the form of constraints on autonomous action.

Professional nursing practice emphasises the importance of partnership in the nurse-patient relationship. The idea of the nurse working therapeutically includes the need for a close interpersonal relationship between both parties. However, while research such as that of Lawler (1991) and Savage (1995) would suggest that nurses aim to build such an approach into their practice focus, it is questionable if the power of older patients has significantly changed despite consumerist ideology and humanistic philosophy.

Research by Porter (1996) suggests that patients have more power and hence more autonomy because of their increased knowledge. Porter argues that as a result, nurses have less power. The data so far in this study would suggest otherwise. It is very obvious that patients have access to information and knowledge. Indeed one of the surprising aspects of the data is the extent of information giving and teaching that takes place between the nurses and patients. However, it has been previously asserted that an increase in knowledge does not necessarily deliver greater autonomy (Bhaskar, 1989) and that many older hospitalised people lack the disposition to exercise autonomous action and are indeed powerless (Clark and Dyer, 1998). Within this data, while nurses spent considerable periods of time exchanging information and attempting to increase patients' knowledge, in all but the more 'trivial' examples (e.g. choosing food from a menu) nurses directed the decisions made. While patients' views were sought out there was a tendency towards paternalism rather than autonomy. Nurses' privileged position in their relationship with patients appears to provide plenty of scope to adopt strategies of inducement, encouragement or persuasion in order to influence patient decision making behaviour. However, the key issue here is whether such authority is being used to initiate actions that are essentially in the patient's best interests. There is a need, it would seem, to distinguish between persuasive tactics that are in the patient's best interests and those that are essentially coercive. A number of principles for action are manifested in this data.

Principles for Action

- Listen to patients and allow them to 'tell their story' as a legitimate part of assessment processes.

- Wherever possible, encourage patients to identify solutions for existing problems and care needs, set within negotiated parameters of risk-taking.
- 'Get to know' patients and establish a negotiated level of engagement before decisions about degrees of risk taking are made.
- For informed decision-making to be facilitated in a patient-centred way, refrain from 'imbuing' decision-making processes with one's own values.
- Suspend the use of prior knowledge about a patient and their social context until they have been enabled to tell their 'story'.
- Recognise that the uniqueness of patients' experiences versus the 'routineness' of nurses' experiences limits a patient-centred approach to decision-making.
- Accord the patient's perceptions of their care situation equal status as those of health care professionals.
- Patients' 'subjective' views of their lives should be respected in decision-making.
- To facilitate patient participation, understand and be confident with the boundaries of one's decision-making potential.
- Adopt a patient-centred approach to risk assessment and risk taking.

7 'Speaking for you or Speaking for me?'

How much input patients had in their care decisions was reflected in the continuous interplay between nurses, other professionals, patients, their families and the culture of the care environments. The phrase 'Speaking for you or Speaking for me' consistently re-emerged in my reflections, as I worked with the data:

Reflection

> Throughout the data, I continuously have an impression of the nurses trying to gauge their language and style of conversation, so that it meets their own needs and those of the patients. I get a sense of the nurses using words to enable patient decision-making, while in reality they are representing their own views, concerns and values. I keep asking myself the question - are they speaking for the patient or for themselves? or from a patient's perspective, I think the phrase 'speaking for you or speaking for me?' captures the essence of what seems to be happening.

The phrase represents the interplay that existed in interactions and the use of language by both professional and lay 'players' in the research to present their own views through the guise of patient decision making, i.e. participants were seen to use language in such a way as to present their own views, but to do so in a way that had the trappings of negotiation. The structures and processes involved in these interactions have already been discussed in Chapter 5. These uses of language are indicative of the 'power games' that were seen to occur in Chapter 6 and represent an overall constraint on patient engagement in care decisions. The manifestation of the interplay that occurred in interactions is represented through three themes:

- Constraint on Autonomous Action.
- Socialization and Enculturation.
- Professionalisation of Relatives.

161

Constraint on Autonomous Action

In this study, constraints on actions were seen to affect the decision-making capacity of nurses and patients. Members of the expert group stressed the importance of considering the context in which nurses worked and the limitations such a context may place on their practice:

Expert Group Interview (Lines 1309-1318)

EX4:   I'm not saying that this is total mitigation um by any means but if one can think of their reality ... so the kind of things that are in their minds and all the other agendas, and other people, and other considerations when they engage in (a) particular encounter.

Participating nurses described various constraints on their practice and in the facilitation of patient decision making that will be discussed in this section. However, there was a consistent view held by all of the participants that the many agendas they have to fulfil in their roles within specific time periods act as the greatest constraint on their practice:

Reflective Conversation - Leslie (Lines 324-336)

L: I've got a focus when I go into work about what I'm going to do and who I've got to please you know, politics around it. Because I'm primary nurse down there and I'm trying to get the Associates through it. They are quite vulnerable with regards to doctors and their power ... and it's a case of me trying to have so many eggs, so many hats on. Um, getting through the organisation of it of where somebody needs to go, (when) do we need the bed by, what are they doing, the whole lot...

Four types of constraint were identified through the following sub-themes:

- Organisational Constraint.
- Routinised Practices.
- Emotional Constraint.
- Lack of 'Synchronicity'.

Organisational Constraint

In this study, organisational constraints are understood as:

factors in the organisation of care and care services that inhibit the operationalisation of 'patient-centred' decisions.

Although there appeared to be an intention among nurses and other professionals to work in a patient centred way, i.e. work in partnership with the patient in making decisions about care, a number of organisational factors prevented such an approach from happening effectively. Organisational constraints were manifested in the form of organisational policies and planning and continuity of care.

Organisational Policies these were seen to work against patient's having control over aspects of their care. These policy restraints occurred both within the immediate care environment and in potential long-term care environments. The most notable example of constraint in the immediate care environments, identified in nurses' interactions with patients, was the planning of 'self-medication' programmes, i.e. patients having control of their medicines, including their storage so that they can take them according to their usual routine rather than the routine of the care environment. While nurses were seen to spend considerable time teaching patients about their medication programmes and enabling them to continue with their usual routine, this was hampered by the policy of the care environments which stipulated that all medicines should be locked in a central cupboard:

Case Study 3/ Interaction 3/ Mrs. Archer

```
105 P:   Can these go on here (2.0) don't see why not do you?
106 N:   No I mean what would probably be the best thing to do
107      would be to present you with your medication each
108      time (0.3) so it would mean that I would actually look
109      after them=
110 P:   =all yours ((patient and nurse laugh))
111N:    but but only (0.3) yes (0.4) but only until you and I*
112 P:                    ⌊you bring them over and you take them*
113      away?
```

In the planning of long-term care, other policy constraints were identified:

Case Study 15/ Interaction 1/ Aidan

```
569 D:                                              ⌊you'll have your
570      own room with your own things round you yeah not too
571      big but big enough yeah* (0.1) it'll be like being in your own
572 S:      ⌊a load of old photographs* on the wall
573      ⌈place in a way
574 S:   ⌊well your own roo:::m your little house (   )
575 P:                                         ⌊you get your own
576      fridge and tha' there=
577 S:   =YEAH yeah=
578 D:   =well you won't need a kitchen will you you'll eat-your meals
579      will be cooked for you
580 P:   =(if I had a) small fridge I could have some food that I could
581      cook with=
582 N:   =it depends on the::::: um:::
583 D:                                ⌊the space I suppose=
584 N:   =it depends on the space it depends on the policy of the
585 P:                                   ⌊yeah
586      home (0.1) but as long as you:: you check with them then
587      usually you can have in there what you want (0.1) a::nd they
588      encourage that they like you to be as personal as you make it
589      (0.1) okay?=
```

This conversation is part of a long interaction between Aidan, members of his family, the nurse and a care manager. The aim of the interaction is to 'encourage' Aidan to choose to live in a residential care home. The confidence and authority with which the family speaks about what is possible in the care home is interesting. In line 580, Aidan suggests that if he could have a small fridge in his room then he could do some cooking for himself. This request is directly in response to the picture of 'normality' that the family has been painting. The patient is not deviating from this theme, but is suggesting that his focus is slightly different. He demonstrates a desire to do 'normal' activities, such as cooking. This says something about the values that he holds and his personal wishes and desires.

The nurse's response to this is a cautious one and this cautious response (line 582) is interrupted by the daughter who suggests that space may be a problem. While this in itself acts as a constraint on Aidan's autonomous desires, the nurse suggests an even more fundamental constraint - the policy of the home (line 584). This assertion illustrates the differences in priorities that are at work in this interaction. Aidan has demonstrated a desire to retain his freedom of choice and action. The nurse and family encourage this, but at the same time they desire for him to go to residential care and have painted a picture of the care home that is supportive of individual autonomy and differences. However, the 'policy of the home' contradicts the ideal picture being painted. One could argue that in life generally, there are rules that must be adhered to and that breaking these rules carries consequences. However, for Aidan, in this case there is an extra set of rules, i.e. those of the individual care home. This is further illustrated in the data example below:

Case Study 15/ Consultant Ward Round/ Aidan

> I'm a <u>bit</u> worried about is (in terms of placement) he used to
> have his drinking friends when they were out of prison
> (0.07) around him ( ) when we were talking to him
>
> N: ⌊yeah
>
> yesterday he was talking about not wanting to loose contact ( ) but I
> would IMAGINE that if em he went somewhere like ((care home
> name))
> (which is sheltered housing with residential care) and then his friends
> came along and they have drinking parties it would not be e:::m very
> satisfactory for either the other residents or indeed for Aidan=

The balancing of organisational and societal rules with individual wishes and desires is a part of living in 'community' (Luhmann, 1997) and of being a citizen (Berlin, 1992). As Feinberg (1989) identified, the ideal of the autonomous person is that of an authentic individual who engages in reflective evaluation of action in the context of being a member of a community. This reflective evaluation of action is consistent with Berlin's idea of 'positive freedom' (Berlin, 1992). However, Willcocks *et al* (1987) argue that for the older person moving to residential care, there are costs and losses, benefits and gains and that it is this equation that the older person has to translate in very personal terms for themselves if life is to be comprehensible. Willcocks *et al* (1987; 52) argue that this reflective evaluation is often hindered by the lack of a contract that clearly spells out this equation. Willcocks *et al's* research found little evidence of discussions about choices in residential care decisions and they concluded that:

It is therefore very difficult, if not impossible, for residents to pick up the threads of everyday life in ways which have meaning for them if the connections between former community life and the new residential life are not preserved and nurtured as part of the admissions procedure.

Others (Collopy *et al*, 1991; Mattiasson and Anderson, 1995 [ii]; Lidz and Arnold, 1990; Lewis, 1984) have all argued for the maintenance of an individual's choices and preferences as central to decisions about long-term care.

Planning and Continuity of Care continuity of care was also an issue for patients. A number of interactions demonstrated the problems experienced in enhancing and maintaining patient independence, because of nurses' failure to work with agreed care plans, as illustrated in the following data examples:

Case Study 6/ Interaction 1/ Mrs. Burke

```
39 P:    =I dressed-no (0.1) not this morning they wouldn't let me
40       because they said they had plenty of other people to
41       take-I had a bath (0.1) and what I wanted to do was to=
42 N:                        ⌊ye:s
43 P:    = dress myself after the bath=
44 N:    =right
45 P:    (0.1) they said "no"=
46 N:     =but you were cajoled into being helped were you?
47 P:                             ⌊they wanted
48       other people to have a bath (0.2) and I was being a
49 N:                         ⌊oh right
50       nuisance=
51 N:    =O:::h n::o
52 P:            ⌊well, no it wasn't-that wasn't the word but they
53 N:                                                       ⌊no
54       wanted me so I had to eh=
55 N:    =but yesterday you dressed yourself
56 P:    (0.1) yes yesterday I dressed myself=
```

Case Study 4/ Interaction 3/ Reg

```
24 N:    =How have you been getting on over the
25       weekend with them?
```

26 P: Well they (0.1) they they didn't let me do it
27   myself yesterday I just-
28 N: ⌊they didn't* let you do it
29   yourself?
30 P: (0.3) I supose they forgot about it=
31 N: =oh right was that all day yesterday?
32 P: Yes (0.4) (   )
33 N: that rather defeats the object doesn't it?
34   (0.7)
35 N: So (0.1) Slow K

Patients' abilities to become independent and thus regain autonomy are hampered by the ability of the nurse to follow the care plan. While a primary nurse adopts a patient centred approach establishing a programme aimed at maximising independence, in her absence this approach appears to be omitted by other staff. Further, patients were seen to make excuses for the other nurse's actions (for example 'Reg' 'they probably forgot'). Here Reg is demonstrating his acceptance of the practice norm that is in place each day. If Reg knows that he is self administering his medications, then why did he accept the giving of them to him? Why did he not tell the nurse that he was self medicating? Does Reg view it as an important activity for him to learn and something that is about returning control to him? It has been argued that in the exercising of their decision-making capacity, patients have a responsibility to perform those activities that facilitate their recovery as quickly as possible (Chervenak and McCullough, 1991). In Reg's case, his mastering of the administration of his own medicines was an important component of his rehabilitation and one that would have enabled the organisation of a discharge package that maximized his independence.

Continuity of care is also an issue in the planning of a time frame for patients to make decisions:

Case Study 15/ Interaction 7/ Aidan

51 N: I'm not here next week so can you get feed back from what
52   he's actually thinking I've asked if he can try and make up
53   his mind by Tuesday so that we've got some feedback for the
54   round e:::m will he have to::: (0.07) apply for funding now
55 ?:   ⌊yes
56   and wait or are they prepared to::=
57 ?:   =I'm not sure what they'll do really you'll have to ask them

Here the nurse identifies that there is a time limit attached to Aidan making a decision about going to residential care. It also highlights the lack of a consistent plan for the organisation of ongoing care arrangements. Throughout all of the data, there was a tendency to make decisions about care arrangements in a very informal way. For patients this could be a particular problem as at no time was there a deliberate intention to spend time with a patient and family putting together all the pieces of the discharge-planning jigsaw. Patients were informed about particular decisions, but no interactions were recorded whereby the nurse recapped the complete plan and the place of particular decisions within that overall plan:

Expert Group Interview (Lines 1368-1380)

EX1:   Is that about how nurses work with other people and make use of that time to help that person move on to the next stage of their journey or their getting well or whatever it is. So it's about knowing the right time to suggest you know, 'do we need to work together to look at how you're going to manage the tablets at home?' 'Have you thought about the stairs because that always happens?' 'Do you think about home yet?'. Knowing these sorts of things rather than somebody else prompting you because they've already been here three weeks, you then need to find out about. And then the nurse's are like trying to pull back that time she's lost and dashing in.

This lack of proactive planning may be a significant factor in the pressure that appeared to exist to make discharge decisions quickly. The urgency of this decision making further prevented patient involvement. Few patients appeared to have an overall discharge goal established and because of this, decisions about discharge were inconsistent and appeared unplanned:

Case Study 9/ Interaction 5/ Sid

94 N: I mean, do you have *((interruption by other patient [0.35]))* yes
95   what I thought was I said to Heidi that I would see how you were
96   over the week end em (0.3) and talk with Meg and see what she
97   felt and what you felt if we felt by Monday that you were strong
98   enough and if you felt confident about the stairs e:m I mean
99   Heidi will be back on Monday so I can talk with her e:m and
100   we felt we could probably let you go e:m (0.2) I mean there
101 P: ⌊yes

102   would perhaps be a pop-in visit to see if you are ok but perhaps
103   not you know I think you might be o:k you've improved a lot
104   haven't you really even just the couple of days I've been off=

Maintaining continuity was also a problem because of staff shortages:

Case Study 3/ Interaction 3/ Mrs. Archer

28 P: (0.2) Now then when are (you going to bath me)=
29 N: =well do you want to get into a more comfortable position? (0.3) I
30   mean we can certainly give you a bath if you are prepared to wait
31   just a little bit longer while we find ourselves as one nurse has not
32   turned up this morning so we'll get to everybody but it may take a
33   little longer (0.2) if you change position I'll just go
34 P: ⌊alright alright
35   and run and get my (   ) and then you can take
36   (something)=

The problem of staff shortages and 'time' to work in a patient centred way was consistently identified as an issue among nurse participants during their reflective conversations. Nicola illustrates this while discussing the time needed to support patients in their understanding of their care plans:

Reflective Conversation - Nicola (Lines 1782-1787)

N: there isn't the time ... in nursing to pursue things the long way round. And I'm actually quite fond of the long route but it's not always, well it's hardly ever possible. ... you know you've got twelve patients you're looking after ... spend too much time with one person it's not-you've got to balance it and if there is any excess then that can be directed towards the person with the most need.

Nicola's assertion concurred with the evidence from the conversational data, whereby interactions appeared to be 'orchestrated' (as discussed in Chapter 6), with nurses not responding to particular cues in order to control the agenda of the conversation. One reason for this could be the pressures of time and workload.

      Savage (1995) has identified the paradox of the dominant ideology of contemporary nursing and that of health care management, in the form of a clash of cultures between a philosophy of humanism as articulated through patient-centredness and the dominance of managerialism in organisational cultures. The dominant focus on shorter lengths of stay and maximizing throughput hinders notions of patient-centredness with an emphasis on patient decision-making, choice and a culture of 'healing'. While this study is set within the context of Primary Nursing as a method of organising nursing work and enabling individual patient decision-making, there is little evidence to suggest that patients in this study were more empowered as a result of this organisational system. Time pressures dominated the perceptions of all the participating nurses in their reflective discussions, thus indicating the degree of conflict between the two competing ideologies (humanism versus managerialism) in contemporary health care.

Routinised Practices

Although participating nurses identified staff shortages and lack of time as reasons for the often lack of opportunity to work in a patient centred way, the issue of routinised practices was evident in the data. Routine practices were in evidence throughout the data sets and many of these have been discussed already in other categories, such as doing the stairs and home visiting. However, the greatest routine that appeared to exist was that of 'assessment'. In the majority of interactions with patients, nurses appeared to have an implicit set of questions that they wished answered and the structure of their interactions suggested a desire not to deviate from this list, even if patients' responses to questions indicated a need to. A routinised approach was seen to act as a constraint on patients' autonomy as it prevented patients from expanding on particular issues. Because of the implicit but routinised assessment approaches adopted by nurses, patients were reliant on nurses to identify the salient features of the conversation and items that needed further expansion. The routine approach adopted, resulted in nurses appearing to miss important 'cues' from patients and failing to respond appropriately to particular utterances (as discussed in Chapter 5).

Case Study 1/ Interaction 1/Jack

72 N: I'm going to ask some questions which perhaps seem a bit
73   irrelevant but we just have to write them down=do you have any
74   allergies as far as you kno:::w=

Case Study 1/ Interaction 1/Jack

133 N: yeah and sight OKAY do you wear glasses-?
134 P: ⌊Well this one eye got no
135   vision at all=
136 N: =no vision in:::=
137 P: =the right eye
138 N: ⌊the right eye (0.2) righ' was that an injury o:::r
139 P: (0.1) no::: it's eh something eh what do they call it C something=
140 N: =O:::H ri:::ght (0.1) °yeah °right=
141 P: =I've been down to the ((Hosp. Name)) and saw a specialist there
142   he said no there's nothing I can do:::=
143 N: =right so you wear glasses for re::ading do you?* right okay and
144 P: ⌊oh yes
145   your speech is okay (0.2) so when you are at home you look after
146 P: ⌊°yes (that's fine)
147   yourself completely do you (0.06) you do your own housework
148 P: ⌊°yeahs
149   your own cooking? your own shopping deal with your own
150 P: ⌊yeahs   ⌊°yeahs
151   finances indepe(h)nde(h)nt ((laugh)) and that't how you want to=
152 P: ⌊°yes   =I would like to=
153 N: =yeahs I'm sure yeah have you been poorly at home before the
154   operation was it becoming difficult for you to (0.06) to do those
155   things::
156 P: (0.1) No I haven't been too:: bad really just occasionally a day
157 N: ⌊no:::
158   you know but nothing much=
159 N: =what did you get? breathless or
160 P: ⌊yeah=
161 N: =yeah (0.1) is it fairly close where you do your own shopping?=
162 P: (0.07) no I go down to the city=
163 N: =do you you go on the bus
164 P: (0.05) yeah I gets across the road where I live (0.05) there's the
165 N: ⌊yeahs
166   bus stop
167 N: ⌊ri:::ght

In both of these interactions with Jack, the nurse outlines that the assessment is a routine part of practice and that although he may have been asked the questions before (he was transferred from another hospital), she needed to 'just write them down'. The assessment process that follows (lines 133-171) is ritualistic and consists of the nurse working from a list of pre-established questions. Her responses to Jack's previous utterances are not designed to seek further clarification or expansion of issues raised. Instead, her responses serve as acknowledgments of what was said and as opportunities to move to the next question.

The routinised approach adopted by nurses in this study is seen to affect patients' decision-making potential because of the way it limits their ability to express particular desires or wants. In addition, it prevents nurses from identifying cues (as discussed in Chapter 5) that may indicate particular needs, wants or values that patients are not conscious of or have difficulty expressing. Further, not responding to cues contributes to a lack of recognition of patients' emotions.

Emotional Constraint

Emotional constraints arose from the perspectives of both the patient and the health care professional. In this study, emotional constraints are understood to be:

> An individual's expressed emotion associated with the care experience that inhibits the individual from acting on care decisions.

These expressions of emotion manifested themselves in the form of:

- patients' anxiety about their care;
- patients' anxiety about long-term care arrangements;
- family emotions;
- professionals' fear of risk taking.

The emotions expressed by older people in this study, related to their anxiety and fear about losing their independence and dignity and feeling embarrassed about their care needs. As a result of these emotional struggles, patients were limited in their ability to exercise freedom of action:

Case Study 5/ Interaction 3/ Molly

125 P: Yes thank you (0.2) and eh Tuesday I go to the X-
126 ray

127 N: (0.1) we've already arranged it (0.8) Twenty First of
128   November at two pm
129 P: ⌊pick me up ⌈here*
130 N: ⌊here* and bring
131   me back thank you and I'm keeping my fingers
132   crossed it's okay=
133 N: =because what they are going to be saying to you
134   is (   )
135 P: I am (0.1) if I can just get over to the toilet little
136   things like that make all the difference instead of
137   having to ring a bell and ask to be taken all the
138   time it's (0.2) it irks me
139 N: (0.2) Yes °infuriating I saw you hopping on there and I
140   thought that was em=
141 P: =oh did you see me-my daughter's with me I won't
142   go unless somebody's with me you see (0.2) she
143   took me round to the toilet
144 N: (0.2) well I saw you hopping and I thought 'gosh
145   that's not easy'

In line 135, Molly demonstrates her frustration with having to ask for help with daily activities - constraint on her autonomy. The nurse's response informed her that she had seen her 'hopping'. The nurse had not finished her explanation, when Molly interjects with a surprise response that the nurse had seen her. She interprets the nurse's response as her being 'caught' doing something that she shouldn't do and goes on to explain that she only did this because her daughter was with her. In lines 144-145, the nurse indicates the misinterpretation made by Molly by empathising with her situation.

Molly's frustration with her situation was manifested in other patients as embarrassment. This was particularly so for Jim who had a problem with incontinence associated with the need for a circumcision to be performed. This had been a long-term problem for him:

Case Study 13/ Interaction 1/ Jim

174 N: °yeah well we need to know a date for (   )
175 P: ⌊I mean
176   it should have been done before (   )=
177 N: =°yeah: °yeah we'll get it all sorted Jim
178 P: (0.06) but that was my fault (for not saying anything about it)

179   before (0.1) I was a bit embarrassed to talk about it to anybody
180   (0.1) I feel I can talk to you now (and I can fill in) Dr Haigh about
181   it and they looked at it then when this other doctor came down
182   (0.07) I don't know where he was from but he came down and said
183   I think (   )=
184 N: =alright then well when Dr Haigh comes in we'll
185   check on we'll see if he's got any dates organised or
186   anything for you alri::ght=
187 P: =(   ) I think I'll feel a lot better when that's done=

Feeling comfortable with the care environment was also an important factor in reducing patients' fear of hospitals and has been highlighted in previous research (Miller and Gwynne, 1972; Genevay and Katz, 1990). Indeed research by Cumming and Henry (1961) demonstrated that older people are often more disturbed by changes in their physical environment than they are about loss of contact with family and friends. More recent research by Willcocks *et al* (1987) further demonstrated the importance of familiarity with environment in an older person's transition to residential care. Patients compared a community hospital with a larger secondary care center and in one case (Sid) refused to go to the larger center to receive care, but instead chose to have it provided in the community hospital:

Case Study 9/ Interaction 1/Sid

367   =she's em she's a GP she works at your practice doesn't she
368 P: ⌊o:h yes she's
369   ⌈a new one just* started yes I do yes I've got two (0.1) GPs
370 N: ⌊do you remember*   ⌊she was nice wasn't she?
371   she said if she I think she was slightly worried about you and I
372   think she felt that if we couldn't get you sorted out in a couple
373   of days that she might get you to the ((Hospital name)) but you
374   weren't very keen on that were you?=
375 P: =no I wouldn't go there no=
376 N: =you wouldn't go right so we have got to try and sort you out
377   here then haven't we=
378 P: =I mean if you want to know anything I'm sure they will tell you
379   and I don't think that I (0.1) well I think that you know as
380   much about aches and pains here as anybody do (0.2) because
381 N: ⌊i:m
382   what I see here are similar to where I am to have to walk
383   etcetera (0.2) but eh no I wouldn't go to I wouldn't leave here

384 N: ⌊i:m yeah
385   (again no)=

The emotional connection of the patient with their family also served as a constraint on patient action. When nurses were encouraging particular decisions by patients, such phrases as 'everyone here *(members of the family)* is concerned about ya...' (case study 15/ interaction 1/line 161/Aidan) and 'they *(the family)* think if you go back to the flat then you might go back to drinking' (case study 15/ interaction 1/line 161/Aidan) acted as emotional constraints. For Aidan, the emotional constraints associated with the family were powerful in influencing his decision to move into residential care:

Case Study 15/ Interaction 1/ Aidan

452 Man: ⌊the
453   situation arose too (0.07) is when he has been drinking and you go
454   and visit him and he's in such a sta::te that he can't talk
455   anyway and all of us have made like shall we say trips of at
456 N: ⌊right
457   least an hour (0.05) travelling two hours travelling to visit
458   you to find you in such a state that you can't even speak to
459   ya so you don't bother to do it again therefore::: we don't
460   visit him=
461 D: =well it reaches a stage where you before you visit* you
462 S: ⌊you don't want to
463   think (0.07) what time of the day it is which day of the week
464   it is if it's pension day we definitely don't go::: and for four
465   days after pension day*
466 DL: ⌊if you find him::
467 N: ⌊you're the one whose missing out on
468   all this=

Professionals were also seen to use emotional constraint as a means of constraining patients' decisions. This was usually instigated as a means of convincing patients to take a particular course of action when they were undecided or wished to take an alternative action that was not the preference of the professional. This expression of emotion was also associated with the professional's concern about risk taking. The expression of such emotional constraints did appear to effect how patients felt about their relationship with health care professionals:

Case Study 9/ Interaction 1/ Sid

```
414 P:   Not while I am as I say I do feel well I don't feel there is
415 N:                                      ⌐im
416      anything wrong with me that warrants an operation you know I
417 N:                                                      ⌐°im
418      may be wrong but (0.1) I mean I know I upset my doctor Dr
419 N:                  ⌐im
420      Simpson (   ) yeah I know I did yes he wanted me ah (0.1) to go
421 N:               ⌐did you?
422      to the ((Hospital name)) for something (0.1) because the Sister at
423      our practice tried to get me to go and I wouldn't go and he said
424      'Sid why won't you go for me' I said 'No not just for you'
425      the (   ) afterwards was very bad you know (0.1) very bad of
426      me you know=
```

Sid highlights how persuasion at an emotional level can be used as a type of *coercion* by professional staff in order to manipulate the decision made (lines 422-426). The type of coercion highlighted in line 424 could be described as *emotional manipulation*. Although Sid defended his case, he identifies his perception of the consequences of having done so, i.e. that he upset his doctor because of his decision. He demonstrates the paradox of asserting autonomous action, but feeling uncomfortable about doing so because of how he perceives the effects of such action on other people and his perceptions of authority. Sid feels that he has upset his doctor and that that was 'very bad' of him. His interaction is therefore constrained by his understanding of the way his activity should be limited by his perceptions of reasonable behaviour.

Lack of 'Synchronicity'

The term 'synchronicity' emerged from the expert group to describe a way in which the 'ideal' nurse-patient relationship and the manifestation of nurse and patient autonomy within that relationship could be conceptualised. Synchronicity is used to encapsulate concepts underpinning contemporary professional nursing practice and the nature of the nurse-patient relationship. It encapsulates such concepts as partnership, empowerment, honesty and empathy. In this study 'synchronicity' means:

the nurse and patient working together in order to achieve a particular goal.

Boykin and Schoenhofer (1993) illustrate the importance of synchronicity in the relationship between nurse and patient. They describe this as the 'dance of carers' that is underpinned by concepts of mutuality, respect, empathy and care. Boykin and Schoenhofer argue that therapeutic caring is like a dance with both parties synchronised through the sharing of a common goal. This relationship establishes a personal-professional connection based on mutual respect and honesty (Genevay and Katz, 1990).

The expert group was critical of the approach used by many of the nurses to facilitate patient involvement in decision-making. The conversation data itself provides some evidence of nurses' aiming to achieve synchronicity with older patients and factors that prevented this from occurring. Participating nurses themselves had some insight into factors that they felt prevented synchronicity in their relationship with patients. This includes issues such as the perceived attitude of older people to hierarchy and authority, time, workload factors and the influence of family. However, the categories that were derived from the data and that were confirmed through the interviews/reflective conversations were:

- Intent and Motivation for Action.
- Knowing the Patient.

Intent and Motivation for Action It was evident that if synchronicity in the nurse-patient relationship was to occur, then the need for nurses to explain their intent and motivation for pursuing particular courses of action was important in enabling patients to understand the parameters of decision making:

Expert Group Interview (Lines 636-642)

EX4:   ... they just aren't that structured in how they go about things. They know they've got so many things to do but it's not necessarily a structured plan in their minds as to how they are going to go about it and it's just 'Oh well I'm here so I'll have a bit of a chat and then I'll, Oh yes I need to do this and I'll ask him about this'.

Few nurses in the study explicitly explained their intent in interactions, with few of the interactions having their purpose explained. For members of the expert group, there was disagreement about the importance of this. While there was general agreement that patients needed to understand why they were being asked particular questions or being offered particular choices, members of the group warned against nurse-patient interaction becoming too 'stylised' and losing its spontaneity. However, being clear about their intent and motivation for action and setting this out clearly at the beginning of an interaction, was also seen as an enabling factor in negotiated decision-making:

Case Study 16/ Interaction 7/ Len

```
6 N:    This afternoon we had u::::m the Ward Round with Dr ((name))
7       and Dr ((name)) who is the Senior Registra::r and she saw
8       your husband (0.1) briefly (0.2) with rega::rd to what your
9       husband's been able to do::: and looking prior to the fa::ll
10      there isn't that much of a deficit now between ability (0.1)
11      a::::nd what I just needed to clarify was that both parties
12      were happy if we started to organise discharge (0.3) a::::h
13      following the operation=there is always a high percentage of
14      success rate with this type of operation to remove the clots
15      a::::nd providing there is no re-bleeding into the area
16      that's been evacuated then there is usually a good success
17      rate for recovery which has shown with you=
```

In this interaction, the nurse clearly describes the background to the request to begin planning for Len's discharge. She provides his wife with information that enables her to see the appropriateness of this request and sets it in the parameters of her husband's abilities.

Negotiation was also seen in the ability of the nurse to be flexible in the organisation of their day:

Case Study 7/ Interaction 2/ Mrs. Day

```
120 N:  ye:ah:: a man with a spanner! ((laughter)) OK then
121     anything you want to ask me or anything no=
122 P:  =yeah I was wondering if you could see if I'm all right
123     °below=
124 N:  =yeah  I'm on 'til nine 'clock now (0.1) o::h right I'll
125 P:                            ⌊don't feel quite
```

```
126     right
127     have a look later then (0.1) are you? OK I'm on until
128 P:                          ⌊I'm a bit worried about it
129     nine o'clock so remind me a bit later if I forget to
130     come and have a look⌈all right* I'll see if I can see
131 P:                       ⌊all right*
132     anything ((laughter))
133 P:   oh ho ho=
134 N:   =I'll get my torch
135 D:   (     ) before we go:: put me mind at rest=
136 N:   =o:h right=
137 P:   =I'll have to ring you then wouldn't I=
138 N:   =e::m yeah (0.1) I could-what time are you going?
139 D:   (0.1) probably not till about half four quarter to five time=
140 N:   =OK I need to go and do some tablets I think if I
141     haven't done it in a bit ring the bell or come and find
142     me OK (0.1) and then we'll send them up to the sitting
143 P:               ⌊I'll come and find you
144     room for a minute and eh eh-then I'll come and
145     have a look all right ok then I'll see you in a bit then
146     all right thank you
```

In ending an interaction with Mrs. Day, the nurse offers her an opportunity
to ask further questions. She requests an examination by the nurse. The
nurse suggests that she would do it later (line 127). Mrs. Day's daughter
intervenes and indicates that she would like to know the results of the
examination before she went home. The nurse outlines to Mrs. Day and
the family the way she would readjust her plan in order to do the
examination and report back to them.

Being flexible was not just about nurses changing their work plans.
It also included the involvement of patients and significant others in these
decisions:

Case Study 11/ Interaction 6/ Mabel

```
599 CM:  (0.1) What about getting to the toilet Mrs ((name))?
600 P:   (0.1) eh?
601 CM: What about getting to the toilet=
602 P:   =oh it's on the level I've got a radiator in the bathroom and
603 CM:                          ⌊i::m
604     the toilet door open and the back kitchen open see then I
```

605 CM: ⌊im

606   shut the middle door so that keeps in heat in

607 CM: (0.1) Are you going to need a commode upstairs?=

608 P: =I don't think so=

609 N: =Mabel you were saying that you use a <u>bucket</u> when you're

610   at home=

611 P: =I do yes for weeing in yes=

612 N: =so would you like a commode instead? in your bedroom

613 P: (0.1) Well yes=

614 N: =it wouldn't be so precarious as hovering over a bucket

615   would it?=

616 P: =no be better than a bucket I wouldn't

617 N: ⌊yes

618 P: Yes

619 CM: Right=

620 P: =see sometimes I get out in the night sometimes I don't=

621 N: =I think if they can provide a commode I'd go for the

622   option of a commode as opposed to a bucket=

623 CM: =⌈absolutely

624 P: ⌊yes yes

This section of the conversation is focused on facilitating Mabel's decision making about her toileting routine. The care manager asks her a direct question in line 601. This is clearly understood by Mabel and she answers the question directly with an appropriate explanation. This explanation also indicates that the toilet is downstairs. The care manager is concerned about Mabel having access to toilet facilities upstairs and asks her if she would need a commode upstairs. Mabel replies that she didn't think so. In line 612, the nurse intervenes on behalf of Mabel and reminds her about her earlier explanation. The nurse offers the commode as an alternative to her current practice and Mabel agrees.

    This is a good example of a focused and framed conversation. Mabel's response to the care manager's question (line 607) is set within her own framework of her current situation, i.e. she does not need a commode because she uses a bucket. The nurse takes a different conversational style, which puts the suggestion of the commode in the context of Mabel's current practice (using a bucket) and therefore makes it seem more like a reasonable option. This highlights the importance of making explicit the framework within which choices and options are set and the way they relate to a patient's current situation and involving them in the resulting decision.

The recognition of patients' usual routines and the framing of decisions within this routine appeared to be effective in involving patients in decisions made. It appeared to enable them to see the relevance of information provided by nurses and the importance or not of this information from their perspective.

Knowing the Patient Judging the appropriate approach to working with patients in a way that made decision-making frameworks explicit requires nurses to 'know the patient' (Jenny and Logan, 1992; Tanner *et al*, 1993). Knowing the patient is not just achieved through an assessment of health/illness history, but it is a cognitive and relational process whereby the nurse identifies salient aspects of the patient and their situation while establishing their professional credibility (Jenny and Logan, 1992; 254). Jenny and Logan highlight the reciprocal nature of 'knowing', in that it is as important for the patient to know the nurse as it is for the nurse to know the patient. The knowing process is influenced by specific-patient attributes (e.g. patient cooperation); the amount of time spent with the patient and the nurse's professional expertise and empathy. Tanner et al (1993) suggest different outcomes for patients through 'knowing'. In particular, they highlight the importance of knowing the patient as a component of skilled clinical judgement that is broader than the assessment of physical systems.

The routinised approaches adopted in patients' assessments by nurses in this study has been highlighted earlier. This routinised approach is seen to prevent knowing the patient from occurring and as a significant factor in the prevention of patient-centred approaches to decision-making. In this study the potential for knowing the patient was more often demonstrable through patients' stories.

Throughout the data, there is evidence of patients using story telling as a means of expressing themselves. These stories appeared to serve two functions:

- an indication of their values that underpinned their lifestyle;
- information about themselves.

What appeared to be an important factor in the nurses getting to know patients was their receptiveness to patients' stories. Throughout the data there is evidence of patients telling stories about their lifestyles in response to discussions about their health state or presenting symptoms:

Case Study 9/ Interaction 1/ Sid

69 P: =I eh (0.2) yeah I was refereeing for ten years
70 N: (0.1) Really! what football?
71 P: (0.08) football* yeah=
72 N: ⌊were you?* =whereabouts local-
73 P: (   )=
74 N: =really! you like your football do you
75 P: (0.1) Not now funny enough since I packed up refereein'=
76 N: =when did you pack up refereein'
77 P: (0.1) oh quite a while ago=
78 N: =did you=
79 P: =yeah quite a while ago since I packed up refereein' I've seen
80   one football match and that* and that was Oxford Boys=
81 N: ⌊is that al::l?*   =was IT?
82 P: °yeah I used* to ref all over the place (near London) (   )
83 N: ⌊goodness*   ⌊goodness
84 P: (0.2) I was a (terror at my trade)=
85 N: =were you=
86 P: =yeah I never (0.1) no game ever got (   )
87 N: (0.1) no?
88 P: No well=
89 N: ⌊always in control were you
90 P: =yes I never ha'a use a pencil and paper or yellow card like
91 N: ⌊yeah   ⌊n:o
92   they do today I used to I used to run up the side (   ) "next
93 N: ⌊n:o   ⌊yes
94   time you do that that's your lot your off' (0.6) I never had it no
95 N: ⌊did you?   ⌊yeah
96   more=
97 N: =that used to be enough did it=
98 P: =yeah that used to be enough and I used to (0.1) go into a
99 N: ⌊yeah
100   dressing room of the football stadium and they used to say
101 N: ⌊yeah
102   "look who we got for a referee a proper so-an'-so"=
103 N: =yeah (0.3) what would you be doing at home at this time of
104   day Sid?

The nurse in this interaction does not intervene in the patient's storytelling until some time into the interaction. In the interaction, Sid demonstrates such values as being meticulous about what he does (line 84), the importance of rules (line 90) and his need to be in control (line 90). Although he demonstrates these values in this storytelling, the nurse does not subsequently recognise the importance of the story, other than from a social history perspective. Indeed the nurse intervenes in the story (line 103) by initiating a topic change that does not directly relate to the story being told.

For one nurse in particular (Ann), knowing the patient was an important factor in determining the way she would work with them:

Reflective Conversation - Ann (Lines 1270-1273)

A: Unless I've got that good rapport with the patient and then I'll sit *(and discuss emotional aspects of care)* but then I think it's because I have that confidence, I know them, I've got that good relationship with them. But that's sort of like a splodge in a big ocean really.

Knowing patients enabled Ann to engage with them and to feel freer to offer a wider range of choices/care options and to take more risks. However, what was concerning about Ann's approach was that her perspective about the patient was determined during the first interaction with him/her and her particular emotional state:

Reflective Conversation - Ann (Lines 1316-1332)

A: ... there are people I'll identify with very very quickly. It's like fitting into a jigsaw. Sometimes I fit very well and sometimes I don't.
BMCC: And what makes the jigsaw fit?
A: Feeling comfortable with that person. For whatever reason, whether it's I've woken up and it's a good day ... and when I first meet them.

This was clearly highlighted in two of the case studies involving Ann. In one case study, Ann knew the patient (Shirley) socially as well as from previous admissions to the hospital. When working with Shirley, Ann was receptive to her interactions and indeed Ann often initiated stories herself as a means of engaging with her. For the other patient (Mabel), Ann did not know her so well and throughout the data, while Mabel told many stories that were indicative of the way she had lived her life so far, these were not utilised by Ann in discussions about her care or in deciding about care options.

The 'friendship' that appeared to exist between the nurse and Shirley was enhanced by the sharing of 'everyday' information by the nurse about herself and life on the ward. Shirley was obviously known to the nurse and the ward and therefore the nurse took the time to talk about changes in the ward that had occurred. This friendship was seen to enable the nurse to approach subjects that in the reflective conversation she found 'difficult'. This was particularly the case regarding discussions about emotion, whereby she discussed emotional concerns more freely and thoughtfully than was evident in the way she addressed emotional needs with other patients.

For Mabel, storytelling acted as a means of illustrating her coping abilities used throughout her life:

Case Study 11/ Interaction 3/ Mabel

```
103 P:   =and I worked until I used to wash my grandson up 'till
104      Christmas=
105 N:   =re::ally: goodness me
106 D:   (0.1) And give him his bowl and his soup=
107 N:   =yea:::h well you've had a busy life haven't you=
108 P:   =and I used to work in a cinema (0.1) for over twenty*
109 N:                              Lo::::h goodness me
110      five years in ((place)) here
111 N:   (0.1) You could teach us youngsters a thing or two then=
112 P:   =yea::h had a letter from the Que:en  (0.1) I got a card from
113 N:                              La:::h
114      the Queen I had a nice letter from the Mayor of ((place))
115      thanking me for you know working there to keep the place
116      open because I was the last one there see we didn't want it
117      shut until he sold it you see (0.1) then the TV took over my
118      responsibility then
```

In this interaction Mabel describes how she had worked all her life and in addition helped care for her grandson (who has a learning disability). The nurse's responses to utterances are not intended as a means of helping Mabel to elaborate on her story or to ask further questions that may be helpful in getting to know her.

Case Study 11/ Interaction 4/ Mabel

```
161 P:   =in fact I'm very seldom in bed well nearly always half past
```

```
162      seven my son - when I'm up my daughter's you see the
163 N:        ⌊right OK
164      weekend he brings a cup of tea in well I don't go off to sleep
165      no more see and by the time I'm dressed it takes me a long
166      while to dress because I have to sit down and take my
167      breath like=
168 N:   =right ok well look Mabel I'll em I'll sort out the sheet and
169      everything (0..8) em I'll just see where your hot cup of tea's
170      coming or hot drink should I say
171 P:   (  ) because I mean my daughter does my washing you see
172 N:                                                    ⌊yeah
173      and sheets and that (0.1) (tearful) and I don't like to be
174      moaned at me too much=
175 N:   =°right do you think you've settled down today in
176      hospital?
```

In contrast to the interactions with Shirley, when Mabel expresses emotions about the way she likes her care (line 171) and eludes to the kind of relationship she has with her daughter, the nurse does not address this and indeed she initiates a topic shift (line 175). In another interaction between the nurse and the doctor it is evident that an opinion of Mabel has already been formed that would account for the nurse not responding to her stories or emotional expressions:

Case Study 11/ Interaction 3/ Mabel

```
20 DR:   (0.2) She's doing that (0.1) she's ⌈going down* she pla::::ys
21 N:                                        ⌊going down*
22       up to being a dying duck an awful lot=
23 N:    =right because her daughter's got a disabled son=
24 DR:   =⌈yes (  )
25 N:     ⌊Yes yeah right=
26 DR:   =they are a very (0.1) strange family difficult family in that
27       they don't particularly like looking after her basically and
28       she lives on her own quite a lot (actually)=
```

While little attempt was made to understand Mabel's needs from her perspective, the use of biography and narrative in the assessment of older peoples' needs is gaining prominence (Dex, 1991; Bertaux, 1981; Agich, 1993; Schofield, 1994). Such authors recognise the importance of narrative approaches in the determination of an individual's values, and approaches to care delivery that are consistent with their values.

What Did Older People Themselves Think?

For the older people who participated in the interviews, forming a good relationship with the nurses was seen as important to their role as 'patient'. However, these older people did not see the role of the nurse as that of supporting them with emotional needs. When asked about the role of the nurse, it was the observable tasks that they described (e.g. washing people and administering medicines). However, they did feel that it was important that the nurse listened to them and their concerns:

Focus Group Interview - Patients

BMC: What do you think the nurse's role is in hospital? What do you expect from a nurse?

J: Well they look after you. They give you pills. They give you medicine and they talk to you if want to ... And then they don't (deal with any of your) personal problems. They never ask you, no.

BMC: So you don't expect to speak to them about personal things do you?

J: Well if there was anything really important, yes I would ... The ones I get to know, yes. The ones I think would be important in actually making those decisions for you.

These perspectives as described by Joan were agreed with by all those participating in the interviews. Again, Edward emphasised the patient's duty:

(Lines 832-833):

E: The duty is not for them (*the nurses*) to make it good for you (*the patient*). I think it's for you to try and make it good for them.

However, in forming a relationship with staff and in the ability of staff to get to know them, they emphasised the importance of being able to 'give something back' in the relationship:

Focus Group Interview - Patients (Lines 994-1008)

K: With the ... nurses you can usually give them something of yourself
       by the way of information or whatever and you know they've come
       to me knowing my job and asked me things ... but um, I've been able
       to help them if they want to know anything they come and ask (me)
       so then I feel I'm giving something in return

From the interviews with patients and the expert nurses, it is clear that
through the adoption of patient-centred approaches to decision-making,
patient participation can be enhanced. Such approaches as making explicit
the reasons for performing particular actions, the parameters of the
decision being made and assessment frameworks were considered to be
important. Flexibility in practice and the organisation of services around
the patient's usual routine are also significant. However, all of this is set
within the context of the nurse-patient relationship. The degree to which
patient involvement was based on the nurse 'knowing the patient' is an
important issue. It was evident in the data that patients who were 'known'
by nurses were more involved in their care and there was evidence of
greater partnership between the nurse and the patient. This raises questions
about how the nurse gets to know patients given the issues that have been
raised about stylised and routinised approaches to assessment that were
adopted by the majority of nurses in this study. Listening and accounting
for 'patients' stories' is considered to be an important factor in getting to
know patients and in the formation of a friendship between them and the
nurse. An important part of that friendship from the patient's perspective
is the ability to give something back in the relationship. For the patients in
the focus group this was an important factor in getting to know the nurses
and establishing a trusting relationship with them.

        While this section has focused on exploring those factors that
restrain patient participation in care decisions, an important consideration
is the socialization and enculturation of both nurses and patients into their
respective roles.

Socialisation and Enculturation

Nurse participants in this study felt that the way patients engaged in interactions with professionals was 'typical' of compliant relationships that older people have with those they consider to be in positions of authority:

Reflective Conversation - Ann (Lines 309-323)

A: ... Perhaps it's their way of life before hand. I think our generation has moved on. We want control, we want to know things, we are not going to accept well you fouled up. You know, we want an explanation. I mean you see more cases of people being sued, you know ... Whereas going back to Jim's (*case study 13*) era, it was yes sir, no sir whatever sir. They never expected an awful lot and I don't think they were ever given that.

This perception of older people influenced Ann's practice and while later discussing her relationship with patients she stated:

Reflective Conversation - Ann (Lines 697-704)

A: I think the age group we work with are very accepting of whatever we say. ... They are just very accepting and I think I've got into that mind where you just give them the facts and you leave them to it. ... I wouldn't say that I have openly thought 'Oh gosh yes we are empowering patients here'. It's not come into my thinking.

Ann suggests that she has developed a 'mind set' of providing information to patients and leaving it to them to decide what to do with it. This concurs with her earlier assertion of letting members of the multidisciplinary team know about a planned discharge and leaving it to them to get on with organising it. This was evident in her practice with patients, in the way that she 'told' them information and used a piecemeal approach to it.

Nurses expressed the view that older people expect and are expected to behave in a particular way in hospital and that the patients in this study demonstrated the way older people conform to the prevailing systems of power and control, because of their individual perceptions of their degree of control (Hugman, 1991; Partridge and Johnston, 1989), learned helplessness (Taylor, 1979), perceptions of their involvement in care decisions (Waterworth and Luker, 1990) and 'locus of control' (i.e.

beliefs about one's control in a situation and the ability to influence the final outcomes) (Folkman, 1984).

Reflective Conversation - Leslie (Lines 265-272)

N: ... You know you get this ... elderly person scenario of 'Now I've got old I'm expected to conform'. A lot of them do it. Very very few have the will and the strength to actually ... carry on being their own individuals.

Members of the expert group were less convinced that the compliance evident in the conversational data was exclusive to older people. They suggested that the rhetoric of patient-centredness doesn't always consider the worldview of the patient. They identified the problems that this raises for older people as consumers of health care and that if this rhetoric is to be made a reality then nurses have got to be sensitive to where the patient is starting from and to consider the relationship over time:

Expert Group Interview (Lines 164-172)

EX1:   Perhaps its more to do with seeing a relationship over time. That those things take place much more in a more structured way in the beginning of a patient's stay ... and then they are shortcut (as the relationship develops) ... and one of the questions is - when is that permission given and how is it given?, because it's not always given explicitly, but that part of the relationship is shortcutted and who initiates that and controls that?

Within the data itself the compliance of older people with professional decision-making and their deference to professional authority was evident. Many of the issues already discussed including the dominance of the professional in interactions; the power of the professional over decisions; the powerlessness of the patient in the professional-patient relationship and the imposition of constraints on patient actions by professionals, all relate to this particular theme. Indeed it could be argued that these issues arise because of the socialization of both the patient and professional (Hugman, 1991; Agich, 1993; Willcocks *et al*, 1987).

The themes that were most significant in the way that patients engaged with professionals, were:

- Deference to Professional Opinion.
- Lack of Skill in Dealing with Emotion.

Deference to Professional Opinion

Throughout the data, patient's allowed the decisions of professionals to dominate their decision-making. This was manifested through a view that the professional's view/opinion was the one that mattered and the seeking of professional approval for choices/decisions expressed:

Case Study 1/ Interaction 1/ Jack

```
332 N:  Yes (0.1) °ri::ght but you want to go home soon because
333     you are worried that if you are not the::re=
334 P:  =well I would like to as quickly as possible=
335 N:  =can we do it by phone calls? would it be possible for us
336     to:::: (0.1) I just* (0.2) yea:::h:: I mean would it help if
337 P:                  ⌊well I think (    )
338     Hazel [friend] came to see you I mean are you just
339     frightened that you might lo:::se (0.05) that you might lose
340     the place or::: (0.1) I mean I just re::ally feel deeply in my
341 P:  ⌊well eh::
342     heart that because you only came yesterday it might be nice
343     if you stayed the weeke::nd so that we could just see that
344     your well enough and strong enough I'd hate you to
345 P:                      ⌊yes yes certainly
346     go out too soo:::n (0.06) e:::m
347 P:                          ⌊I'll stop over the week end
348     then is that what you want?=
349 N:  =I could ring Hazel and you could talk to Hazel on the
350     phone I can get you a telephone that you could ring her
351     and talk to her=
352 P:  =oh thank you
```

Jack collaborates unquestioningly through the series of sequences that occur. While he does attempt to exert authority at various stages of the conversation, in an attempt to state his preference to go home, he does not sustain this resistance. Instead he cooperates with the answers and explanations offered and on most occasions thanks the nurse. Indeed, although Jack does not achieve his expressed wish to go home that weekend, he expresses gratitude to the nurse.

Further examples of patients' need to comply with professional opinion are evident in the data. In the interaction below, Sid demonstrates the paradox of his desire for one outcome, but his willingness to give way to professional control:

Case Study 9/ Interaction 7/ Sid

```
111 N:  right okay then (0.2) are you sure you are okay with that=
112 P:  =yes=
113 N:  =with Wednesday?=
114 P:  =yes anything that (you say) because I wouldn't go against you
115     because as I said to you
116 N:                          ⌊yes I know but I don't want you to be
117     unhappy and get low because you are not going home=
```

The opinion of the doctor was also seen to matter to patients in influencing their views and opinions:

Case Study 11/ Interaction 1/ Mabel

```
349 N:  =but Mabel you'd like to go home on Mo:nday
350 P:  E::h?=
351 N:  =you'd like to go home on Monday?
352 P:  Well it's all according see (0.1) it's all according Dr Jackson
353 N:                                                  ⌊yeah I
354     think what we'll do we'll get Jackson Dr Jackson to pop out
355     and check you over tomorrow=
```

In this interaction the nurse reminds Mabel of a choice she has already expressed - to go home on Monday (line 349). However, in line 352 Mabel highlights how that choice is dependent on the opinion of her General Practitioner and his decision. Such deference to professional opinion and the inappropriateness of the language of consumerism is illustrated through this example:

Case Study 11/ Interaction 6/ Mabel

```
646 CM:  (0.3) You go to bed about half past nine you said-you like
647      to go to bed at ⌈half past nine
648 P:                  ⌊about half past nine yes=
649 CM:  ={It might be* a bit earlier than that we'll see
650 P:   ⌊(   )
651 N:   (0.2) The lady might come in a bit earlier than that Mabel=
```

```
652 P:  =(   ) matter she can sit down see as long as she can tuck me
653     up in bed=
654 N:  =yeah
655 P:  I've got me bedside lamp see=
656 N:  =yeah okay=
657 P:  =oh yes it's all according to suits her=
658 N:  =okay (0.2)
659 CM: You will have to pay a little bit for this care Mrs Smith=
660 P:  =I thinks so yes=
661 N:  =yes and you have to fill a form in
662 P:  (0.1) Ye::s=
663 N:  =can you fill a form in or would you
664 P:                                     ⌊well yes my daughter
665     will help me to sign it
```

In this conversation, the care manager begins by stating Mabel's preferred time for going to bed. Mabel confirms that half past nine is the time she likes to go to bed. The care manager then informs Mabel that it is likely that the carer will come in earlier and therefore she will have to go to bed earlier. Mabel continues to demonstrate her sense of powerlessness to control the situation and agrees to the compromise (line 657). The nurse in line 658 reinforces this subservience. In line 659, the care manager informs Mabel that she will have to pay 'a little bit' for her care. She agrees to this. The fact that Mabel's care is means tested resulting in her having to pay for it, places her in the 'classic' definition of customer, i.e. she is purchasing something as a consumer. However, it is interesting that although she is paying for the care, she has not got consumer power in her position as patient. She was not offered a range of options to choose from and indeed was asked to compromise some of her usual routine in order to accommodate the routine of the organisation. This predicament that Mabel found herself in is consistent with Holliday's (1992) view of consumerism in health care - that it represents a partial but incomplete move from paternalism to autonomy.

Deference to professional opinion and decisions in preference to their own could be seen as the older person needing to please the nurse as suggested by Edward (patient interviewee):

Individual Interview - Edward (Lines 1231-1263)

P: I, (lie in the bed) and somebody comes along and has a chat ... I think it's a question of attitudes. Without a doubt, a question of attitudes ... I always, well I accept they've got more on their plate than I have. You know, I've got something wrong with me. All right that's why I'm in there. But by golly they've got you know 20 people up and down the ward that got something wrong with them. Either worse or the same as me you know. But they've got to look after all of them.

It was not uncommon for patients to ask if a decision met with the professional's approval as illustrated by this example:

Case Study 7/ Interaction 3/ Mrs. Day

```
23 P:    =I mean she's done a lot (   ) Germaine helps her
24       you kno::w (0.2) she can't do everything so my son=
25 N:            Lyeah yeah                            Lno
26 N:    im right
27       =said he would go and his wife they go shopping
28       every Friday night to Sainsbury's so-is that all right
29       with you=
30 N:    =⌈that's fine
31 P:    Lit's not that I don't like it here
```

Mrs. Day has been providing the nurse with a detailed account of the arrangements made for her going home. While she has articulated her plans clearly, she still felt the need to ask the nurse if the arrangements met with her approval. The nurse responds positively. However, Mrs. Day feels the need to explain to the nurse that it is not because she does not like it in the hospital and to explain her reasons for going home at the time she has chosen.

Lack of Skill in Dealing with Emotion

The way in which nurses facilitated patient decision-making and its subsequent effects on the ability of patients to initiate actions, has already been discussed in other categories so far. However, a significant issue that emerged in a number of the case studies and one in which the expert group felt was a particular issue of nurses' socialization was that of nurses' abilities to deal with patients' emotions:

Expert Group Interview (Lines 723-729)

EX4:   ... I think that (*risk taking*) may have been an element in why the emotions were contained because you know maybe they felt they didn't want to deal with them, didn't have the time to deal with them, maybe didn't have the skill to deal with it if they were to help that person to ... open the gates for the person to say exactly what was the source of the emotion...

While a 'lack of skill' was seen as the most prohibitive factor in nurses dealing with patients' emotions, other factors to do with the way nurses focus on the physical aspects of practice and, in particular, on 'the mechanics of discharge planning' were also seen as influential.

The most explicit and consistent example of this in the data was that of Jim (Case Study 13). He was clearly distressed by his health state and continuously expressed his emotions about how he was feeling. Throughout the interactions, he focused on his emotions. Although the nurse acknowledged this at various stages throughout the interactions, there is little evidence of her wanting to understand more fully what lay behind many of the views and feelings he expressed:

Case Study 13/ Interaction 6/ Jim

```
41 N:    (17.0) what's worrying you now Jim (0.2) the idea
42       of an operation (0.1) no (0.1) being in hospital?
43       (0.4) or is it all the palaver that's going with this?
44 P:    (0.3) ((crying)) (   )
45 N:    Look
46 P:    ((crying)) (oh if only they didn't have to) do this
47 N:    okay:: (0.3) you've been getting on well with the
48       conveens haven't you at night?=
49 P:    =yes (that's what's) worrying me
50 N:    (0.2) it's worrying you?
51 P:    (   ) there=
52 N:    °yeah: they'll do all that for you love (0.3) they'll do
53       all that for you  (0.4) what I'll do on Monday I'll
54       ring ((name) Ward and have a chat with someone
55       up there I'll speak to Dr Haigh and we'll go from
56       there Jim  alright? (0.1) now in the meantime the
57 P:                          Lyes
58       diarrhoea's resolved hasn't it?=
```

The nurse did not seek to understand the source of Jim's concerns about his pending surgery (circumcision). It seems that Jim had been labeled as a 'worrier' and 'overly anxious' and therefore his expressions of anxiety were trivialised and not seen as important or relevant to the progress of his care. The nurse avoided asking him direct questions about his expressions of anxiety. A previous discussion in the Multi Disciplinary Team (MDT) meeting highlighted the team's view - that if the physical aspects of care were sorted out then his worries would reduce. The nurse in her reflective conversation confirmed this selected approach:

Reflective Conversation - Ann (Lines 428-443)

A: ... what was driving me was, he'd had hip surgery that had gone wrong you know, and I knew he was going back in for surgery and I think he thought, well you know, it's bound to go wrong given the luck I've had ... and I wanted it right. ... but I think the major one in my mind, in my subconscious was 'Well it's always gone wrong for you Jim and let's try for this not to go wrong'.

However, although this motive as described by the nurse, may have been the driving force behind subsequent actions, the teams reaction to Jim's expression of emotion did appear to lack skill and understanding:

Case Study 13/ Interaction 7/ Jim

```
237 N:  =I think once the tablets have kicked in Jim and
238     once you are home
239 P:                          ⌊yeah yeah yeah (  ) saying that
240     last night=
241 DN: (  ) coming to day ca:::re?=
242 N:  =Tuesdays and Thursdays as normal=
243 DN: =Tuesday Thursday ri:::ght so tha:t's fi::ne so
244     starting next week thank you okay:::?=
245 N:  =yea::::h (0.07) okay then Jim?=
246 P:  =(yes I'm) alright yea:::h (0.1) if I could buck myself
247 N:                          ⌊mo::rning
248     up I would
249 DN: (0.1) you've got to you've got to be optimistic Jim
250     (  ) it's no good sort o' going ro::und sort of
251 Wife:                                      ⌊if he's
252     like that I shall need them I think=
```

253 DN: =ye(h)s (   ) ((DN & Wife laugh))
254 P: (0.7) (it's not natural to keep on crying like tha' all
255   the time is it) (0.1) I mean I went down there this
256   morning (and felt rotten) (   ) like a lot of wind but
257   it was wet wind (0.2) it's still there
258 DN: (0.8) °i::m you eating sort of normal sort of diet=˙
259 N: =he's eating a normal diet he's eating what he
260   normally ha::s:=

Jim's care package failed soon after his discharge and he was re-admitted in a critically ill state, brought on by dehydration and his inability to cope. It was evident that this care package/discharge would not work because of his lack of inner coping resources. The focus in his discharge planning was not patient-centred but instead was routined and ritualised. The nurse made a decision that going home was the best thing for him, without considering his coping resources. While respecting patient autonomy may not be about 'the patient makes all the decisions independently', respect for autonomy could entail recognition of a patient's emotional state and the effect this might have on decision-making capacity (Collopy *et al*, 1991). In Jim's case, the nurse was focused on practical issues of discharge planning but not on the management of transition (Golan,1981; Cotter *et al*, 1998), a focus that would require a different care planning perspective - a perspective that would be based on the individual's particular needs based on his coping abilities. It was interesting that the nurse had identified the patient's source of anxiety (as indicated in a multidisciplinary meeting) and yet did not initiate any supportive actions to treat the anxiety. Instead she believed that going home would sort this out.

By focusing on discharge planning it is possible to identify the mechanistic approach to care that was adopted by many of the nurses in this study and that as a result, patients found it difficult to exercise their decision making capacity. The need to consider the particular meaning of change in an individual's life is widely recognised in the literature (Chick and Meleis, 1986; Golan, 1981; Selder, 1989). An individual's ability to cope with their changing circumstances can be seen to be important in this research, in enabling older people to maximise their coping abilities.

What Did Older People Themselves Think?

In their focus group discussion, older people themselves confirmed the compliant nature of patients. Having listened to 'vignettes' devised from criteria established by the expert group, members of the focus group (all female) and the individual interviewee (male) recounted their stories of being a patient. All of them expressed satisfaction with their experience of hospitalization and were pleased to be able to 'hand over' decision making to other people (professionals). Because of their physical incapacity, they felt that they 'had to' leave decision-making to others.

However, when questioned further about this, they all expressed a desire to be fully informed and consulted over decisions about their care and expected that to happen. For these older people, that position of wanting to be consulted, but yet being happy for others to make the final decision, reflected the way they lived their lives generally and concurred with other research evidence (*for example*, Fulford *et al*, 1996; Blanchard *et al*, 1988; Beiseker and Beiseker, 1990). Some of them talked about their relationships with their husbands and although their husbands may make the final decision, they always discussed the options and 'had a say'. One member of the group however (Karen) expressed dissatisfaction with not being involved in the decisions about her ongoing care arrangements:

Focus Group Interview - Patient's (Lines 584-622)

K: Well it was all very weird. I didn't quite know whether I was following what my husband wanted or whether it was the home carers. I still don't know ... He (*husband*) seemed to have a lot to say in the matter.

BMC: How does that make you feel?

K: Awful

BMC: In what way?

K: Well in as much as I'm always had to run the table you know. Have to do for others and that and my husband seems to well, he can always go one better. And he thinks this that and the next thing so I shut up.

BMC: Right. So in a way you've had to sort of give way to how you've worked all your life really?

K: Yes Yes Yes Yes

BMC: And do you find that difficult to cope with?

K: I do I find it very hard.

However, focus group members did not feel it necessary to complain about any of their care as they felt that it was a case of 'knuckling down and getting on with it' (Karen) and complying and accepting the hospital's rules and procedures:

Focus Group Interview - Patients (Lines 294-312)

K: Um, one sort of had to obey the rules as it were

BMC: In what way?

K: Well the nurses would want this and want that and your meals are served at certain times and well its just, I just got down and got on with it.

BMC: Right. Did you get involved in planning how your care would happen or how you were going to live the rest of your life and things?

S: Oh no!

and later they expanded on this view:

Focus Group Interview - Patients (Lines 990-997)

J: and there is no need to complain.

BMC: Right.

K: Yes, I feel like this lady does, there is no need for us to complain about any of the nurses. Not really because she like me thinks, 'Oh you young people, you want it all your own way'.

Indeed in his interview, Edward considered it the patient's duty to keep the nurse happy and that this was an important role of the patient in the nurse/patient relationship:

Individual Interview – Edward

E: There are some people who do nothing else but ring the bell and they want this, they want that, they want the toilet you know, every 5 minutes

BMC: Mmm

E: Now that, I don't go along with

BMC: Right

E: If I want to go to the toilet and I see she's busy well I hang on 10 minutes you know

BMC: Mmm

E: I, I don't accept that ah she's there to run backwards and forwards you know. 'Cos that gets them annoyed

BMC: Mmm

E: If they're skipping backwards and forwards

BMC: Yes

E: No you treat them as human beings don't you?

E: I think it's a duty that you-they're performing a duty you know whether they like it or whether they don't you know, they are performing a duty

BMC: Mmm

E: Because they are there for so many hours. I think it's your (*the patient's*) duty to try and make that as happy for them (*the nurses*) as you can, before they go home.

In relation to their role as patients, these older people clearly felt that they did not have an explicit say in the way their care was delivered. Even Edward who described in detail a series of events that resulted in him taking his own discharge did not feel that he could change this situation. In various ways, the focus group members implied frustration at not being in control of their lives. However, they accorded this lack of control to their physical disabilities. As a result, they did not see any way that they could be involved in planning for their continuing care needs and that therefore such decisions should be left to the professionals and to members of their family.

     Issues have been discussed in previous sections regarding the structures and processes of nurse-patient interactions, the power relationship between nurses and patients and constraints that inhibit effective patient-centred practice. However, it is evident from the data in this section that attitudes and beliefs of both nurses and patients play a significant role in interactions between them. Nurses appeared to be working within a framework that reinforced stereotypical perceptions of older age. Such perceptions raise important intergenerational factors that may inhibit nurses from practising in a patient-centred way with older people. As Jefferys (1997;86) writes:

> I am now more aware of a degree of deference paid to me, which I ascribe to my age. In one sense this is gratifying, but in another it seems a distancing device, telling me that I am understandably no longer quite 'one of them'.

Both participating patients and members of the patients' focus group demonstrated many of the stereotypes that the nurses suggested were dominant in older people. Such attitudes as deference to professional opinion, lack of expectations from their care experiences, and an understanding of the duty of the patient to perform a particular role that complies with professionals' expectations were all evident in the data.

There is little evidence in the data of professional staff working with older people to empower them to have a say in their care through the removal of established constraints and stereotypes. While older people who were interviewed were indifferent to making decisions about their care, they all stressed a strong desire to be part of the decision making process and to be consulted about decisions being made. If a patient-centred philosophy is to be instilled into practice, then such prevailing stereotypes as those evidenced in this data would need to be eroded.

One of the factors to be considered is that of the role that relatives play in care decisions. Throughout the data so far, interactions between professionals, patients and relatives have been identified as significant in patient participation in decision-making.

The Professionalisation of Relatives

Not all case studies had relatives involved in their care. However, wherever they were involved there appeared to be a problem in balancing the autonomy of the patient with the involvement of the family. The power of the family in decision-making concerning future care arrangements in particular, was a consistent and significant theme throughout the data. Families were engaged in decision making throughout a patient's hospital stay. Family members were given explicit authority by nurses to engage in decision-making. This authority was exerted even prior to patients' views, wishes and perceptions being established. In some cases, family members were involved in initial assessment discussions with patients and in a number of cases they influenced the outcomes of the initial assessment and shaped the nature of ongoing decisions about care arrangements. During data analysis, the phrase '*the professionalisation of relatives*' was a consistent re-emerging reflection and the expert group supported my understandings and sense of importance of this phrase as a data theme.

Reflection

> I find it strange the way in which the opinions and views of relatives are given precedence over those of the patients themselves. While it is important to consider the views of relatives, I find it hard to accept that the relative should be treated as 'always right' and the patient 'always wrong'. It seems as if the nurses are unable to challenge the perspective of relatives or are afraid to do so for fear of the consequences. It appears to me that the relatives are being treated like a 'fellow professional' and as such act as another layer of authority that the patient has to negotiate with.

In all cases, nurses demonstrated clear difficulties in balancing the wishes of patients with the wishes of family members. Relatives' views, wishes and perceptions were acted upon at the expense of a patient's. This raised significant issues about the ability of nurses to act as an advocate for patients and to negotiate 'best care options' in such situations. The difficulties that nurses' experience in advocating for patients has been well documented (Snowball, 1996) and the appropriateness of nurses assuming advocacy roles on behalf of patients has been called into question (Porter, 1992).

Nurse participants described the problems they experienced in representing a patient's views alongside those of their relatives. They did not find it surprising that the data reflected a dominance of relatives' views and wishes at the expense of patients and they suggested that working in a measured way with patients and their relatives was one of the most difficult aspects of their role:

Reflective Conversation - Leslie (Lines 411-437)

L: He *(Aidan: Case Study 15)* didn't seem to have the guts to defend himself ... And that ... I think is why he lost his case ... He wasn't strong enough to put his own view forward and there were so many of them ganging up on him that even though he was saying 'Oh I want to go home', he didn't have the strength to say 'I want to go home'.

BMC: Did you feel ganged up on as well?

L: Yeah

BMC: Right. Because I wondered why at various points you didn't act on his behalf?

L: Um, I didn't think that they were listening to me ... Because there was one or two occasions where I tried to say something sort of you know on his defence and it was just sort of thrown down.

Another nurse (Laura) offered her perception of why working with relatives in a way that is supportive of the patient is so difficult:

Reflective Conversation - Laura (Lines 348-359)

L: ... Perhaps you are almost ... more willing to keep the peace with the relatives than the patient sometimes ... because they're in a bed. They are in your, under you, you know and you have got this power and the relatives are on the outside and very often stronger.

From Laura's perspective, the patient is powerless because 'they are in a bed' and because they are under the power of the nurse, while the relatives are not affected by such power and are therefore more able to make decisions freely and dominate the decision-making process.

Sometimes this work was made more difficult by the patients themselves who did not always have a clear view of what their goal was. On some occasions, although patients expressed an opinion, they would later be seen to change their mind or take a different perspective in subsequent conversations. However, for the expert group this was a further example of nurses not 'allowing' patients to retain their hopes, dreams and aspirations and of nurses not taking the time to establish what preferences patients might have from a range of possible options.

Two case studies (Case Study 11-Mabel and Case Study 15-Aidan) particularly highlight the involvement of relatives in decision making. In the case of Mabel, she had demonstrated through the stories she told the nurse that she had been an independent and determined person who had developed her own coping mechanisms. However, even though Mabel had demonstrated coping ability, at no time did the nurse use this information to establish how she wanted her care to be managed. In both the case of Mabel and Aidan, the nurses had formed an initial perception of them based on prior conversations with members of their families and from case records:

Case Study 11/ Interaction 1/ Mabel

16 N: Right now I've just gone through things with your daughter
17   about the day centre you go to three times a week all right
18   and then you stay with your daughter x number of times and
19   your care manager is Kathy Sugden well I'll let Kathy
20   know that you are here=

```
21 P:    =yes=
65 N:    =right °right your daughter was just saying that she didn't
66       feel that you'd be able to go back to your own home
67 P:                                              ⌊no
68 N:    (0.3) Do you think you would be able to go back home to
69       yo::ur house if we put in some help? (0.2) what do you
70       think
```

For Aidan, a perception had already been formed about his care needs from discussion with members of his family and transfer information from the previous hospital:

Case Study 15/ Interaction 1/ Aidan

```
161 N:   but the problems are everyone here is concerned about ya
162      a::::nd they've highlighted to me that there's problems that
163      they think if you go back to the flat then you might go back
164      to drinking (0.2) and your health suffers and that's I think
165      I'm right in saying that that's what everybody's concerned
166      about (0.1) now I'm here to help you decide (0.1) what you
167      want to do and I can guide you (0.1) but you have to
168      make up your own mind at the end of the day it's your
169      decision (0.2) but what I'd like you to do is listen to
170      everybody and just take in what the::y (0.1) what their
171      concerns are showing and what they think might be su::itable
172      (0.2) okay now I had a message form the ((Hosp. name))
173      before you came down to say that you might be considering
174      residential care but when I asked you the day after you came
175      in you were saying no you wanted to go back to your flat
176      (0.3) now is there any reason why  you either I got the
177      wrong message or why you changed your mind?
```

For both patients, their expressed wishes were overridden by the wishes and perceptions of their relatives. Mabel expressed on a number of occasions that she did not need help in the evenings and that she only needed help in the mornings to get down the stairs. However, this was overridden by the perceptions of her daughter:

Case Study 11/Interaction 5/ Mabel

```
6 N:     Right you've spoken to the daughter
```

7 CM: Right yes what do you want to know=

8 N: =you spoke to her daughter and:::

9 CM: Em she thinks she's going to need help mornings and

10   evenings=

11 N: =right

234 CM: (0.2) °okay well shall we have somebody come in for you in

235   the mor::ning?

236 P: Yes=

237 CM: =and in the evenings to help you get to be::d=

238 P: =they'd have to have the key wouldn't they?

239 CM: Yeah probably=

240 P: =yes I've got a chain on the door but I shan't put it on=

241 CM: =no no can you come to the door to let them in?

242 P: (0.1) Well I'll have to come down stairs

243 CM: (0.3) I see yes:: so (0.1) so has your daughter got a key?

244 P: ( ) Well they could come in the (back) I could come

245   downstairs I get exhausted that's all

246 CM: ⌈( )

247 P: ⌊(I'm alright to) come downstairs because I could hold the

248   banisters in the front there and one at the back and I count

249   the stairs (0.1) thirteen=

A difficult balancing act needed to be played out in Mabel's care planning. In previous interactions the General Practitioner indicated that Mabel's daughter needed a break from her caring role, something that Mabel agreed with. However, although this agenda was clearly under consideration, it was never made explicit to Mabel and interactions focused on gaining her agreement to care, each morning and evening. The prime reason for this appeared to be that of relieving her daughter of this responsibility, again something that Mabel appeared to agree with. However, the fact that this discussion was never made explicit to her, only served to confuse her involvement in decision making, as she repeatedly reiterated what she was able to do in response to suggested care packages. This suggested that her understanding of the need for care was in relationship to her functional ability rather than as a process for relieving her daughter of caring responsibilities.

This attitude towards Mabel's inability to fully engage in decision-making was highlighted in an interaction about respite care between the nurse and the care manager:

Note: In the following interaction Stefan is Mabel's grandson who has learning disabilities. Green Fields is the name of a residential care home.

Case Study 11/ Interaction 6/ Mabel

394 N: Would you like (0.05) would you like to consider the idea
395   of giving your daughter a regular little <u>rest</u> once every
396   couple of months?
397 P: You would have to talk to her first=
398 N: =but what do you think about it?=
399 P: =oh I think she ought to get help I think myself she should
400   have help she's had a lot of washing with Stefan you see I
401   *(nurse and care manager whispering in background)*
402   mean she - washing and ironing there's always a bag full of
403   ironing but I mean it would help her=
404 CM: =what we are thinking of is what about you going
405   somewhere while your daughter has a rest?=
406 P: =eh?=
407 CM: =we're thinking about the idea of you going <u>somewhere</u>
408 P: What for?=
409 N: =for a little holiday=
410 CM: =while your daughter has a rest
411 P: Where would I go=
412 N: ⌐regularly
413 CM: Lwell you could go to Green Fields or somewhere like
411   that=
415 P: =well I've got relations in Ho:ve
416 CM: (0.3) In in
417 P: LI've got a grand daughter there=
418 N: =ye::s=
419 CM: =o(h)h she's thinki(h)ng holiday as in "Brig(h)hton *(laughs)*
420 P: I've got two grand daughters I've got grand sons=
421 CM: =well that's a long way to go no we were thinking more of=
422 P: =Brighton ( ) really where they live like ( )

The interactional asymmetry that exists in this conversation clearly disempowers Mabel and prevents her playing a full role in the conversational agenda. The way the nurse and care manager approached this situation lacked clear planning and consideration of her understanding of phrases such as 'little holiday'. The approach used serves to confuse her. The description of respite care as 'a little holiday' does not provide Mabel with enough information to be able to engage with the decision-making and the professionals' response to her interpretation (laughter) of their account would appear to be inappropriate.

Similar issues arise for Aidan and his family with regard to decision-making about him moving to a residential care area. The nurse emphasised on a number of occasions that the final decision had to be Aidan's, yet all of the discussions about this option were dominated by his family painting a bleak picture of his home circumstances and their unsuitability for him. A continuous theme dominated the case study of Aidan being offered choices, him making a choice and then professional staff and his family disagreeing with the choice made and recommending an alternative. The fact that Aidan had terminated a previous home care package meant that this option was not considered on this occasion. The family recognised that they needed Aidan's agreement to move to a residential care home:

Case Study 15/ Interaction 1/ Aidan

```
277 D:  =you see Ai:dan tried last year with Dr ((name)) at
278     ((place name)) he said was there any way we could get him into
279     residential care and he said not (0.05) unless (0.05) Aidan
280     (0.05) says (0.05)YES and he wouldn't say yes=
281 S:  =he has to agree to it ⌈he's got to say yes
282 D:                         ⌊we we couldn't do* anything abou::t
283     it (0.2) you know he just wouldn't-there was no way we
284     could get round it=
```

However, on this occasion, the family's approach was to face Aidan with all the reasons why he was unable to cope as a way of making him see his need for residential care:

Case Study 15/ Interaction 1/ Aidan

```
331 P:  =°yeah but I don't want to be curtailed altogether you know
332     if I want a drink (then I want t'be able to ) get one
333     (0.2) which I know a lot of people in ((place name)) won't get
334     me one=
335 S:  =no because you don't just take one=
336 D:  =you kno::w why though don't you?=
337 S:  =you have a bottle bottle bottle bottles it's one after another
338     (0.1) it's not just one is it?=
339 DL: =it's seven or eight bottles a wee:::k not just one a week=
```

340 S: =if there was a situation Dad whereupon you could have a
341   dri::nk (0.1) to have a bottle on the table for example and
342 P: ⌊ye::ah
343   have one a day one drink if that bottle lasted you a week
344   perhaps which is normal or for a person of your situation
345   perhaps you'd have say three or four drinks in a day but not
346   two bottles in a day which is what you've been dri::nking
347   (0.1) two bottles of whisky a day=
348 P: =°no no I don't drink not that much=
349 S: =I've seen the empties
350 D: ⌊you do dad=
351 S: =believe me I've seen the empties (0.3)he's had bags full of
352 DL: ⌊(   ) keeps throwing
353   them all ou:::t
354 S: empty bottles=
355 D: =well it hasn't taken it has it?=
356 S: =anyway that's we don' wanna go into tha' part that's not
357   what we're talking about right now but that's-its easier for
358   you to get your drink in the flat (0.1) too easy and you need
359   a situation whereupon you can keep away from the drink for
360   a certain amount of time so you can get over tha' that
361   attitude=
362 P: =I CAN DO IT (   )=
363 S: =YOU CAN'T=

At no time did the nurse intervene in this confrontation and indeed at a later multidisciplinary meeting, reasons for Aidan's drinking pattern were discussed by the nurse and other members of the health care team. However, none of these were addressed as options in the care package that could be developed. Insights that were presented about Aidan and his ability to cope, included grieving for his wife; loneliness; boredom and peer influence. The fact that these causes were identified suggests that an alternative approach to his rehabilitation could have been taken that focused on his grief and on 'occupation'. The plan focused on seeking alternative accommodation as the answer to his problems, without helping to resolve any of the underlying causative stimuli. A detailed exploration of his lifestyle could have identified particular interests that could be used as the basis of a plan that included counselling and occupational therapy. Aidan appeared to have lost his sense of control, dignity and identity with self (Kitwood, 1997). Moving to a residential care home would not re-instill these attributes, but indeed could add to a sense of worthlessness.

An alternative approach such as this may also have helped his family who were clearly concerned about Aidan's well-being. It is important to consider their context. It is likely that the family had experienced difficulties over a long period of time with their father because of his drinking habits. Therefore it is likely that they were frustrated by their inability to do something to change the situation for him. They were probably being motivated by a desire for his safety and well-being and the provision of the best possible care for him.

In asserting this view, it suggests that older people who have a 'risky lifestyle' do not have a right to live with that risk and that it is okay for family members and professional staff to make choices on the person's behalf on the basis that they know what is best for the patient. Jecker (1991) and others (Barker, 1991; High, 1991; Coulton, 1990; Langner, 1995) all emphasise the importance of families in care decisions with older people. Brody (1978) suggests that family members act as a forum for 'trying on' and 'bouncing off' ideas. Brody argues that a patient cannot know what values he/she holds until they go through a process of 'trying on' various values stances and 'bouncing them off' the opinions and reactions of others he/she cares about. Brody argues that it is through this process that a patient's values emerge. High (1991) and Jecker (1991) argue that autonomy as individualism excludes consideration of the family in decision-making and ignores the interdependency of family members. However, Barker (1991) emphasises the importance of recognising the hidden agendas of family members, who may want to ensure particular courses of actions for the older person because of fears of loss and a need to make retribution for previous problems and failings.

What Did Older People Themselves Think?

Those older people who participated in the interviews acknowledged the participation of their relatives in decisions about their care. For the majority of them they felt that it was okay for members of their family to be involved in decisions as long as they were involved in the discussions:

Focus Group Interview - Patients

K: No I think it's most important that the patient or whoever should be in line just to why the questions are being asked and what purpose you know...

Individual Interview - Edward

E: Up to a point I suppose ah, up to a point the relative has got to assume responsibility haven't they? ... My wife, because she did that, she would always come to me and say what she'd done. She wouldn't, she wouldn't allow any talk behind me back...

The involvement of the older person in decision making with the family appeared to match the kind of involvement the person had in their everyday life. In one case (Joan) her husband had always made the 'important' decisions in their relationship and this carried on after she had a stroke and needed continuous care. For another (Sylvia) she and her husband had always shared decision making and following the death of her husband, decisions about her care were shared with her son, who became her support in life. While Sylvia acknowledged the importance of her son's support, she also described the need for her son to support her decision, i.e. to stay at home and receive care rather than move to residential care. Later when asked about this, she described how she had raised this as an option, how her son had said 'oh no you don't want to do that if you can help it' (line 1360) and she was glad that he had said that as she didn't want to move to residential care, but thought it would be more convenient for him. This again highlights the deference of older people to the opinion of others and the potential/actual influence of members of the family on their care decisions.

However, not all of the participants were satisfied that their involvement in care decisions happened as they wished. Karen felt that she was not always involved in decisions and that she found this difficult to cope with - 'I do find it very hard' (line 617). She described how her daughter had tried to influence her into moving to a nursing home. Karen was angry at this and expressed her determination to her family to remain at home. Karen's views concurred with evidence from the conversational data, which suggests that older people need energy and determination in order to actively maintain their involvement in their care decisions.

However, the importance of having a family member who understands their beliefs and values was seen as essential to these older people achieving the choices they desired in decisions about ongoing care arrangements:

K: You can't beat it you've got a family; you've brought them up. I often talk about when I had my babies or when my babies were young or this or that and the next thing. And I know my husband must get tired of me hearing me saying things like that. He probably does. But that is my life; it has been I mean I've had them now for fifty years.

BMC: OK. And you Joan, if you were asked to go to a nursing home and you didn't want to, would you fight it off?

J: I wouldn't want to go no. I wouldn't want to go.

BMC: And would your family listen to you?

J: Yes that's where my husband would help me you see ... Yes my daughter, she lives a long way away but she knows what I want.

Family involvement in care appears to be a complex tripartite negotiation process between the patient, professional and family member(s). However, the issues of honesty, negotiation and consideration of the older person's beliefs and values appear to be important considerations in decision-making. For the older people who were interviewed, the important issue does not appear to be that of them being the decision-maker, but instead it does appear to be a consideration of their beliefs and values in the making of the decision - irrespective of who makes it. This position of 'involvement in decision-making' but not the 'final arbiter' of decisions is referred to in the literature as a distinction between 'decisional autonomy' and 'executional autonomy' (Collopy, 1988). Having autonomy then, does not mean being able to execute decisions made. However, it does hold central the importance of the older person's involvement with decision-making. This distinction between engagement with decision-making and the execution of decisions is widely supported in the literature (*for example* Kadushin and Kulys, 1994; Abramson *et al*, 1993; High,1991).

Principles for Action

- Be explicit about the intent and motivation for action and the parameters within which decisions are set.
- Maximise patients' independence through the balancing of patient narrative with established care policies and procedures.

- Make decisions within a framework of 'negotiation' with clearly established care goals that are regularly reinforced and reviewed.
- Make time to help patients to integrate 'new' care decisions, options etc. into their already established care programme.
- Acknowledge and facilitate patients' emotional responses as an important part of facilitating patient participation.
- Create opportunities for reciprocity in relationships with patients.
- Do not allow 'age related' perceptions of an individual's ability to limit patient participation.
- Help patients to see beyond their own limited expectations of their involvement in care and their deference to others.
- Continuously reinforce the value of patients' decisions.
- Facilitate patients' 'emotional coping ability' in order to enhance their independence.
- Recognise that while patients want to be consulted about care decisions they do not always want to be the final arbiter of decisions.
- Recognise that older people should have their beliefs and values considered in the making of decisions but being the final arbiter of decisions is not of prime importance.

Conclusions

Through the analysis of nurses' and other health care professionals' interactions with patients, it has been possible to identify complex interactional processes in practice that may enable an inductively derived understanding of autonomy with older people in health care settings. The foundation for the development of this understanding has been that of 'language' and the structure of conversational processes. The data has predominantly focused on issues and factors that limit a rights based understanding of autonomy. This approach has raised issues about power and control, the appropriateness of objectivity in planning one's future, constraints on individual action, the effects of socialisation processes, the role of relatives in care decisions and the possibility of partnership between nurses and older patients. It could be concluded that the nature and structure of institutions inhibit an older person's autonomy and that nurses' autonomy will always be limited because of the constraints of institutional structures. However, the question remains - is it the context or processes of care delivery that enhance or inhibit patient autonomy? It is to this question that Chapter 8 turns. In order to do this, the derived principles for action have been developed into 'themes' that will be used to explore the data from the practice of the community and expert nurses. These themes will be explored in Chapter 8 in order to identify the defining attributes of autonomy.

8 Context, Expertise and Identified Principles for Action

Introduction

The data collected through the case studies so far has identified the constraining nature of nursing practice on the autonomy of older people in hospital. Five themes were used to illustrate the processes of engagement utilised by nurses and other health care workers with patients - Communicative Style; Power; Constraint on Autonomous Action; Socialisation and Enculturation and the Professionalisation of Relatives.

Identifying 'Principles for Action' from the data analysis, i.e. factors/issues that need to be considered if a patient-centred approach to practice built on contemporary issues of partnership and empowerment is to be realised, ended each theme. These were derived from the analysis of the data as presented in Chapters 5 to 7.

All principles for action identified in each theme were then listed and grouped according to their common focus. Five new themes were identified that represented all of the individual principles for action contained in the data. These themes will be utilised as a framework for analysing the data generated by the expert nurse and clinical nurse specialist. These are:

- Informed Flexibility.
- Sympathetic Presence.
- Negotiation.
- Mutuality.
- Transparency.

Definitions/Descriptions of Themes and Data Presentation

The data from the practice of an expert nurse and a clinical nurse specialist in the community are being presented to see if the removal of some of the contextual inhibiting factors or increased expertise would make a difference to the way a patient-centred approach to involvement in care and decision-making occurs, i.e. would these five themes be present in their positive form, rather than as constraining factors. Data will be presented that illustrates the articulation of these themes in the interactions between the clinical nurse specialist, the expert gerontological nurse and their patients. By doing this the attributes of, and antecedents to, patient-centred decision-making will be identified and their relationship with an alternative perspective of patient autonomy explored in the context of the centrality of patients' values.

Informed Flexibility

Theme Definition The facilitation of decision-making through information sharing and the integration of new information into established perspectives and care practices.

Throughout the interactions in the data previously presented, nurses were unsystematic in their approach to information giving and the sharing of information. There was little evidence of nurses recounting previous information shared and the way in which this was used to make decisions. Little time was taken to check out patients' understanding of information shared with them and the relevance of this information to their care plans. This in part was due to the stylised and ritualistic approach to conversational approaches adopted by nurses and their inability to frame questions appropriately in a way that was meaningful for older people. Patients were expected to conform to established routines in practice.

In contrast, both the expert hospital nurse and the community nurse specialist adopted discursive styles that enabled patient participation in decision-making:

Pam/Interaction 1/lines 196-220

```
196 P:   =he hadn't even got the sense to nick the bloody bottom
197 N:                                                        Lto
198      let it through I'm sorry to interrupt your story because it's
199      very interesting and perhaps I'll come back and hear some
200      more of it la::ter=
201 P:   =I'm writing a book about some of the things that have been
202      goin' on and you wait and buy the book
203 N:   ((laughs)) well that's alright ee're happy to wait and buy the
204      book then is it all right if I have a look at your ca::re plan?
205 P:                                                        LO:::H
```

206   no go ahead YES
207   (0.04) your notes to sort of help me work out what you-you
208   know how to proceed for the rest of the shift right okay=
209 P: =OH YEAHS=
210 N: =I'll put it back when I've finished=
211 P: =yeah (   )
212 N: Have they? right=
213 P: =I wasn't aware that was my property or anythin'=
214 N: =well they are your notes you can look at them anytime that
215   you want=
216 P: =well that was a change of policy wasn't it?=
217 N: =and you can well it's a bit different to the co::uncil I think
218   but you can have a look at them and re::ad them and if there
219   is anything that you want to ask or anything that you don't
220   agree with then feel free

In this interaction, the nurse is discussing plans for the day with the patient. Throughout the interaction, the patient sets the conversation agenda as he offers detailed descriptions of conflict with a neighbour and the local Council. The nurse does not interrupt this story, but instead uses open affirming responses that offer the patient permission to continue with the story. In line 197, the nurse interrupts the patient's story, but again does this in a way that demonstrates an interest in what he was saying and that indicates she could hear more of it later. In line 204, the nurse asks the patient's permission to look at the care plan in order to help her plan the day. The patient expresses surprise at the request (line 205), thus suggesting a perceived restriction on his participation rights. The nurse's response (lines 214-220) explains the lack of restriction on his participation. This interaction also highlights the theme of 'informed flexibility'. The nurse engages with the patient, listening to his story and affirming the value of the story to the care context:

Pam/Interaction 1/lines 153-173

153   then I was informed that should be cha::rged with
154   assault on Mister ((name)) (0.1) I claimed it was self defence
155   they said oh no it wasn't self defence it was
156   re::taliation because it took fifteen seconds at least between
157   his blow and
158 N: ⌊and you hitting him back yeah m:::m
159 P: (0.2) that's the law of this country and that's the kind of
160   justice we get

```
161 N:   (0.2) and meanwhile you're lying here with plenty of time to
162      think about all this aren't you?
163 P:   (0.1) well::: you say plenty of time left there's one above
164      there (0.07) who I believe exists (0.1) he's the one who
165 N:        ⌊m:m              ⌊yep
166      directs how much time I've got to think about this=
167 N:   =°right
168 P:   (0.1) if o::::nly you'll give me time to see this BLOODY
169      government kicked out and me achieve a victory over
170      ((County Name)) District Council=
171 N:   =so they are the two things you want to achieve?=
172 P:   =yeah=
173 N:   =right=
```

In line 161, the nurse's response illustrates her concern for the patient and the importance of this story to his overall rehabilitation. The nurse acknowledges the importance of this story to him and the fact that it is currently so important to him. Later in line 171, the nurse does not react to the strength of feeling expressed by the patient, but again is concerned with the patient's goals. While the nurse clearly has time restrictions in place, as indicated by her interruption to the patient's story in line 197, she does not project this in her interaction, but instead is conscious of the need to plan her day based on the care needs described in the care plan.

The clinical nurse specialist continuously operated from an approach based on informed flexibility. In her initial meeting with the patient, she clearly set the basis of her relationship with him and his wife:

Case Study 14 (Ray)/Interaction 1/lines 19-27

```
19 N:   =yeah(h)s ju(h)st like yo(h)u ((laughter))!  Doctor
20      Ma:tthews suggested that maybe the time had co::me for
21      you to   start on insulin (0.2) BUT (0.1) what they wanted
22      me to do was to come out and talk to you both about it
23      (and how you fe::el about it) and to explain why they
24      think that might be an idea
25 P:   (0.3) yeah=
26 N:   =I will not force you into doing a:::nything you don't
27      want to do (  )
28 P:   Yeahs yeah=
29 N:   =⌈Explain
30 P:    ⌊(we fully) realise that
31 N:   (0.3) are you aware that your blood sugars have been
```

32   getting higher?=

The nurse explains her motives for visiting Ray and his wife and in line 26 explains the degree of flexibility in decision-making that is possible. The nurse's approach continues in this way throughout the interaction. The nurse sets the conversation agenda (lines 22-24 and 31) and establishes the goal of the interaction. Her questioning style is direct, but flexible enough to enable the patient to tell his story and ask specific questions:

Case Study 14/Ray/Interaction 1/lines 334-344

334 P: (   ) (0.4) but tell me something all these other tablets
335   this is what I say (0.1) look I think (the diabetic) (   )
336   well we start off with (this insulin) on a very low dose
337 N: ⌊yeah?
338   (0.2) well the next time its a case of o::h well this is not
339   be:tter so we will have to do it twi:ce a day ( ) and then
340   the same thing again I don't respond to this treatment so
341   then three: ti::mes a day (0.1) and then* its mo::re and
342 N: ⌊they won't ( )
343   mo:re
344 N: (0.2) let me re-assure you (0.2) there are two options

Ray responds to the nurse's previous utterance with a question about his tablets and the insulin injections. The nurse responds directly to this question and provides him with a detailed explanation. Throughout their interactions, the nurse empowered Ray to gain knowledge about his condition and care needs through the facilitation of his understanding. She did this through direct questioning, directly responding to Ray's questions with full and comprehensive explanations and the provision of additional information:

Case Study 14/ Ray/Interaction 1/lines 421-445

421 N: yea::h (0.2) one thing I think it would ( ) I can't
422   guarantee it but I'm prett::::y sure that if we can get
423   your blo::od sugar levels back down to normal you
424   will have an aw::ful lot more get up and go=
425 P: =°yeah (0.3) (   ) even if I haven't got it as you get
426   older (Jean don't know what to do with me)
427 N: (0.1) no I know (0.3) what would you like to do? (0.2)
428   do you want to thi::nk about it?=

429 P: =yeah:::=
430 N: =okay ((nurse & wife laugh)) (0.2) I've got for: you a
431   book which (0.2) I know I sound like I'm trying to
432   persuade you but I'm gen::uinely not I'm just trying to
433   give you all the information ((giggle)) (0.1) but this is a
434 P: Lyes but
435   book about people who changed from tablets to
436   i::nsulin (0.2)and it gives you a bit: of information about
437 P: Lo::h yes?
438   why:: (0.1) you've got a high blood sugar and that's
439   what the symptoms are (0.1) feeling very ( ) tired
440   feeling a bit irritable some people get thirsty and spend a
441   lot of time in the loo (0.1) yeah::? those are the
442   symptoms of a high blood sugar and as you can see from
443   here yours is eighte:::en nearly nineteen and should
444   really be in an ideal world between four and eight so its
445   quite a lot (too high)=

In later interactions, the nurse builds on previously established information and knowledge in order to integrate new information:

Case Study 14/Ray/Interaction 2/lines 398-423

398 N: (0.2) now because you've got on with this extremely
399   well (0.2) what I'll show you is how to do the actual
400   injection (0.06) today because my plan was so that you
401 P: Lyeah   Lokay
402   didn't have to learn two completely ne::w things
403 P: L( ) she recognises
404   that I'm a bit dim=
405 N: =NO its not that it it doesn't matter its (0.06) anybody
406   regardless of age intelligence(0.1) people do not
407   remember information if they are given too much all at
408   one go=
409 P: =no no=
410 N: =its got noth(h)ing to d(h)o wit(h)h - you aren't dim at
411   all ((laughter)) nothing to do with either your dimness
412   ((laughter)) or your age nobody learns things if you give
413 P: Lno::
414   them too much information at one go so I'm taking it
415   gently=
416 P: =oh good
417 N: (0.1) but because you aren't dim and you've gra::sped

418   this re::ally well (0.07) <u>yeah</u>=
419 P: =ye::ah I think I've got this off well I can always have a
420   look anyway=
421 N: =yeah I'll show you how to do just the injection not how
422   to get the insulin in the syringe just the injection=

In line 398 the nurse positively affirms Ray's progress with understanding his condition and treatment options and in line 402 illustrates the staged and incremental approach to information giving being adopted. The patient interprets this incremental approach as him 'being a bit dim'. The nurse's response is direct and offers an explanation for the approach being adopted. While the nurse has a routinised approach, i.e. a policy of not giving too much information in one go, this routine is adapted to maximise understanding, independence and to suit the particular progress of the patient.

Sympathetic Presence

Theme Definition an engagement that recognises the uniqueness and value of the individual, by appropriately responding to cues that maximise coping resources through recognition of important agendas in daily life.

    Both the expert nurse and the clinical nurse specialist adopted discursive styles that were focused on the individual patient and their agendas. Although both nurses clearly had an agenda that they were following when engaged with patients, they illustrated an explicit consciousness of patients' responses to previous utterances as a means of focusing next questions:

Pam/Interaction 3/lines 76-104

76 P: =I've got one or two horses there=
77 N: =°o::h right °okay=
78 P: =eighteen to be precise=
79 N: =eighteen yeah a bit more than one or two yeah someone's
80   looking after them (   )
81 P: (I've been) getting a bit worried about them that's why I
82   started getting dressed to get up=
83 N: =right=
84 P: =that's the thing I'm not suppose to do, to jump in (and go
85   out)
86 N: (0.1) °no::=
87 P: =but the nurses at the Rathbone were clever enough to

```
88        realise that if they sent me home (     ) back in I reckon
89  N:    (0.3) °we:::ll how long do you think you're going to stay
90        here?
91  P:    (0.1) well my (0.06) well they first said I thought about two
92        or three days and then talking to (0.1) Sharon? is it Sharon
93        yesterday afternoon (0.1) I said about a week (0.1) after
94  N:                              ⌊im im
95        being here (now) three or four months would be nice
96        ((laughs))
97  N:    ((laughs)) r(h)eally
98  P:    all this lovely food  and attention=
99  N:    =°yeah well perhaps that's a message that's to say to you
100       that you're not quite (0.06) well yet and you need a little bit
101       of time?=
102 P:    =yeah=
103 N:    =to give yourself a bit of time to heal? (0.2) it takes it out of
104       you doesn't it?=
```

In this interaction, the patient has been telling the nurse about his condition prior to this admission to hospital. The patient makes links between aspects of his lifestyle and his perceptions of previous care decisions (e.g. his horses and the reason for his transfer from the DGH (line87)). The nurse responds to previous utterances with questions that seek to gain an understanding of the patient's perceptions (line 89). In line 89, the nurse asks the patient how long he thinks he will stay in hospital. The patient's response indicates his satisfaction with his care. In line 99, the nurse's response is aimed at helping the patient to understand his need for care. The approach used to providing this information is cautious and questioning. The nurse suggests a possible explanation, based on her interpretation of the patient's story. In this way, the nurse acknowledges the need for sensitivity in her questioning style and the power of language.

In a later interaction, the nurse demonstrates sensitivity to a patient's emotional coping ability. In doing this, the nurse does not overtly constrain the patient's actions, but sensitively works with the patient's understanding, in order to eventually reach a decision:

Pam/Interaction 6/lines 27-61

```
27 N:    =do you want to get into your night clothes?
28 P:    (0.2) I don't know whether I o::ught to I got to go (0.1) is it
29       tomorrow you say=
30 N:    =oh for your appointment tomorrow morning that's not
```

31   until sort of u::m I think your appointments about ten

32   o'clock isn't it?=

33 P: =is it?=

34 N: =so someone could help you get dressed in the mo::rning

35 P: ⌊yeahs

36   (0.1) there'll be someone here to help you (0.2) what I was

37 P: ⌊yeah

38   thinking of <u>tonight</u> was um are you wanting to settle down

39   now for the night or do you just want to lie:: on your bed?=

40 P: =yeahs

41 N: (0.3) which one was it?

42 P: (0.2) eh?=

43 N: =did you em did you want to just lie on top of your bed or

44   do you want to get undressed ready for bed?=

45 P: =well I don't know whether I ought to get under (0.2) well

46   well well I ought to go ready to go on that on that

47   a:::mbulance=

48 N: =oh OH I see OH no you don't need to worry about that just

49   yet (0.1) because it's u:m about it's about um seven

50 P: ⌊(don't I)

51   o'clo::ck and you are not going until tomorrow morning

52   (0.2) so if you get undressed tonight someone will help you

53   with your clothes in the morning to make sure you are ready

54   in plenty of <u>time</u>

55 P: (0.1) °oh (0.2) °oh °I °hope °so=

56 N: =yes there will there'll definitely be someone to help you

57   (0.4) so if we make sure there is someone to help you in the

58   morning do you want to get undressed? (0.1) and into your

59 P: ⌊°yeah

60   night wear? (0.1) a:::lright=

61 P: ⌊°yeah   =(so get it off get it all off)=

In this interaction the nurse had noticed that the patient looked anxious and approached her to ask if she needed her help. The patient identified that she wanted to go to bed. In this section of the interaction, the nurse asks the patient if she would like to get into her nightclothes. The patient's response highlights the reason for her anxiety, i.e. if she gets undressed she won't be ready on time for the ambulance next morning. The nurse handles the patient's concern with sensitivity. Her questioning style is focused on enabling the patient to make a decision (line 34). Through these questions, the nurse identifies the reason for the patient's anxiety and offers reassurance in the form of a clear explanation about how she would be helped the next morning. The approach adopted by the nurse enables the removal of emotional constraint and facilitates the making of an appropriate decision.

The clinical nurse specialist adopted a similar approach through an 'open' and exploratory style of conversation:

Case Study 14/Ray/Interaction 1/lines 81-102

```
81 N:   (0.1) tell me how (that feels) how are you feeling=
82 P:   =pretty good except that I haven't got a lot of "get up
83      and go:::"=
84 N:   =right=
85 P:   =I mean (with this eh) (     ) takes a bit of getting used
86      to start sort of (wo::ds) you know=
87 N:   =then would you say that you were lacking in energy?=
88 P:   =yes
89 N:   (0.1) right (0.2) now has that been getting worse as your
90      blood sugars have been going hi::gher
91 P:   (0.2) well I haven't noticed any diff::erence=
92 N:   =right (0.3) one reason for feeling tired and lacking in
93      energy and not having enough "get up and go:::" is high
94      blood sugar levels=
95 P:   =yes
96 N:   (0.1) now according to the letter (0.1)  they did a blood
97      sugar in the clinic and that was eighteen point six
98 P:   (0.1) °yeah=
99 N:   =do you know what normal is?=
100 P:  =no=
101 N:  =right a nor:::mal blood sugar is anywhere between four
102     and eight
```

In this section of the interaction, the nurse asks an open question (line 81) and then supports Ray telling his story about his condition through the asking of further open and exploratory questions. Through this approach, the nurse also facilitates the integration of new information into Ray's storytelling as a means of ongoing assessment. This approach was used consistently throughout each interaction - for example:

```
286 N:  Well we can do that one that's any easy one (  ) can you
287     just tell me more about why you've not been on Insulin
```

By adopting this approach, the nurse facilitated a shared conversation agenda and reduced the potentially powerful impact of some of the information that she needed to provide. By adopting an exploratory approach, she enabled the integration of Ray's perceptions and views with her experience and knowledge. The nurse worked with Ray to remove constraints on his decision-making:

Case Study 14/Ray/Interaction 2/lines 473-496

```
473 Wife: =and I ( ) be worried about him but because he's a
474       stubborn old so and so you know it don't matter what
475 N:                         ⌊((laughter))
476       you say 'Oh ( )'=
477 N:   =WELL (0.2) nobody can make you do anything you
478       don't want to do and I know you are not keen but I
479       honestly honestly think you'll feel heaps better you'll
480       actually feel so: much better when we get the insulin
481       amount right that loads of people have said to me in the
482       past 'I wish I'd done this earlier'=
483 P:   =have they?=
484 N:   =its like a new lease of life=
485 P:   =yeah o::h goo::d well I've got something to look
486      ⌈forward* to at last
487 N:   ⌊it won't* (0.1) it won't be over night yeah it won't be
488       magical over night Ray but a few weeks up to a month
489 P:                        ⌊no
490       and I think you'll start feeling
491 P:                         ⌊you think it would drop
492       in a mo::nth do you?=
493 N:   =yeah I think
494 P:              ⌊the insulin=
495 N:   =yes I think we'll get you your blood sugar much nearer
496       normal
```

In this interaction, the patient's wife sets the agenda for the conversation through her expression of concern about her husband. The nurse responds with an explanation that continues to emphasise Ray's right to make a decision that he is happy with. However, she 'frames' the boundaries of the decision by providing more information that enables Ray to make a more informed decision. This information-giving strategy enables patient decision-making by ensuring that Ray is in possession of all necessary information in order to make an appropriate decision. Thus he is not constrained by a lack of information or knowledge.

Negotiation

Theme Definition patient participation through a culture of care that values the views of the patient as a legitimate basis for decision-making while recognising that being the final arbiter of decisions is of secondary importance.

Both the nurse expert and the clinical nurse specialist used negotiation frameworks as an implicit component of their conversation approach. Through their conversation style, they both facilitated patients' ownership of their health care decisions. Patients were consulted about care decisions through their interactions. For Pam (nurse expert) the seeking of permission from the patient before initiating an action was an explicit part of her decision-making framework:

Pam/Interaction 3/lines 127-147

```
127 N:  =((laughs)) °right okay um do you mind if I have a look at
128     your notes? just so I can find out what's you know what
129     care you've been having and
130 P                             ⌊quite a lot=
131 N:  =quite a lot °okay
132 P:  (0.1) I do have thirty two tablets a day=
133 N:  =a:::h right (0.2) have a look at your tablet card then (19.0)
134     are you taking your own tablets or have we got them? and
135     are we putting them out for you?=
136 P:  =you put them ⌈out
137 N:                ⌊we're putting them out just at the minute
138     right=
139 P:  =to be honest (I got a bit of a fright) (  )
140 N:  okay=
141 P:  =about ha:::lf of them I was having before I went into
142     hospital (0.1) a lot of the:: well all the antibiotics are from
143     the hospital
144 N:  (0.05) right and you say that made you a bit a bit sort of
145     puzzled has it?=
146 P:  =yeah=
147 N:  =yeah
```

Pam asks permission from the patient to look in his notes and offers a reason for wanting to do this. The reason offered by her enables the patient to provide more information (line 132) that assists Pam with focusing on his 'tablet card'. She continues to adopt an open questioning style (line

134), thus reinforcing the patient's ownership of his health care decisions. This style further enables the patient to explain how he feels (line 139).

Pam rarely alters her negotiation style and continuously engages the patient in the decisions made:

Pam/Interaction 3/lines 155-175

```
155 N:   Right (0.1) well if you if you need me to do anything for you
156      or to help you with anything then just either ring the bell or
157      come and find me (0.1) u:::m (0.2) right=
158 P:   =there's only two things I disagree with=
159 N:   =what's that?=
160 P:   (this cold water)=
161 N:   =OH you don't well I'll see if I can get you just ordinary tap
162      water?=
163 P:   =and=
164 N:   =what's the other thing?=
165 P:   =well I like a bath everyday but (like I told Mary) I thought
166      it would be all right just to call Mary to get me out (but
167      it's not fair to call on her)
168 N:   Yeah it's a bit different to home is it?
169 P:   Yeah
170 N:   Yeah
171 P:   (        ) I got terrific strength in my arms but not a lot
172      (else)=
173 N:   =right okay well I'm working tomorrow morning so I can
174      help you get out the bath if you want a bath tomorrow
175      morning? that will be fine
```

In line 155 Pam gives the patient explicit permission to seek assistance from her. The patient immediately responds with two issues that he has problems with. The nurse responds positively to the patient's request for different drinking water and encourages his expression of the second issue of concern (line 164). The patient explains about his bathing routine and the nurse empathises with his perception (line 168). In line 173 the nurse offers the patient the help he needs, but continues to place the final decision with him. While she offers him assistance with the bath, she suggests that his need for a bath should be his decision.

The clinical nurse specialist adopted a similar approach to negotiation. In all of the interactions with Ray, the conversation agenda was continuously shared between him, his wife and the nurse. The nurse always responded to the views expressed by the patient and his wife and used these expressions to:

- provide more advice:

Case Study 14/Ray/Interaction 1/lines 244-252

244 N: (0.1) well what ever else happens how's about I make
245   another appointment and I bring the meter to show you=
246 Wife: =°yeah=
247 N: =⌈YEA:H?
248 P: ⌊yes=
249 N: =because whatever the decision today that will help I
250   think will it?
251 P: (0.1) yes=
252 N: =are you happy with that?

- provide more information:

Interaction 1/lines 427-445

427 N: (0.1) no I know (0.3) what would you like to do? (0.2)
428   do you want to thi::nk about it?=
429 P: =yeah:::=
430 N: =okay ((nurse & wife laugh)) (0.2) I've got for: you a
431   book which (0.2) I know I sound like I'm trying to
432   persuade you but I'm gen::uinely not I'm just trying to
433   give you all the information ((giggle)) (0.1) but this is a
434 P: ⌊yes but
435   book about people who changed from tablets to
436   i::nsulin (0.2)and it gives you a bit: of information about
437 P: ⌊o::h yes?
438   why:: (0.1) you've got a high blood sugar and that's
439   what the symptoms are (0.1) feeling very ( ) tired
440   feeling a bit irritable some people get thirsty and spend a
441   lot of time in the loo (0.1) yeah::? those are the
442   symptoms of a high blood sugar and as you can see from
443   here yours is eighte:::en nearly nineteen and should
444   really be in an ideal world between four and eight so its
445   quite a lot (too high)=

- demonstrate a particular aspect of care:

Interaction 1/lines 610-624

```
610 N:  =right well we'll make an appointment to do that
611     before we move on would you like me to just do a
612     demonstration (0.1) in depth and without the actual
613     insulin so you know what it feels like or would you
614     rather not=
615 P:  =no I'm not very kee::n ⌈(      )
616 N:                         ⌊Not keen (0.2) we'll leave it
617            then=
618 P:  =yeah=
619 N:  =oka:::y? (0.1) ri:::ght (0.2) the other thing I'm going to
620     offer you (   ) was a little information pack about (the
621     injections) (0.2) would you like that or would you rather
622 P:             ⌊yes
623     (    )=
624 P:  =yes yes we'll have a look
```

Mutuality

Theme Definition the recognition of the others' values as being of equal importance in decision-making.

Valuing the perceptions of patients was consistently identified as an important component of assisted patient decision-making. The problems of the professionals' values being seen as more legitimate than those of patients were identified as a reason for the lack of facilitated decision-making by nurses and the overriding of patients' preferences and views. In addition, it was recognised that patients were expected to have had an 'objective' view of their lives, i.e. to be able to appreciate the difficulties the future held for them and to make appropriately related decisions.

While the data recorded by the expert nurse and clinical nurse specialist did not focus so dominantly on discharge planning or residential care decisions, there was substantial evidence in the data of both nurses planning care from the patients' perspectives:

Pam/Interaction 9/lines 159-188

```
159 P:  (0.1) (this shingles is affecting) it's affecting me::::
160 N:                                              ⌊°mm
161     gradually I'm getting very depressed=
162 N:  =right (0.1) what about e::m sorry to interrupt you but do
163     you think perhaps that (0.05) would you be better off if you
```

164   had a bit more company?
165 P: (0.06) NO-NO-NO I'm a lo:::ner=
166 N: =oh you don't want company right
167 P: ⌊(   ) my daughter my
168   other daughter wanted to take my grandson from London to
169   see me and my grandson from-(they'd like to) take the great
170   grand children lovely children (0.1) they will be coming up
171   here toda:::y °oh dear (0.1) no I'm better off without
172   ((name)) looks after me:: (12.0) it's all very well this I'm
173   feeling <u>sorry</u> for my::self=
174 N: =are you?=
175 P: =yes=
176 N: =i:::m I'm not surprised
177 P: (0.4) couple of weeks ago ((turning of pages)) (   ) you
178   know crying (0.1) at least one of the nurses a temporary
179   nurse just (   ) basically I said I <u>haven't</u> cried so much
180   since my hu::::sband died=
181 N: =°right=
182 P: =I I said (I wasn't) cryi::ng for him (0.1) basically (Ididn't
183   mind that much) (   ) we were supposed to be an ideal
184 N: ⌊((laughter))
185   couple but (0.1) every day over (   ) he (   ) the good of
186   his opinion except he was <u>BO::::RING</u>=
187 N: =he was boring was he? but presumably you didn't realise
188   that when you married him?=

In line 159 the patient identifies that she is feeling depressed. The nurse's response is to offer to move the patient to an area of the ward where she would have more company (line 162). In line 165, the patient responds with 'force' and highlights that she is a loner. In line 172 a 12 second silence occurs and the nurse waits for the patient to continue without the need to interject. The patient suggests that she is feeling sorry for herself. The nurse does not try to close down the patient's utterance, but instead asks another open question and follows this with an affirmation of the patient's feelings, thus demonstrating the legitimacy of her views (line 176). This affirmation enables the patient to further express her feelings and to continue with her story about her values.

For the clinical nurse specialist, the patient's beliefs, values, views and perceptions were central to all interactions and care decisions. At no time did the nurse seek to change the patient's views through the expression of her beliefs and values as being of greater importance. Instead she used negotiation processes set within an information-giving framework as a means of enabling informed decision-making. She continuously reinforced the importance of the patient making decisions and reiterated these when new information was being offered:

Case Study 14/Ray/Interaction 1/lines 799-809

```
799 N:   (0.1) now did I give you my ⌈phone number
780 P:                               ⌊I know you're doing it for
781      my benefit re:::ally I mean its no advantage for you::=
782 N:   =not at all::: ((nurse and wife laugh)) (0.4) but then what
783      I think is best for people may not be what they think is
784      best (for them) so it's got really to be your decision we:
785      can't make (the decision) for you=
786 P:   =no (0.2) but I do feel though that this eh (sugar) would
787      do be:::tter  if we could get a definite re:::ad out you
788 N:                              ⌊yeah
789      know=
```

In the previous conversation, the nurse had been explaining to Ray her motives for wanting him to commence insulin therapy, but he was reluctant. In this conversation the nurse makes explicit her beliefs about the importance of patients making the care decision. She clearly explains the importance of the patient's perceptions as a part of the decision-making process. In line 806, Ray continues to highlight his belief that if the blood sugar recordings were more accurate then there may not be a need for insulin. The nurse does not disagree with this perception, but instead makes arrangements for the necessary equipment to be provided.

This conversation clearly highlights the skills of the nurse in recognising the centrality of the patient's values in care decisions. Although, she may have the technical knowledge and understanding about the reasons for his high blood sugar levels, she does not attempt to coerce Ray into agreeing with her and reaching a decision to commence insulin therapy. Instead, she suspends this knowledge and works with his perception and provides the necessary equipment. Ray is not made to feel that he holds a misperception or that his decision is wrong. In this way the nurse does not expect Ray to hold an objective view of his life, but instead is prepared to work with the perception that he holds. In later interactions, he understands the need to commence insulin therapy, but only after he exhausted other potential solutions.

Transparency

Theme Definition the making explicit of intentions and motivations for action and the boundaries within which care decisions are set.

In the previous section, the clinical nurse specialist makes explicit her beliefs and values about what would be best for the patient. However, she also makes explicit to the patient that his views, perceptions and values are of equal importance and demonstrates this through her ability to work with the agenda established by him. This transparency of intentions and motivations was evident throughout the data of both the clinical nurse specialist and the nurse expert.

In relation to this theme, the data from the nurse expert predominantly focused on her making explicit her intent and motivation for action, as illustrated in the example below:

Pam/Interaction 6/lines 4-13

```
4  N:   You alright there Esme? (0.1) are you alright there?
5  P:                    ⌊E::H?                    ⌊yeahs
6        (0.2) I wondered if you were trying to catch me eye
7        befo::re? (0.1) you were looking across in my di::rection::
8        ⌈and I wondered* if you were trying-you we:::re (0.1) can I
9  P:   ⌊yes I was
10       do anything to help you?=
11 P:   =yes put me to bed=
12 N:   =put you to be(h)d? alright then (0.1) have you finished
13       your SU::PPER:?=
```

The nurse engages with the patient's gaze and identifies it as an expression of need. She makes her perception clear to the patient and the patient affirms that she was trying 'to catch her eye'. The nurse's response is in the form of an open question 'Is there anything I can do to help you?'. This form of approach was explicit throughout her interactions with patients and enabled the setting of the conversation agenda and the establishment of decision-making boundaries.

Being transparent about her intent and motivation for actions was also commonplace with the clinical nurse specialist. In establishing the agenda for action, she made explicit the boundaries within which decisions would be set and her motivations:

Case Study 14/Ray/Interaction 1/lines 108-119

108 Wife: (he's not too long going on the insulin) but I think its
109   probably because he's always falling asleep=
110 N: =is he yeah (0.2) it's most likely to be due to the high
111   blood sugars I'm afraid
112 Wife: (   ) wouldn't know what to do (   )
113 N: right (0.2) if your husband went on to insulin (0.1)
114   number one I do my best to make sure that hypos don't
115   happen (0.2) but I would also teach you what they are
116 Wife: ⌊yeah
117   when they might happen and what to do if they
118   do:: happen (0.3) and (0.1) what do you think happens
119   in a hypo

Later in this interaction, the nurse clearly explains the complications associated with diabetes:

Case Study 14/Ray/Interaction 1/lines 312-332

312 N: (0.1) there's a sli::ght problem Ray with that (0.1) in as
313   much as (0.1) that various complications in diabetes that
314   you are talking about the damage to the feet and the
315   damage to the ey::es come after a long ti::me of high
316   blood sugars (0.1) once the damage has happened (0.2)
317   then controlling your blood sugars unfortunately doesn't
318   fix it doesn't make it better=
319 P: =doesn't it? it doesn't go ba:ck=
320 N: =it doesn't go back to where it wa::s (0.3) those so:::rts
321 P: ⌊oh
322   of problems tend to happen after a lo:ng time and I mean
323   ye:ars of hi::gher then normal blood sugars (0.2) and
324 P: ⌊yeah   ⌊yeah
325   once they have happened you can't make them better
326   again by then getting the blood sugars down (0.1) I
327 P: ⌊oh
328   wish it worked that way but it doesn't unfortunately
329   so one of the re::asons the doctors are keen is to
330   prevent problems with the eyes and the feet and other
331   bits and pieces ((laughter)) i(h)n th(h)e f(h)uture
332   ((Dog barks))

The nurse is explicit in her description of the associated complications. She does not attempt to 'soften' the explicitness of the description offered, but instead provides full details. This explicit description could be associated with the nurse's motivation to encourage Ray to commence insulin therapy. Later in this interaction she makes it explicit that that is what she wants to happen. Unlike nurses in other case studies, she does not attempt to hide her agenda for action and makes it explicit to the patient that this is her motivation:

Case Study 14/Ray/Interaction 1/lines 772-777

```
772 N:  (0.1) I have to tell you I will work at trying to persuade
773     you=
774 P:  =I know I reckon you're employed by (   )
775 N:  ((laughter)) by whom? Evans?=
776 P:  =Evans you know they make all the insulin=
777 N:  they don't in Britain any more=
```

The nurse continues to provide a reason for this motivation:

```
790 N:  (0.4) the reason I'm trying to persuade you ((giggle)) is
791     that I have a re:::ally big feeling that you will feel so
792     much more energetic ((giggle)) but then it is really
793     your choice honestly=
794 P:  =yeah  (0.4) well we'll have a think about it=
795 N:        ⌊yeah ((laughter))   =o::ka:y (0.1) you will
796     honestly start (   ) if you're still unsure when I see you
797     next time then Ill leave it I won't push it: okay?=
```

The nurse explains to Ray that his presenting symptoms would be relieved by the use of insulin. However, she continues to emphasise the importance of him making the choice once he has considered all the information provided.

Like the nurse expert, the clinical nurse specialist also made explicit what she would write in records:

Case Study 14/Ray/Interaction 2/lines1281-1284

```
1281 P: (0.1) Can you (grant) me to take it along to the do::ctor
1282    and see him about it and (   ) you know I decided to go
1283    on insulin=
```

1284 N: =well I'm going to write him a letter=
1285 P: =oh are you=
1286 N: =saying (0.1) I saw Mr Maxwell and I'll give him a mini
1287   history of what has happened

The interactions in this case study were much longer than those of the other case studies. Each interaction constituted one visit by the clinical nurses specialist to the patient in his own home and lasted one hour. The patient in this case study also demonstrated considerable knowledge about his condition and symptoms and was therefore able to engage in lengthy interactions with the nurse. This created a different problem for the nurse - that of controlling her time. However, she did not hide from the patient, the pressures on her time or to bring interactions to a close prematurely. Instead she was explicit about the time available:

Case Study 14/Ray/Interaction 2/lines 1216-1220

1216 P: =yeah (0.2) are you pushed this morning I mean are we
1217   getting on too fast for your time to go and see
1218   somebody else=
1219 N: =I've got to see somebody else I can give you another
1220   five minutes or so=

In a later conversation, the nurse explains her motivation for putting a time limit on her input with the patient:

Case Study 14/Ray/Interaction 2/lines 1760-1779 (W = wife)

1760 N: =Ray's actually picking things up incredibly quickly with
1761 W: └yeah
1762   other folk I go a lot more slowly and I'm trying to
1763   actually slow him down a bit ((laughter)) because
1764   otherwise I could be here all day and you'd still be
1765   asking me things ((laughter))
1766 P: Yeah yeah ((laughter))
1767 N: I don't mind it's just that I have got to go somewhere
1768   else=
1769 P: =yeah ah well °yeah
1770 N: └yeah? (0.2) but em (0.1) we'll go through
1771   that again we'll go through the new finger pricker and
1772   we'll go through pens on Monday and I'll bring with me
1773   the insulin cartridges for the pens so we might do some

1774 revision see how much you've remembered from today
1775 P: ⌊yeah
1776 I've got a feeling you'll have remembered an awful lot
1777 we'll see how you are getting on with the meter and how
1778 P: ⌊yeah
1779 and how you are getting on with the injections=

In line 1764, the nurse explains how Ray's level of engagement necessitates her limiting the input she offers. Although she is responding to the wife's previous utterances, she directs her response to Ray. However, she recognises that this could be interpreted as a criticism and therefore follows up her previous utterance with an explanation as to why there is a time limit. She then affirms Ray's progress with him in preparation for the next visit. This transparency enables the nurses to balance the individuality of the care situation with their overall workload. This is in direct contrast to the other case studies, where nurses engaged in a series of interactions aimed at closing conversations and limiting their input into patients' care. This resulted in an approach that appeared deceptive and inconsistent.

Summary and Conclusions

The interactions of the expert nurse and clinical nurse specialist are significantly different from those of other nurse participants. Their interactions provide some indication of the way in which the identified principles for action can be operationalised in order to develop a patient-focused approach to practice.

Both practitioners demonstrate identified attributes of expert practice. Key attributes of expert practice include, holistic practice knowledge (Benner *et al*, 1996), saliency (Benner, 1994[ii]), knowing the patient (Jenny and Logan, 1992), moral agency (Benner and Wrubel, 1989) and skilled know-how (Carlson *et al*, 1989). They identify the salient features of interactions and demonstrate deliberateness in their responses. This is predominantly articulated through the principle of 'sympathetic presence'. They focus on the individual needs of each patient by identifying appropriate cues and engaging in a dialogue that sought to establish implied meaning of cues in order to respond appropriately. In addition they paid attention to the agendas of the patients and adopted flexibility in their practice in order to meet their needs.

Unlike much of the interaction of other nurse participants, the clinical nurse specialist and the expert nurse did not focus on the resolution of individual and disconnected problems. Instead, they focused on the individual patient's overall condition and coping resources through processes of 'negotiation' and 'informed flexibility'. Focusing on their agendas rather than those of the nurses' facilitated patient decision-making. Information was offered at a pace appropriate to the coping resources of individual patients and their perspectives on care practices. They further articulated an ability to engage at a level appropriate to the individual patients and were open to deal with the circumstances presented in the particular situations. Unlike other nurse participants, they did not attempt to direct the agenda from their perspectives, but instead used patients' responses to determine next questions. In the context of expert practice, both practitioners demonstrated the characteristic of being attuned to the particular situation that was shaped by patient responses without the overt reliance on conscious deliberation.

Both nurses negotiated care plans and while they offered particular care inputs, these were usually negotiated with the patient. On those occasions when the nurses needed to recommend particular actions, they usually offered choice in the way these actions would be undertaken. This was clearly demonstrated by the clinical nurse specialist who engaged in a lengthy process of negotiation with regard to the administration of 'insulin injections'. The patient's values were clearly recognised as important and 'mutuality' was demonstrated in the engagement between the nurse and patient. Both participants articulated their values in the situation and there was evidence of the patients respecting the nurses' values as part of their decision-making process. This seems to suggest that in those situations where patients' values are respected that they may be more receptive to advice and information from the nurse.

Both nurses demonstrated the principle of 'transparency' and made explicit their intentions and motivations for care decisions. In the context of expert practice, they demonstrated 'moral agency'. While the expert nurse practised in a hospital environment, there was little evidence of the organisational culture acting as a constraint on decision-making and both nurses demonstrated expertise in their practice. It can be concluded that the expertise of the nurse does have an effect on the way a patient-centred approach to decision-making is operationalised. While context can also be seen to constrain autonomy, it has been highlighted that practice which is expert in nature can minimise the impact of such organisational constraints.

9 Autonomy as Authentic Consciousness

Introduction

Given the constraints identified in previous chapters, it is difficult to hold a concept of autonomy for older people in hospital as an individualistic right to do what one wants. The research data has identified complex interactional processes occurring in the relationship between nurses, patients, patients' families and other health care professionals that prevent an individualistic concept of autonomy from prevailing.

In this chapter, some of these issues will be revisited in the light of the evidence presented through the data of the nurse expert and the community based clinical nurse specialist. The discourse in this data has been shown to be significantly different from that of other case studies and it was concluded that both the context of care and the expertise of the nurse do have a significant impact on the way autonomy is manifested in practice with older people. Using the themes generated from the 'Principles for Action', an alternative presentation of autonomy will be explored, based on Heidegger's (1990) theory of 'authentic consciousness'. It will be proposed that autonomy as authentic consciousness represents a values based understanding of the concept of autonomy, whereby the patient's values are held central to all decision making. It will further be proposed that autonomy as authentic consciousness is best articulated through the concept of a 'life plan' as articulated through patients' narratives (Meyers, 1989).

The Problem of Autonomy and Older Hospitalised People

The idea of the autonomous person being a self-reliant individual who functions independently of the context of his or her situation (an individualistic perspective), operates from a definition of autonomy as 'individual freedom to act'. This view is based on the original Greek word autos (meaning 'self') and nomos (meaning 'rule' 'governance' or 'law'), with the literal meaning of 'the having or making of one's own laws'. For the older person as a consumer of health care, appeals to autonomy are usually made then, when there is conflict among competing decisions and choices.

Gadow (1980) raises the important question of the relevance of such a position for older people. She suggests that professional consumerism is only a sophisticated form of paternalism, which insists that, in the interests of individual autonomy, people are required to make important decisions alone, such as those of long-term care arrangements or the acceptance or refusal of treatment. The dominant discourse in this approach is that of individual rights, and in particular, the individual's right to 'self-determination'. Having rights is a fundamental component of a liberal society and as Agich (1993) argues, having rights as an individual in receipt of health care is an important 'counterweight' against the impersonal decision making of health care institutions and health professionals who hold a disproportionate share of power. Autonomy as 'individual rights', focuses on a universalist understanding of autonomy as a strict and determinate absolute and is consistent with both the Kantian ideal of 'perfect duties' (i.e. duties of commission stated as descriptions of acts - not to lie, not to steal etcetera) (Sullivan, 1990) and Childress' (1982) description of autonomy as a 'side constraint', i.e. something that limits possible actions or as Gorovitz (1988; 183) articulates - '*(the belief) that it is obligatory to leave people alone unless we have powerful reasons for not doing so*'. In addition, a focus on autonomy from an individualistic rights perspective raises the problems of reflection on desires as described by Dworkin (1991) and discussed earlier in chapter 3.

If an individual has a right, then he or she equally has the right not to exercise that right. To do this successfully the individual reflects on their authentic desires that are based on universal principles that have been critically reflected upon and integrated into their life. However, as was identified earlier in chapter 3 the identification of desires that are authentically one's own and the problems of conflicting desires (Thalberg, 1989; Childress, 1982 and Norman, 1993) render the idea of personal autonomy an unachievable goal. In addition, for hospitalised older people the capacity to undertake such reflection at a time when they are most vulnerable limits an older person's ability to be autonomous.

It is clear from the data that a 'rights' perspective of autonomy designed to protect individuals from interference by others, is inconsistent with the experience of the older people in this study. There is little evidence in the data of older people exercising freedom of choice as consumers of health care. As was seen in this research, many of the nurses adopted a position of 'information giving' as their dominant mode of operation. Their focus was that of providing information as a part of their commitment to patient participation. However, the lack of a clear framework in which such information was contained and the dominant role of professionals in decision making, resulted in such information acting as another form of control that served to reinforce decisions already made by professionals, rather than a means of enabling decision making by patients themselves. The conversational style of nurses, including their control of the conversation agenda and the conversation focus, prevented patients from determining care outcomes for themselves. Nurses were clearly at an advantage over patients, because of their ability to identify salient features of conversations and integrate these into their already established 'picture' of the patient. However, while it is easy to label such approaches as those identified in the data as paternalistic and controlling, it is difficult to anticipate an alternative model from a rights perspective of autonomy. Given that the rights perspective demands that an individual has the necessary competence to choose between competing choices and that an essential component of this is the possession of all the necessary information needed to make such a decision, then personal autonomy for older hospitalised people would appear to be an unachievable ideal.

In addition, it has been identified that patients have a limited understanding of the health care system compared to that of health care professionals. Within this research, this fact alone was seen to place nursing staff at an advantage over patients, enabling them to make plans according to their understanding, for example, regarding the availability of community services and how to access them. In terms of the relationship between nurses and patients, this clearly placed nurses at an advantage in terms of their ability to make decisions about care provision and it would appear to be an impossible ideal to expect an equal level of knowledge and understanding from patients in order for them to exercise their individual autonomy. In addition, the differing discursive rights of nurses and patients manifested through both 'internal constraints' (factors that reduce or eliminate the capacity for an older person to claim autonomy) and 'external constraints' (legal, moral and institutional overriding of autonomy for reasons perceived to be in the best interests of the individual) (Fry, 1991) creates an imbalance of power in the nurse-patient relationship that can be seen to erode individual autonomy. In this research, internal constraints such as the expectations of older people from services, their expectations of nurses, their perceptions of the role of the nurse and nurses' attitudes towards older people, were all seen to be factors in the prevention of patients exercising their rights. In addition, external constraints such as the organisation of care, the use of language as a form of control, routinised and ritualistic approaches to practice and the prevention of risk taking by patients further eroded individual autonomy. Fry (1991) creates a distinction between autonomy as a 'prima facie principle' as articulated by such authors as Beauchamp and Childress (1983) and discussed in this research as a 'universal principle' and autonomy as an 'ideal' as articulated by Dworkin (1991) and discussed in this research as 'a capacity'.

Fry argues that in health care decision-making for older people, both the principle and the ideal of autonomy are woven together, i.e. a universal principle of autonomy based on an individual's rights is held central to decision-making and patients have the capacity or not to articulate those rights. For older hospitalised people, as seen in this research data, this principle may be hard to operationalise because of illness, decreasing mental and physical ability and institutional rules and obligations. Because of these constraining factors, even the ideal of autonomy may be lost because the capacity to make independent choices is constrained or judged to be limited or non-existent (Fry, 1991).

As highlighted above, arguing against an individual rights concept of autonomy places older hospitalised people in the vulnerable position of being considered to be non-autonomous and therefore legitimise surrogate decision-making (Buchanan and Brock, 1989). Kitwood (1997) has argued that in the field of dementia care, older people with dementing illness are assumed not to be autonomous because of their inability to make decisions and exercise freedom of choice. Kitwood argues that because autonomy in such cases is understood as a capacity based on individual competence, then health care professionals (and others) are justified in making decisions on their behalf. Within this research however, similar processes of surrogacy appeared to be in practice. As was identified in the data, an implicit assessment of individuals' competence for decision making appeared to be in operation - implicit, because the interpretations of individuals decision-making capacity was rarely discussed with patients themselves. Implicit views of patients' competence in decision-making were manifested through the acceptance of the views of family members and other 'objective' assessments as more important than the perceptions of patients themselves. If individuals are rational, fully informed and independent decision makers (as implied in a rights perspective of autonomy) then such decision-making has to be performed by others when individuals are unable to do so for themselves (Agich, 1993). Because of the many internal and external constraining factors identified in this research, then the adoption of a surrogate decision-making perspective is probably inevitable. However a distinction should be made between 'decisional autonomy' and 'executional autonomy' - that is, a distinction between the ability and freedom to make choices and the ability and freedom to carry out and implement choices (Collopy, 1988). Just because an individual does not have the capacity to carry out a decision does not mean that they do not have a right to be involved in the decision-making itself - a position supported by others such as Kitwood (1997). The role of the nurse is that of maintaining and facilitating decisional autonomy when capacity for executional autonomy is reduced or threatened. What is interesting in this research is that while none of the patients participating were deemed to be mentally incompetent (as judged by the results of a mental health assessment), their capacity for executional autonomy was reduced by both internal and external constraining factors. What appeared to be happening is that the value of the patients' well being was defined by the health care team, rather than the patients themselves (Fry, 1991). As a result, the nurse changed position from one of advocate for maximising decisional autonomy to one of 'risk controller'. This was evidenced by such practices as 'doing the stairs', home visits and decisions about the need for residential care. Inevitably, conflict of well being versus autonomy arose.

The role that families played in care decisions can also be legitimised within this perspective. It has been argued (Buchanan and Brock, 1989) that someone closely involved with a patient, other than a health care professional, is in the best position to advocate and make surrogate decisions for them. Indeed such a position is strongly favoured by such organisations as The Centre for Policy in Ageing (Dunning, 1995) which argues strongly in favour of advocates working with older patients to protect them from the power and control of professional care staff. What is evident in this research is the power of family members themselves to assume a superior stance over patients in decision-making and the deference of nurses to family members. This has been referred to in this research as 'the professionalisation of relatives' and represents a paradox in proposals for surrogate decision-making. Studies such as that by High (1991) argue that family members are the most appropriate surrogate decision-makers and that older people themselves prefer family members to represent them. Others, such as that of Uhlmann, Pearlman and Cain (1988) and Zweibel and Cassel (1989) conclude that families are poor substitute decision-makers for elderly relatives. The case for family members involvement in decision-making is well rehearsed in the literature (High, 1991; Barker, 1991; Fry, 1991; Jecker, 1991; Coulton, 1990; Kadushin and Kulys, 1994) and essentially is based on the premise that family members are important sources of information about their relatives' values and previous life choices and often confirm values expressed by patients in conversations with nurses. However Fry (1991) adds a word of caution and highlights the fact that some family members do not know their relatives' values. Jecker (1991; 202) suggests that children may lack the interest or skill to be active players in parents' health care:

> Overwhelmed by its demands, they may reject filial responsibility altogether, they may form coalitions with health professionals that ignore or discount ageing parents, they may push for overtreatment of relatives out of guilt or insist on undertreatment to escape onerous financial or emotional burdens.

While raising this cautious note Jecker (1991) does recognise the important role of family members in care decisions. However, as was evidenced in this research, the place of family members in decision-making set within an individual rights perspective of autonomy is problematic. The primary nurses in this study placed greater emphasis and importance on decisions made by family members, resulting in the erosion of patients' rights to make individual self-determined decisions. As a result, patients' individual autonomy was eroded. Fry (1991) argues from a Rawlsian (Rawls, 1992) perspective of justice that, if family members are to be seen as the 'objective' evidence providers in the assessment of older patients' needs, then there is a need for a differing conception of justice than that of 'rights', as the acceptance of such evidence erodes the older person's right to self-determined decision-making.

However, an important factor that was consistently evident throughout the primary nurses' data was clarity of decision-making. In comparison to the data of the expert nurse and clinical nurse specialist, there was little evidence of the primary nurses clearly framing the nature of the problem or need and articulating a range of possible or potential solutions. Instead, they appeared to engage in a disconnected series of decisions that all had a common purpose of achieving a particular goal, without clear definition of the goal, clear and consistent explanation to the patient and family or a clear plan that was regularly reinforced with the patient and family. In addition, patients were seen to change their minds about their desire for potential care outcomes. While the lack of a clear decision-making framework by the primary nurses and other professionals affected the way care outcomes were achieved, the issue of patients being expected to have an 'objective' view of their lives and thence have clarity about desired outcomes is important to consider.

Autonomy as 'second-order reflection', as discussed in chapter 3 (Frankfurt, 1989; Dworkin, 1989, 1991; Feinberg, 1989) necessitates the hierarchical ordering of desires. An autonomous choice is one that is authentically one's own, that is, it is conceived of one's own reflections and ordering of desires. However Benn (1976) adds a note of 'reality' to the ideal of the self-determining reflective person. Benn argues that at its most basic level, this approach seems to be oblivious of the fact that as a member of society and communities, persons are often 'slaves to convention' and make uncritical choices from established social norms. In relation to making choices about care in hospital, then older people are 'slaves to convention' as much in this setting as any other part of society. In addition policy changes to the delivery of health and social care enforce convention in decisions. Making choices about long-term care is an important example for older people and was particularly evident in this research. While the 'rhetoric of choice' prevails in health and social care policy (Hope, 1996), particularly regarding older peoples' right to choose their long term care arrangements, in reality this ideal is impossible to fully achieve, because state provision of long term care places limits on the choices available to older people. Choices about the place of care delivery, the amount of care provided and the amount of money paid for care provision are all constrained by government policy and financial provision. Choices can be made within these parameters. Primary nurses and care managers in this research were seen to operate within these limitations also and therefore limit choices offered to those that complied with these parameters. This was in contrast to the expert nurse and clinical nurse specialist, who offered choices freely. However, it was also evident that even when older people themselves were paying for their care provision, and in this sense operating within a proper notion of being a consumer, limits were also placed on their choices in terms of quantity of care provided and methods of provision. These factors highlight the 'community' and 'cultural' nature of autonomy. That is the standards and values employed by a person are not of an individual's creation, but are taken from one's culture and development (Norman, 1993; Collopy *et al*, 1991).

The expectation to have an 'objective' view about one's life also fails to recognise that making choices in everyday life is 'monotonous' and a process that we are on the whole 'oblivious of' (Agich, 1993). As Bergmann (1977; 77) asserts:

choice does not hover only between two alternatives; there is rarely just a simple fork, a stark either/or; rather, at every step, we could have moved in countless possible directions whether we realize it or not.

However, in this research, the objectification of older hospitalised people's lives that was expected when making decisions about long-term care arrangements, failed to recognise the multifaceted potential of available options. Instead a 'simple fork' of stark either/or choices was in operation. What it means to be a 'person' in relation to the concept of autonomy has been discussed in chapter 3. As Frankfurt (1989) argued, a key component of being a person is that of being capable to want to be different in preferences and purposes from what we are, or in Berlin's (1992) positive concept of freedom, being conscious of oneself as a thinking, willing, active being, bearing responsibility for one's own choices and being able to explain them through reference to one's own ideas and purposes. While Berlin's concept of freedom is located within an individualistic concept of autonomy, it does emphasise the importance of older people having the freedom to make decisions for themselves. To reiterate Meyers (1989) argument, everybody starts off with an equal capacity to be autonomous (an inborn potential), but individuals learn to exercise it through social experience.

This idea of autonomy as 'interconnectedness' is well established in the literature (*for example* Tronto, 1993; Agich, 1993; Gadow, 1980; Gilligan, 1982) and is based on the premise that people are sometimes autonomous, sometimes dependent and sometimes provide care to those who are dependent (Tronto, 1993). Therefore people are best described as 'interdependent'. Tronto argues that current individualistic notions of autonomy as independence places autonomy and dependence at either end of a continuum. Dependency in some aspects of life does not lead to dependency in all aspects of life. In rejecting an individualistic concept of autonomy Agich (1993) supports the basic tenet of this argument.

The older hospitalised person is dependent on others in a way that is atypical for most other adults. The way such dependency is managed can lead to feelings of either hope and trust or despair and mistrust, as the older person attempts to accommodate the dependence associated with the incapacity as well as needing to rely on caregivers for help in dealing with the initial state of dependence. Dependence associated with disability among older people can lead to infantilization, as the person finds themselves needing supervision and help with essential activities of daily living (Agich, 1993). While located within this perspective of dependency the older person is expected to 'recover' and resume normal or newly defined social roles. As Agich (1993; 96) suggests:

> Given the expectation of recovery and resumption of normal social role activities associated with being sick in our society, it is a constant source of frustration for sick elders, since this usually powerful expression of hope is recognized as pallid and counterfeit. Talk of recovery or doing better can understandably be perceived as mockery or ridicule by an elder who has not adapted to this new state.

An individual's well being is identified by the health care team (Fry, 1991) based on objective diagnostic measurement and professional perceptions including the type and amount of care extended. However, the seriousness of an illness is not measured in such an objective way by older people themselves (Kitwood, 1997; Seedhouse, 1986; Bowling, 1995). The seriousness of an illness is also judged by how much care the older person is willing to accept (Agich, 1993). With the ageing process, the image of the body as an object becomes more of a reality. The alienation experienced as a result of deteriorating physical circumstances offers a daily tangible reminder of the body's limitations to the outside. Such feelings of alienation can result in the individual seeing themselves as less of a person and more like an object, whereby the feelings of alienation within an ageing body limits the person's connection with the outside world (Gadow, 1991). As we age, we need to be able to adapt to the different demands made upon us (Sacks, 1991). The problem is less that of dependence itself, but more about the meaning of dependence to the particular older person and the way such a meaning is facilitated.

In this research, the primary nurses' focus on physical care delivery and the technical management of the discharge plan resulted in a failure to recognise the importance of the transition through dependence that patients were engaged in. In addition, the lack of attention to the emotional 'cues' and expressions of patients resulted in an objectification of their lives. In contrast to the Community Clinical Nurse Specialist who took the lead from the patient and his wife, primary nurses in this research engaged in routinised practices that prevented their recognition of cues being offered by patients and a failure to respond appropriately. This was particularly evidenced in the themes of '*emotional constraints*' and '*lack of skill in dealing with emotion*'.

The routinised and ritualistic approaches to practice that were identified in the data and that prevented a patient centred approach, raised issues about paternalistic practice among primary nurses. The complexity of the interactions between these nurses, patients and their families blurred the boundaries of paternalism and beneficence. The concept of paternalism, with its conceptual roots embedded in parental care for their children, including the making of decisions on their behalf, is rarely considered in positive terms in health care literature.

The idea of respecting the patient's right to self-determination has resulted in a shift in thinking about the role of the patient in health care decision-making and a move towards a 'patient-centred' practice philosophy. Buchanan and Brock (1989) argue that in the large majority of cases, persons are rightly considered to be competent to make health care decisions for themselves, and their decision-making authority ought to be respected by others with no necessity for examining their competence further in the instance at hand. This right to and respect for self-determination in patient care is central to notions of ·patient-centred practice. In doing so, paternalism is rejected as a motivation for action and individual decision-making is respected.

However, it must be remembered that an interaction is not an exclusive three-way encounter between the practitioner, patient and disease. In the world of market economies in health care, a major concern of the practitioner is financial. Even if the practitioner believes that she *knows* what is best for the patient, it may not be possible to proceed in that way because of various organisational constraints. This situation is in evidence in this research and was a dominant focus of discussions during reflective conversations with nurse participants. Throughout these reflective conversations the issue of 'time' was raised. However, there was evidence in the data of an apparent lack of skill in balancing competing aims in practice that further exacerbated the lack of time available to them. This was manifested in the data as lack of negotiation, multiple attempts at closure of conversations, control of conversation agendas, failure to respond to cues and the deferring of decision-making. In this research there was evidence of nurses' perceived need to protect patients' well being acting as a constraint on patient autonomy. The results of this research concur with those of Fried *et al* (1993). Primary nurses were unsure about the limits of their responsibility and accountability for discharge plans. As a result, they were seen to over-compensate for potential 'risky' decisions and considered a 'failed discharge' to be as a result of a bad decision, rather than an unsuccessful risk.

In an understanding of autonomy as the right to self-determination, there is the danger of promoting an ideal whereby the patient is *always* right and any intervention in a patient's decision is paternalistic. Within this research, there was evidence of patients being unsure about the most appropriate decision to make (for reasons already identified). Many cases could be constructed, where the patient would not be the best judge of their own well-being, for example, the older person wanting to remain in their own home even though it is unsuitable for their continued care. In this research, case study 15 (Aidan) represented a particular example of this. While the data analysis focused on the way Aidan's decision to move to residential care was considered coercive and paternalistic, Aidan's ability to cope on his own could be questioned. However, even this case does not present a sufficient argument for a return to paternalism, but instead represents a particular approach to consensus decision making, described by McKinstry (1992) as the doctor (*or health care practitioner* (my alteration)) as agent:

> In this relationship, the doctor does not see him or herself as being in charge, but considers the patient as the final arbiter of all important decisions.

The central tenet of the relationship is honesty and is influenced by such issues as communication skills, knowledge and experience of the nurse, the patient's knowledge and experience, the patient's personality, the nature of the problem and the time available for consultation. When considered against the data in this research (for example case study 15 - Aidan), there is opportunity for a beneficence model of decision-making as opposed to paternalism being in place. Agich (1993) argues that often the difference between the two approaches is a failure to communicate. In Aidan's case (and other case studies) this can be seen to be a fundamental issue. Throughout the data in this research, it was difficult to tell if decisions reached were those that patients would choose for themselves or if indeed nurses were going against patients' authentic desires. This lack of clarity existed because of nurses' (predominantly) failure to communicate effectively with patients, including keeping them fully informed about progress of care outcomes, changes to the context of decisions, barriers to patients' expressed preferences and choices, or the views of other members of the multidisciplinary team. Beauchamp and Childress (1983) assert that:

> the communication between a health professional and a patient should prevent ignorance from constraining autonomous choice, whether ignorance is present from a lack of information or a lack of comprehension.

The complexity of many health care decisions (as is often presented as the argument against consumerism, patients' access to their health records and patient participation in decision-making), coupled with the stresses and fears of illness, with its related anxiety, dependency and regressive tendencies, means that a patient's ordinary decision-making abilities are often significantly diminished. Buchanan and Brock (1989) argue that if the patient holds the ultimate responsibility for their health care decisions, then their treatment choices may fail to serve their well being as conceived by the patient. Thus they argue, the same value of patient well being that requires patients' participation in their own health care decisions may sometimes also require persons to be protected from the harmful consequences to them of their own choices. When considered in practice, the risk to autonomous decision-making by patients from paternalistic health care workers is significant. Siegler (1977) and Szasz and Hollender (1956) assert that the means of preventing such action is by having a clear picture of what the patient really values about their life and how they make sense of the things happening to them. In the exercise of their decision-making capacity, patients bring an individual approach to their concept of their own well-being. Health means different things to different people (Seedhouse, 1986) and is accorded various degrees of importance by individuals - therefore there is no one single intervention for a particular condition that is best for everyone. While certain procedures may be more appropriate than others in particular cases, it is the individuality of the particular case that determines the most appropriate approach. For this reason, health care decision-making ought to take a joint approach from practitioner and patient, as each brings knowledge and experience that the other lacks, yet which is necessary for decisions that will best serve the patient's well-being (Buchanan and Brock, 1989).

So far, the ideal of the liberal notion of autonomy from an individualistic rights based perspective has been presented as an untenable representation of autonomy for older hospitalised people. The complex relationship between nurses, patients, their families and other health care workers as well as the complexity of health and social care decision-making and internal and external constraining factors have been shown to prevent such a concept of autonomy being a viable option. Factors presented in the data are seen to work against older people executing autonomous decisions as consumers of health care. However, it has also been demonstrated that just because an older person lacks the capacity to execute an autonomous decision, this does not mean that they do not have the capacity to exercise decisional autonomy. It is the erosion of decisional autonomy that has been the consistent problem throughout the research data. Indeed what was evident in the data is the extent to which patients weren't involved in decisions, resulting in paternalistic nursing practice. The importance of patients' values in decision-making has been a consistent theme throughout the discussions so far. It is from this perspective that an understanding of autonomy as 'authentic consciousness' with older hospitalised people will now be proposed.

The Concept of Authentic Consciousness

> To be an autonomous agent does not mean that, at bottom, one is independently self-sustaining and capable of critical-reflective reasoning, but rather that the world as an object of experience is held in dynamic relationship by the intentional nature of consciousness itself (Agich, 1993; 120).

In the previous section the problems associated with the adoption of an individualistic rights based conception of autonomy have been identified. One of the central arguments against such a conception was that of the rejection of an atomistic understanding of persons, i.e. as rational agents capable of independent decision-making. In rejecting such a position, autonomy as 'second-order reflection' (Dworkin, 1991) was considered to be particularly problematic when the dominant ideology is that of individualism. It was recognised that such a demand for older hospitalised people is an unrealistic ideal and one that can only serve to justify paternalistic practice. Fundamentally, if therapeutic nursing is dependent on the individual relationship between a nurse and a patient, then attempting to base therapeutic nursing practice on an individualistic concept of autonomy can be seen to be flawed.

However, if the ideal of reflection on one's desires as a means of facilitating autonomous decision-making is removed from an individualistic philosophy and placed within a philosophy of interconnectedness and partnership, then an alternative understanding of autonomy can be achieved and the potential for paternalistic practice minimised. Within the literature, there is a growing recognition of a conceptual understanding of autonomy that recognises the interdependence and interconnectedness of individuals in society, which at the same time respects the uniqueness of persons (*for example* Agich, 1993; Meyers, 1989; Gilligan, 1982; Gadow, 1980; Kitwood, 1997).

The word 'authentic' is often used in discussions about autonomous decision-making (*for example* Kant (Sullivan, 1990); Christman, 1989; Childress, 1982 and Dworkin, 1991). Dworkin (1991) for example argues that to be autonomous a person must have desires that can authentically be considered one's own, with processes of socialisation in society recognised as a necessary part of developing an authentic mode of consciousness and a unique set of values (*for example* Meyers, 1989). An individual's life is always embedded in the culture of the communities from which identity is derived (MacIntyre, 1992). People have a past, present and future and to detach oneself from the past serves to deform the present and plans for the future.

For older people, the recognition of their history acknowledges their social, psychological and cultural biography and that in acknowledging this biography, development continues through their life-span, '*forming the tapestry of one's life*' (Selder, 1989), i.e. that their life continues to be in transition. Transitions can be seen as passages from one life phase, condition, or status to another, incorporating elements of process (*how the transition is managed*), time span (*the time it takes to move to a new state*) and perception (*beliefs and values about the transition and the desire for it to occur*) (Chick and Meleis, 1986). Therefore a transition will occur if a change or disruption to a person's reality necessitates a reorganisation of that reality (Selder, 1989). Reality refers to the everyday world. It is imbued with personal meanings, beliefs and values that are essential to the way the person 'sees' themselves and the way their world is constructed. While many aspects of an individual's reality may be shared with others so that common understandings can exist in order to form a sense of community, it is the individuality of our personal meanings that determines 'who I am'. A person's reality is characterised by relatively stable patterns over time. Within those patterns, the person makes distinctions concerning what reality is and is not. The distinctions made are the threads that are woven uniquely into the tapestry of one's life (Selder, 1989). It is this tapestry of meaning that creates the foundation on which the structures of one's life are built. When the threads of such a tapestry are severed and torn, as occurs through major life events such as illness and disability, then a once stable foundation becomes unstable and the structures of one's life fall. The disruption that ensues extends from the first anticipation of transition until stability in the new reality is achieved (Chick and Meleis, 1986).

From this perception of the older person being in transition and continuous development throughout the life span, it is clear that the idea of authentic person being a free agent who hasn't been tainted by socialisation is not a viable option. As MacIntyre (1992; 221) suggests:

> Without these moral particularities to begin from, there would never be anywhere to begin; but it is in moving forward from such particularity that the search for the good, for the universal, consists.

When applied to a nursing context, Gilligan's (1982) notion of autonomy as 'attachment' suggests that a patient's true potential can be fulfilled if there is an attachment between the nurse and the patient that is based on the patient's unique value system. For Gilligan, each person is emersed in a web of ongoing relationships and being 'in relation' to another is a fundamental part of human existence. Persons are defined by their historical connections and relationships and the aim is not to abstract universalised principles from the particular in order to achieve a 'totally impersonal standpoint' (Kohlberg, 1981). A moral relationship is not about how one impersonal person reacts towards another (impersonal person). Instead the essence of morality is located in the inter-relationship of the subjectivity that both individuals bring to the relationship. To care for a person in this way entails a necessity to know the other. The nurse must take into account the particular person that the patient is, the particular relationship that exists between them and the patient and the particular understandings and expectations implicit in the relationship (Blum, 1982). Such an understanding is achieved through an understanding of the person's authentic values:

> By authentic is meant a way of reaching decisions which are truly one's own - decisions that express all that one believes important about oneself and the world, the entire complexity of one's values (Gadow, 1980; 85).

The nurse knowing about another's authentic values requires caring about the other in a way which appreciates an understanding of each patient as an individual human being, in a particular relationship with herself. Such a particular caring knowledge of patients is necessary in order to determine the particular course of action to take from a variety of potential options. Merely applying a universal principle such as 'do no harm' (UKCC, 1992) or 'do not tell lies' does not inform the nurse what 'harm' means to the particular patient in the particular situation.

Heidegger (1990; 345) recognises the connectedness of persons, but argues that authenticity would be completely misunderstood if it was seen to consist of simply taking up possibilities which have been proposed and recommended, and seizing hold of them. Heidegger argues that only those options that are seen to 'belong' should be considered. What Heidegger appears to be suggesting here is that only those options that fit one's overall values base should be considered as possible options for action. It could be argued that Heidegger is advocating a similar position as Dworkin (1991) in terms of reflection on desires. However, he does not propose a hierarchical ordering of desires, but instead encourages individuals to be mindful of the whole of their lives, by paying attention to the lives of each other. In this way, Heidegger clearly argues against individualism and recognises the importance of considering the effects of autonomous actions on the lives of others. As such, Heidegger's idea of authenticity is consistent with 'community' and 'cultural' perspectives of autonomy (Norman, 1993; Collopy *et al*, 1991).

Heidegger describes his ontological perspective of 'being' through the analogy of a 'workshop' in which tasks are performed. His perspective has particular relevance for older people. Using this analogy Heidegger (1990; 102) describes how a workshop has no place for something that is 'unusable':

> when we concern ourselves with something, the entities which are most closely ready-to-hand may be met as something, unusable, not properly adapted for the use we have decided upon.

Here, the older disabled person is reduced to an object (Gadow, 1991), no longer able to fulfill a role in life. Heidegger goes on to describe how the unusable equipment just lies there as a 'thing' ready to be used but without the ability to function, i.e. the patients viewing themselves as objects without a role to play in life.

This harsh account of older age clearly has implications for the care of older people in hospital. The effects of institutionalisation (Goffman, 1961) have been well documented and others such as Sacks (1991) and Gadow (1991) have demonstrated the impact of older people being reduced to things or objects. Research in the rehabilitation of older people consistently demonstrates the importance of purposeful activities in their lives (Waters and Luker, 1996; Ellul *et al*, 1993; Nolan, 1998; McCormack and Whitehead, 1981; Turner, 1993) as a means of maintaining their connection with their world.

Just because something cannot be used for its original purpose does not mean that it is devoid of any purpose whatsoever - '*The damage to the equipment is still not a mere alteration of a thing*' (Heidegger, 1990; 103). Unless we continue to see the damaged equipment as having meaning, then the equipment that we do accord a usefulness to loses some of its meaning - '*it reveals itself as something just present-at-hand and no more, which cannot be budged without the thing that is missing*' (Heidegger, 1990; 103). Here, the accumulative life experience that the older person brings to a given situation imbues meaning on the situation itself and current practice. The worth of older people, then, is more than an instrumental worth, but represents the positive notion of freedom articulated by Berlin (1992) as thinking, willing and active beings.

A person's authenticity is composed of 'signs' (Heidegger, 1990; 108):

> Among signs there are symptoms, warning signals, signs of things that have happened already, signs by which things are recognized; these have different ways of indicating, regardless of what may be serving as such a sign.

'Signs' represent our lives, i.e. beliefs, values and life experiences. We can treat these either as detached things (as argued in notions of universal principles) that have little significance, or as central to our lives. It is not enough to just take note of another's beliefs, values, views and experiences. They must be integrated into the being in the world for that individual. Being conscious of another's beliefs and values does not tell the nurse what to do, but rather it orientates the nurse to a particular way of being. (I interpret this as meaning, the recognition of beliefs and values does not provide a prescription for action, but instead guides the nurse towards the most appropriate approach for action based on the individual's life experience.) As Gadow (1980) argues, the recognition of the other's beliefs and values allows the older person and the nurse to have the kind of caring relationship that they want to have, appropriate to the context of care. Codes and obligations remain important, but only in the sense of supporting the interconnectedness between the nurse and patient. In recognition of this interconnectedness, the individuality of both parties is made explicit in the relationship. Such an approach requires commitment on the part of the nurse to want to engage in such a relationship and on behalf of the patient to accept it. The nurse cannot impose a particular way of practising on the patient, but instead must be sensitive to his or her individual perspective.

Taking note of 'signs' enables the nurse to place actions in context or as MacIntyre (1992; 210) suggests, '*the act of utterance becomes intelligible by finding its place in a narrative*'. For an individual's values to have meaning they need to be placed in the context of their lives, as we only become aware of our values when they are challenged either positively or negatively (Heidegger, 1990; 112). Without clarifying the meaning of a value in its original context, then it may be difficult to move it from something that is available to us, to something that guides action. If a value cannot be clarified, that doesn't mean it doesn't exist but other values may be needed to access it. For example, even if I value my right to determine decisions for myself, it may not be possible for another person to understand the importance of that value to me until other values have been clarified, such as those I hold about humanism and the importance of fairness and justice in society.

Taking note of 'signs' enables the facilitation of decision-making from the patient's perspective, i.e. facilitate their authenticity. Heidegger argues that when the maintenance of another's authenticity is not a priority in caring practices then there is a danger of stepping into the place of the other and solving the problems or meeting the needs on behalf of the other. Heidegger calls such *practice 'defective solicitude'*, for one becomes dominant and the other is made dependent, thus reducing the other to a thing. In a 'freedom-gaining' relationship (Barker, 1991), one looks ahead with the other to help him or her understand what lies ahead and to develop appropriate coping mechanisms. There are times when such a partnership may not be possible and that one may have to 'leap ahead' of the other in order to facilitate the other's authentic consciousness. The goal remains that of helping the other recognise what he needs for himself and to develop a mechanism for the other to cope successfully on their own. One steps back to enable the other to deploy his or her strategies, but steps forward to support in times of weakness, leaving the other free to determine his or her own fate (Barker, 1991:191; Heidegger, 1990:159). This concept of authenticity concurs with current philosophies of 'personhood' (Kitwood, 1997) within a nurse-patient relationship that requires involvement, risk taking, stepping back to create space and stepping forwards in times of vulnerability. From the data, the key issue appears to be the ability of the nurse to move between these differing modes of 'being' in the relationship in order to reach the best patient outcome.

So, authentic consciousness is understood as a consideration of the whole of one's life in order to sustain meaning in life. Authentic consciousness is not a hierarchical ordering of possible desires, but instead is the clarification of one's values in order to maximise one's potential for growth and development. It is based on the clarification of values and the recognition of the importance of these values in decision-making. The role of the other in a caring relationship is to enable the clarification of values in order to maximise opportunities for growth and the making of authentic decisions, i.e. decisions that are representative of one's life as a whole. For older people, when autonomy is understood as authentic consciousness, the potential for the reduction of the person to a 'thing' is eroded and personhood is maintained.

The 'Life Plan' as a Representation of Authentic Consciousness

Viewing autonomy as authentic consciousness starts from the position that everyone possesses autonomy as an 'inborn potential', but that individuals learn how to exercise it through social experience (Meyers, 1989). Meyers considers autonomy to be a 'competency'. Autonomous people must be able to pose and answer the question - what do I really want, need, care about, believe, value, etcetera? (*self-discovery*); they must be able to act on the answer (*self-direction*) and they must be able to correct themselves when they get the answer wrong (*self-definition*) (Meyers, 1989; 76). To do this, people must have 'autonomy competency' - the repertory of coordinated skills that makes self-discovery, self-definition and self-direction possible.

At first, it might appear incongruous to propose this approach, with its emphasis on reflection on desires and the skill to act, as a means for articulating authentic consciousness. However, a number of underpinning principles of this approach make it consistent with the overall findings from this research. Firstly, it is based on the premise that virtually everybody has the inborn potential necessary for autonomy, but that they learn how to conduct their lives through processes of socialisation. For older people in general (but older hospitalised people in particular) the effects of socialisation have been identified as a significant factor on the way they experience health care. However, as adults, they have the same inborn potential as all other adults and are affected by socialisation in the same way as other adults in a similar culture. This leads to the second consideration - that because various internal and external constraints may be in place that prevent an individual's full potential from being realised, this does not mean that they do not have the potential for autonomy. Because Meyers' position is established from recognition of the impact of socialisation, then she is not proposing an atomistic perspective of persons, but instead recognises that people may need assistance in determining the most appropriate course of action. Thirdly, this approach demands that the nurse's role in the care of older people focuses on facilitating an individual's authentic consciousness, so that their full potential can be realised and their capacity to exercise autonomous action maximised through facilitating the erosion of constraining factors.

The representation of individual authentic consciousness is through a 'life plan'. A life plan is not merely a list of objectives with a plan and strategies for carrying them out - a mechanical list. A life plan is a presentation of what a person wants to do in life (Meyers, 1989: 49). It enables reflection on life goals within the context of achieving integration in ones' life. Life plans evolve over time, with new experiences that are consistent with one's life plan being integrated into it in order to create future goals and projects. A life plan would include at least one activity that the person wants to pursue, or a value that the person wants to advance or an emotional bond that the person wants to sustain. As most people have a variety of activities, values and emotions that they would wish to be identified with, then typically a life plan would consist of an ordering of assorted desires and concerns and some ordering of their priority, so that they can invest time and energy appropriately:

> ... it recognizes that the authentic self is dynamic and explains how individuals can gain control over their selves, along with their conduct. ... The self of the person who exercises autonomy competency, then, is an authentic self - a self-chosen identity rooted in the individual's most abiding feelings and firmest convictions, yet subject to the critical perspective autonomy competency affords (Meyers, 1989; 61).

So, for example, the older person considering the option of moving to residential care, may list values such as retention of their independence, family contact, contact with friends and colleagues, being able to attend religious services in their local church, being able to eat what they want and when they want it, as values that they hold central to their decision-making. However, maintaining contact with their family may be the overriding desire and therefore assumes greater importance than other desires. In choosing suitable residential care, this desire would be given greatest priority.

However, as already identified, throughout the life span, individuals continually grow, develop and experience transition and so there is always the potential for a new direction in life to be taken. So long as this new direction is consistent with the individual's authentic consciousness, then the evolving-self can be accommodated within this approach. If a person's life plan contains conflicting traits and goals, then the individual can be paralysed by confusion and ambivalence and would rarely be able to act with confidence that the action satisfactorily represents his or her true self (Meyers, 1989). Self-definition (reflection) on the effectiveness of decisions is always considered against authentic consciousness.

In terms of making choices within a life plan, Meyers adopts Rawls (1992) perspective on rational choice. The making of choices has two components - rational choice and deliberative rationality.

For a choice to be rational, a person must know what sorts of things are important to them, must evaluate the relative intensity of their desires, must order their preferences consistently and must envisage alternative plans for action (Rawls, 1992; 418-419). These principles enable people to opt for the plan that will enable the achievement of more 'ends' than other potential plans and for the one that is most likely to succeed. While Rawls argues from a rational perspective that decisions should be postponed until all necessary information has been availed of, he does also recognise that being aware of the dominant values in one's life and aiming to achieve unity and consistency of values, should enable the making of decisions based on what they intuitively know is best for them (Rawls, 1992; 412). In the making of rational choice, the principle of adopting the plan which maximises the expected net balance of satisfactions is the one to be chosen, that is, the person should choose the course that is most likely to achieve their most important aims (Rawls, 1992; 416).

Deliberative rationality is the choosing of the plan that is most consistent with one's overall values and other principles, such as, being consistent with the dominant theme in one's decisions and the avoidance of inconsistency (Rawls, 1992; 417). However, Meyers rightly argues that without others' interpretations of choices, then the process of deliberation is reduced to an individualistic self-referential process. Without the consideration of others' perspectives then an atomistic view of autonomy re-emerges and the effects of socialisation ignored.

Life plans are formed through, memory, reflection, imagination and through conversation with others. Through reflection on an individual's values, individual traits and broad ambitions, various options for action are outlined. Evaluation of an option is undertaken based on its consistency with overall values, its potential for achieving more 'ends' than other potential plans, the one that is most likely to succeed, but most importantly, the one that is most likely to achieve their most important aims. It may be necessary to divide an option up into particular segments to enable thorough reflection and evaluation. The person can explore how they would feel about particular outcomes from choosing that option or how they would behave if that outcome was chosen. Their attraction to or aversion from the potential outcomes and behaviours and their strength of feeling about these provides a yardstick for assessment of options.

Meyers (1989; 83) argues that unless people are able to carry out their desired life-plans, then their deliberations will be wasted. She suggests that both 'resistance' and 'resolve' are required to do this - resistance of unwarranted pressure from other individuals and resolve in one's determination to act on his or her own judgements. However, the data in this research has identified how difficult it is for older people in hospital to sustain their resistance and resolve in the making of autonomous decisions. In recognising this issue as the single most important factor in enabling autonomy as authentic consciousness becoming a reality, then the role of the nurse as a facilitator of authentic consciousness will be explored in chapter ten.

Conclusions

This chapter has criticised the ideal of the liberal notion of autonomy from an individualistic rights based perspective as an untenable representation of autonomy for older hospitalised people. The complex relationship between nurses, patients, their families and other health care workers as well as the complexity of health and social care decision-making and internal and external constraining factors have been shown to prevent such a concept of autonomy being a viable option. The importance of patients' values in decision-making has been a consistent theme throughout the discussions and it is from this perspective that an understanding of patient autonomy as 'authentic consciousness' with older hospitalised people has been proposed. Authentic consciousness is understood as a consideration of the whole of one's life in order to sustain meaning in life based on the clarification of one's values in order to maximise one's potential for growth and development. The recognition of these values as central to decision-making is emphasised in the facilitation of autonomy with older people. Authentic consciousness with the centrality of values is most appropriately conceptualised through a 'life plan' - a presentation of what a person wants to do in life. Such a plan enables the clarification of values, identify consistent themes in decision-making and plan future action. The interactive nature of life-plans prevents an atomistic understanding of autonomy from being perpetuated.

From this perspective, the role of the 'other' in a caring relationship is to enable the clarification of values in order to maximise opportunities for growth and the making of authentic decisions, i.e. decisions that are representative of one's life as a whole. For older people, when autonomy is understood as authentic consciousness, the potential for the reduction of the person to a 'thing' is eroded and personhood is maintained. However, as was identified in this research, the internal and external constraining factors that exist in practice work against such an approach being adopted. Therefore, Chapter 10 will explore key principles necessary for practice if autonomy as authentic consciousness is to be realised.

10 The Nurse as Facilitator of Authentic Consciousness

Introduction

This chapter will explore the idea of the nurse as a facilitator of authentic consciousness. The themes of informed flexibility; sympathetic presence; negotiation; mutuality and transparency, identified in chapter 8 that have been used to articulate the 'Principles for Action' derived from the data will be presented as 'Imperfect Duties', i.e. maxims that guide action, but account for context, individual preference and values. It will be proposed in this chapter that these imperfect duties can form the basis of an approach to person-centred practice that enables the facilitation of an older person's authentic consciousness. Using the developmental themes derived from the focus group interview with expert nurses, recommendations for changes to nursing practice with older people will be made, so that such an approach could be adopted in practice.

The Care Situation

In the facilitation of authentic consciousness, freedom of self-determination is seen as a fundamental and valuable human right. This however, is not the negative view of freedom as criticised in Chapter 9. Instead it is based on the interdependent and interconnected relationship of persons and the belief that individuals sometimes need assistance with decision-making (Gadow, 1980; 85):

> individuals be assisted by nursing to authentically exercise their freedom of self-determination. By authentic is meant a way of reaching decisions which are truly one's own-decisions that express all that one believes important about oneself and the world, the entire complexity of one's values.

Working in this way requires a centrality of values, including the clarification of contradictions and conflicts. It requires the re-examination of values in the context of the new care situation that the person is in or moving to (Benner and Wrubel, 1989). To work in this way requires a connectedness (Gilligan, 1982) between the nurse and the patient and a consideration of the patient as a whole person.

The care situation focuses on the facilitation of an individual's authentic consciousness through the consideration of his or her values, experiences, moral principles and organisational concerns. Each individual patient interaction denotes a care situation. If each care situation is approached as a unique interaction and that the focus is on the interaction with that patient at that time, then ethical standards can be maintained based on the individual's life plan, with broader political factors acting as influences rather than controls. However, total connectedness with a patient can lead to 'ethical blindness' (Benner and Wrubel, 1989) and in order to balance the intensity of an individual relationship with a reflective approach to decision making, the nurse needs to move between three 'stances' when working with patients (after Heidegger, 1990). These stances represent different levels of engagement (connectedness) between the nurse and patient.

Engagement (Ready-to-Hand) in this stance the patient and nurse are connected in the relationship. The nurse and patient are extensions of each other's being and a care partnership exists. Collaborative decision-making takes place and the values of both nurse and patient are present at an unconscious level in the giving and receiving of care. The nurse may be aware of political, environmental and cultural pressures that impact upon the way she gives care, but she interprets and prioritises the salient features of such pressures and integrates these into her practice. However, a dilemma may arise in the care relationship that effects the way the nurse and patient are able to work together.

As a result *partial disengagement (Unready-to-Hand)* occurs while the nurse takes stock of the situation and formulates the problem. In this stance, an unusual (novel) situation occurs that interrupts the interconnected working between the nurse and patient. Whatever the cause, the relationship between the nurse and patient is altered and the nurse may lose the maximum grasp that was available while engaged with the patient (Benner and Wrubel, 1989).

Such disengagement then requires a period of contemplation and, for a period of time, *complete disengagement (Present-to-Hand)* occurs. In this stance the nurse contemplates the available options from a more objective stance. The nurse re-assesses the values that underpin the relationship and decision-making. The nurse may use available mechanisms to decide on appropriate action and to reconnect the relationship. Such mechanisms as supported reflective practice (Johns, 1997; 1998), clinical supervision (Bishop, 1998) and case reviews (Robbins, 1996) all help achieve this goal. While the nurse continues to work with the patient in seeking the most satisfactory resolution, the connectedness in the relationship is broken until such time as a resolution can be found that is coherent with the values of the patient.

A skilled nurse will be able to adopt these different stances at different times with the patient and were indeed evident in the practice of the expert nurse and the clinical nurse specialist. Each stance may be short lived, but what is important is for the nurse to be able to move between these positions in order to stand back from the relationship with the patient, contemplate options and establish the most appropriate resolution. In contemplating options and choices three factors have been identified from the analysis thus far, that are considered important in the creation of an environment that facilitates authentic consciousness:

- The Patient's Values.
- The Nurse's Values and Expertise.
- The Context of Care.

The Patient's Values

It has been argued thus far that having a clear picture of what the patient values about his life and how he makes sense of what is happening to him is needed. This provides a standard against which the practitioner can compare current decisions and behaviours of the patient with those values and preferences made in life in general and which form the basis of a life plan (Meyers, 1989).

As has been highlighted in the data analysis, the meaning of life for older people is not demonstrated through the tedium of superficial daily life (Katz, 1990). Latimer (1997) and Agich (1993) (*for example*) warn against the exclusive reliance on general and functional abilities as the mode of assessing an individual's capacity for autonomous action.

Approaches to patient assessment that include a 'biographical account' using narrative and story, is one method of establishing a baseline value history and establishing a life-plan. There is wide recognition of the value of biography in social gerontology (Dex, 1991; Bertaux, 1981 *for example*), particularly as a means of understanding older people in terms of what older age means to them. Biographical approaches emphasise an understanding of older people's own definition of their needs through their accounts of their lives and planning services to meet these definitions of need (Bornat, 1994). While in the 1970's Johnson (1976) argued for an approach to the assessment of needs based on individual life histories, it is only recently, that there has been an increasing emphasis on the value of this approach (Johnson, 1991).

Primary nurses in this research afforded low priority to story telling by patients as compared with the approach adopted by the clinical nurse specialist. They were seen to dismiss these stories as irrelevant to the conversation agenda or treat them as stories, that is, as fictional tales that had little relevance to the particular interaction. Both the expert nurse and clinical nurse specialist however, were seen to adopt a differing approach and integrated patients stories in the conversation agenda and utilised their interpretations of stories to evaluate previous utterances and formulate next questions. These two differing approaches by the nurses in this study, illustrate two common approaches to storytelling in the care of older people (Agich, 1993). The first approach treats stories as accounts of the past that objectively happened to the individual up to the present. The aim is discovery of what 'really' happened to the person and according to Agich (1993; 91), it represents a technical approach to biography that is aimed at depicting an objective account of an older person's life story:

> The knower is simply assumed to be the passive net that gathers the true facts of the past, or, at worse, as someone who distorts what really happened. Once it is taken for granted that an individual has a real past that occurred and is knowable, it becomes mostly a technical affair to know someone's past, personal history, or life story.

The second approach, the one that has greatest relevance to the facilitation of an individual's authentic consciousness, is an understanding of biography as an interpretative process. Agich (1993) is critical of technical approaches to biography and he argues that the uniqueness and individuality of stories is often overlooked. Life stories are not constructions of a past that is 'out there', separate from the individual's current experiences and that has been discovered through the process of story telling. Instead, constructing a biography is an interpretative process that involves the conferring of meaning about oneself and the whole of one's life course. The purpose of the story is to make sense of the present in light of the past. Whether the account is objective or a subjective construction of a reality is not important, as it is the account developed in the present with the purpose of making sense of things. However, Agich warns against professional interpretations of biographies that produce accounts from a nursing or medical perspective. An interpretation of a biography should be that of the biographer.

This approach is currently evidenced through approaches to reminiscence and life review which attempt to aide an understanding of the meaning of life, through a wish to find in the experience of older people, elements of strength and positive affirmation (Moody, 1991). Even though life around the person may have little meaning or significance, through individual life review, the person may discover meaning in *his or her* own life. Assisting the individual to find this meaning may help them to tolerate the incongruity of their current situation and create a future. As Moody (1991) asserts, if my life is intelligible, my life has purpose and my hopes and desires ultimately can be satisfied, then happiness can be found.

An individual interpretative biographical approach to the assessment of need and the planning of care inputs can be seen to be essential to the development of a life plan. The foundation of the life plan approach is an understanding of the individual's life values. Understanding the individual's interpretation of their current situation from the basis of their interpretation of their past, provides one of the most important modes of access to what is important to them (Agich, 1993; 92):

> Life stories indicate the things that people value most; they tell us who the person is and with what they most identify.

Respecting the individual beliefs and values of the patient rejects the concept of paternalism and prepares the way for a model of decision making based on the individual's authentic consciousness. Basing care decisions on the patient's value history could be deemed idealist and in an ideal notion of autonomy places the nurse in a powerless position, whereby only those decisions that are made by the patient and that are consistent with their value history could be followed. Indeed it is argued (Fulford, 1997) that such a position reduces (nursing) to responding to the requests and demands of patients without a need to consider broader professional and sociological implications. However as argued in chapter 9, in reality many cases could be constructed where the patient would not be the best judge of their own well-being, e.g. the older person who insists on returning to their own home even though it is uninhabitable. However, even cases such as these do not present a sufficient argument for paternalistic decision making by nurses. In collaborative decision-making, the nurse does not see herself as being in charge, but places the patient's values (or their advocate) central in determining a resolution in important decisions. The central tenet of the relationship is honesty and is influenced by communication skills, knowledge and experience of the patient, the patient's knowledge and experience, the patient's personality, the nature of the problem and the time available for the decision to be made. While certain approaches may be more appropriate than others in particular cases, it is the individuality of the particular case that determines the way forward. For this reason, decision-making ought to take a joint approach between practitioner and patient, as each brings knowledge and experience that the other lacks, yet which is necessary for decisions that will best serve the patient's well-being (Buchanan and Brock, 1989; 30):

> In the exercise of their right to give informed consent, then, patients commonly decide in ways that they believe will best promote their well-being as they conceive it.

Working with authentic consciousness allows patients to have the relationship that they want to have with a nurse. Therefore the adoption of a passive role by a patient does not equate with a lack of autonomy, but instead is a confirmation of the patient's autonomy based on his or her values history. However, as current research indicates, professional carers need to be open to listening and hearing the stories of older people and valuing this activity as an important part of care giving (Goldsmith, 1996, *for example*).

The Nurse's Values and Expertise

Although the language of partnership is commonplace and as discussed earlier, nurses are encouraged to 'soften' their professional presentation to the patient, it remains unusual for nurses to present their own views as a component of the array of information that patients are given to assist their decisions. While the patient's values should be the decisive ones (Gadow, 1990) the nurse's values also contribute to the process. Indeed it could be argued that if a connected relationship exists between the nurse and patient, then it is especially important that the nurse's values are expressed - particularly when they conflict with the patient's values. If the nurse is truly working in partnership with the patient then there is no reason why the expression of such values should be coercive. Instead, the disclosure of the nurse's values may help the patient to understand particular approaches taken by the nurse and it may offer the patient an alternative view when considering their own values. Such an approach, however, requires skilled and sensitive communication on the part of the nurse and an ability to judge when is the most appropriate time for disclosure. For example, it would be inappropriate to pre-judge an elderly person's partner as 'uncaring' should that person express the desire not to carry on a caring role. However, it may be appropriate to express the importance of family relationships in the lives of older people as a means of helping the carer to see another perspective. Disclosure of values by the nurse is not to persuade the patient or inform them of most appropriate action. It is however, as argued by Gadow (1990) a demonstration to the patient that the nurse considers values important not as a way of impersonally prescribing action, but as a professional commitment to ethical reflection.

The nurse can offer an alternative perspective that complements the perspective of the patient. In addition, it has been argued that the atomistic perspective of autonomy with its emphasis on individualistic reflection on decisions and actions is only a partial perspective, as it fails to consider implications of decisions that may not be a part of the individual's reality. Therefore, the expression of values by the nurse serves to complete the partial perspective of the patient, with a focus that is formed from experience and knowledge of typical cases (Gadow, 1990). Indeed the need for ethical reflection by the nurse is paramount in effective decision-making (Johns, 1998) and the development of clinical expertise (Manley and McCormack, 1997). A care environment, that provides opportunities for practitioners to learn from their practice, explore and clarify their values and develop expertise in supporting patient-centred ethical decision making, can enable the development of expertise in patient-centred practice (Manley and McCormack, 1997). These factors will be explored further, later in this chapter.

The Context of Care

The context in which care is provided has the greatest potential to enhance or limit the facilitation of authentic consciousness as identified through the data in this research. When facilitating autonomous decision-making, nurses find they not only balance competing care values, but often they find it necessary to consider organisational values too. Nurses are not free to exert autonomous moral authority and on occasions they may find themselves having to accept a forced choice (Yarling and McElmurry, 1990). Nurses are not free to fulfill a moral obligation to the patient without considering organisational and professional implications (Johns, 1995). In contemporary health care, the fundamental moral predicament of nurses is that while they are expected to engage in autonomous decision-making (Manthey, 1980), they are often deprived of the freedom to exercise moral authority (Johnstone, 1989).

The context in which care is provided offers particular challenges to nurses in contemporary health care. Research by Savage (1995) challenges the possibilities of patient-centred care, because the values articulated through the internal market directly oppose the humanistic care values that underpin patient-centredness. 'New Nursing' (Salvage, 1990), with its emphasis on connectedness between the nurse and patient that can only be sustained in a continuous skilled nurse-patient relationship, and the language of the market, that emphasises cost effectiveness, efficiency, and productivity, are considered to be direct opposites. However, it is all too easy to become distracted by the political tensions of care and the forces that appear to work against effective patient-centred practice. It is precisely because of these forces that there is a need to clarify principles that underpin an approach to patient-centered practice that is based on a facilitation of another's authentic consciousness.

The Place of Imperfect Duties

The term 'imperfect duties' is derived from Kant (Sullivan, 1990). In the development of his universal theory and the categorical imperative, Kant made a distinction between perfect and imperfect duties. Perfect duties are strict and enforceable. Principles can be morally 'forced' to honour the duty prescribed. Being moral entails compliance with valid rights, no matter whether doing so conflicts with other moral goods or other values.

In contrast, imperfect duties are '*wide, broad and limited*' - '*they leave us a play-room for free choice in following the law*' (Sullivan, 1990; 52) as there is no means of offering an exhaustive and a priori account of how the duties are to be fulfilled. Such duties as compassion, concern, benevolence, respect and care would all be imperfect duties. One cannot force someone to be caring. Instead, imperfect duties rely on the moral character of the individual, or what Kitson (1987) refers to as '*a moral attitude*'. Kant views such duties as 'imperfect' because in ethical decision-making one may have to decide between competing duties and account must be taken of the context in which decisions are made. Nurses should not only focus on developing moral reasoning and decision-making skills, but also on developing moral sensitivity and an individual sense of moral responsibility. In this sense, the importance of education for moral reasoning and for the character traits that are desired in a relationship such as that between a nurse and patient is paramount.

In Chapter 9, the importance of context in decision-making and the problems of a 'rights' based approach to autonomy have been articulated. It was argued that the complex relationship between nurses, patients, their families and other health care workers as well as the complexity of health and social care decision-making and internal and external constraining factors prevent such a concept of autonomy being a viable option. In addition, the importance of patients' values in decision-making was identified as a significant issue in the research data and it is from this perspective that an understanding of autonomy as authentic consciousness with older hospitalised people has been proposed. While this approach emphasises the centrality of a patient's values in decision-making, five 'imperfect duties' (derived from a thematic analysis of the 'Principles for Action') are considered to be important to the operationalisation of this approach - informed flexibility; sympathetic presence; negotiation; mutuality and transparency. These duties will be presented in the following way:

- Definition of the duty;
- Description of its meaning;
- Key attributes;
- Enabling factors.

and organised into the conceptual framework illustrated in Figure 8.

Figure 8: **Autonomy as Authentic Consciousness - Conceptual Framework**

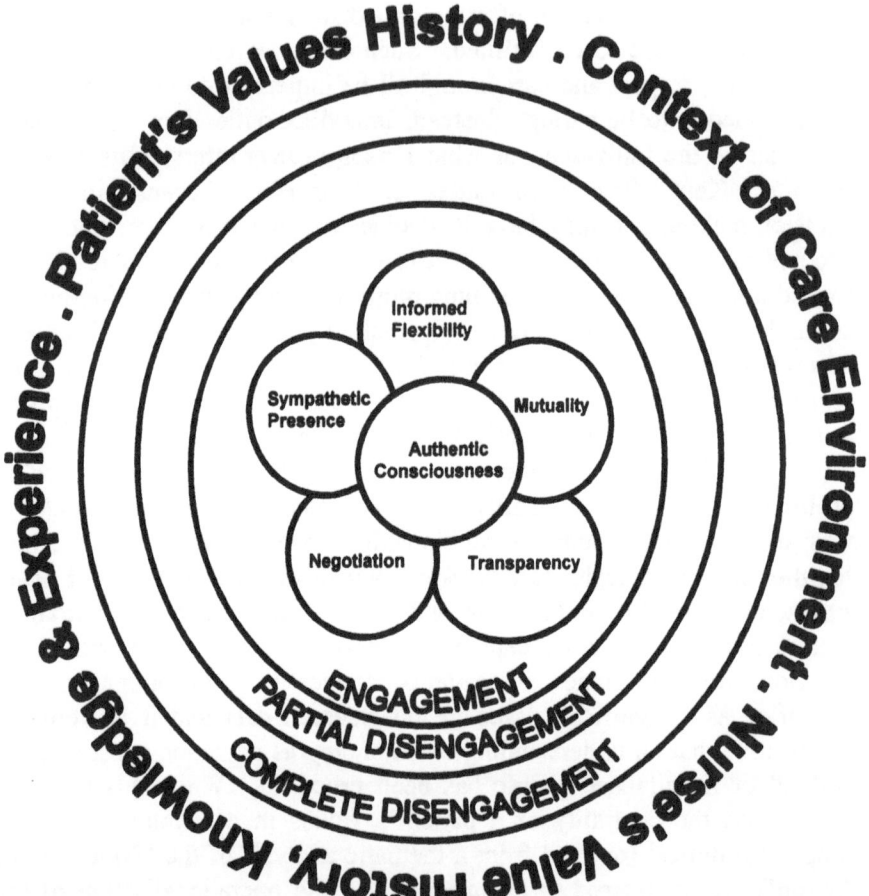

Informed Flexibility

Definition   The facilitation of decision-making through information sharing and the integration of new information into established perspectives and care practices.

Description This research suggests that 'doing for' people is what nurses do best and is supported by other studies such as that of Waters and Luker (1996). However, the negative connotations that are associated with such activity usually equate with paternalistic nursing practice, whereby the older person is passive and the nurse is active. It often implies that the nurse is in the best position to make decisions for the patient and can therefore perform the activity on behalf of that person. However, this does not imply passivity on the part of the patient. Wade (1983) describes an approach to care that is characterised by consultation and involvement of the patients in their care programme. Their adulthood is recognised and every effort is made to maximise their physical and mental independence. Having a clear goal of care that is understood by the patient, family and significant others is central to this approach. This active involvement provides a form of rehabilitation that is aimed at improving functional independence, improving competence in self-care activities, preventing secondary complications, and promoting psychological well-being, confidence and self-esteem (RCN, 1993). Continuing assessment of people's needs should include an evaluation of how the person could or does function in a socially productive manner, in addition to the typical focus on problems, pathology and losses (Hutchinson and Bahr, 1991).

Restoration of self-worth through the experience of respect from others can bring about a form of healing in itself. Confirming another's self-worth, also includes recognising the health potential of the person irrespective of their current health state. Health seen as 'potential' (Seedhouse, 1986) prevents fatalism in approaches to care, demonstrated through negative nursing behaviours of apathy and neglect, with the underlying assumption being that as older people are unwilling/unable to change old behaviours or learn new ones, health promotion is not relevant (RCN, 1993).

Key Attributes;

- Information provided in a way that is relevant to the patient's ability to understand it and in a way that is meaningful to their life plan.
- Having a clear goal of care that aims to maximise the individual's capacity to achieve independence.
- Facilitation of knowledge and understanding of care processes, that empowers the individual to gain further knowledge in the context of their life experiences and altered levels of independence.
- Regular reinforcement of care decisions, integration of new information and formulation of new decisions in partnership with the patient.
- Recognition of the uniqueness of the patient's hospital experience.

Enabling Factors;

- Nurses' conversational competence - having a repertoire of conversational approaches and the ability to appropriately frame questions.
- Flexibility in the organisation of services and non-routinised approaches to care practices.
- Care policies and procedures that aim to maximise independence.

Sympathetic Presence

Definition   An engagement that recognises the uniqueness and value of the individual, by appropriately responding to cues that maximise coping resources through the recognition of important agendas in daily life.

Description the environment of the care setting should avoid making premature assumptions about people. The setting should offer a stability in which the person can find his or her unique individuality within it. An objective understanding of the ageing body, an understanding of the individual's subjective interpretation of their own ageing journey and the individual meanings attached contributes to a sense of wholeness and allows the nurse to enter the subjective world of the older person to meet care needs. Acceptance of the older person's life ways is perhaps one of the most humanistic qualities shown in nursing care. The older person is mindful of the many roles played during life and the losses suffered over the years.

To have a nurse show, through acceptance of the person, an empathic understanding of the patient's losses and present limitations, is to establish a therapeutic relationship which is directed at gaining an effective outcome from care that is centred on the person's needs and life perspectives. This understanding of the person's self-worth directs the nurse towards flexibility in nursing care that seeks to preserve the integrity of the person. It also, through the appreciation of the individual's uniqueness, makes explicit to the nurse, the limits beyond which the person cannot be taken and prevents the setting of unrealistic objectives. If nursing older people is to be directed towards a humanistic philosophy, then as many opportunities as possible should be made available for the older person to exercise freedom of choice, take risks, express opinions, make decisions and be listened to! The according of such respect to the older person can in itself offer an approach to the 'healing' of the body and the restoration of individual self-worth. As Taylor (1992; 110) proclaimed:

> As older women we are a considerable force once we own our strength. We can use it by becoming teachers. Acknowledge that you have a sense of destiny, that you know who you are and have something to say, Say it! You may be a film-maker or a writer. You may want to stand on a box and shout about it, you may make a basket or weave a rug. At whatever level, be a teacher - an exemplar. Say I have done something worthwhile with my life and I count.

Key Attributes;

- Acknowledgement of the individual's 'emotional coping ability' and the facilitation of emotional responses to their experiences.
- The setting of a conversational agenda that acknowledges the centrality of the patient's life history as an expression of their values that underpin care plans.
- The recognition of the nurse's role in the prevention of constraints that negate autonomous decision-making.

Enabling Factors;

- Recognition of the power of language and the effects of language on the autonomy of the other.
- The use of an appropriate questioning style that facilitates the setting of a patient-centred conversation agenda.
- Non-ageist decision making.

Negotiation

Definition   Patient participation through a culture of care that values the views of the patient as a legitimate basis for decision-making while recognising that being the final arbiter of decisions is of secondary importance.

Description the importance of approaching assessment from the patient's perspective is paramount. If the focus of assessment of older people's needs is based purely on the functional assessment of activities of daily living, then an understanding of the person's uniqueness can never be gained. Is that person really just a collection of body systems that all meet together conveniently, and on the basis that one or more of them has malfunctioned, thus requires care? ... or alternatively is that person a unique individual who has marked out a unique journey in order to reach this stage of their life and now requires help to move on to the next stage? By taking a biographical approach to assessment the nurse can establish a 'picture' that is individual and unique. A person's biography can be seen as an account of a number of separate but related life events that have influenced and directed the person's life. It is the history that gives meaning to the values of the individual and provides the explanations that are needed when crises occur and care decisions are being chosen (Johnson, 1991). Indeed Schofield (1994) suggests that an experienced nurse will be able to recognise when biographical details are important to clarify concerns in care, thereby identifying the appropriate focus of care and the maintenance of the person's integrity.

Key Attributes;

- Patients' ownership of health solutions for care decisions set within a framework of collaboration.

- Facilitation of patients' life reviews as a means of establishing the values that need to be held central to care decisions.
- The involvement of the family and significant others in the provision of information necessary for negotiated decision-making.

Enabling Factors;

- Working within a collaborative framework that values the 'subjective' views of the patient equally with other 'objective' measures.
- Establishing a negotiation framework that seeks to clarify the patient's values in the situation and that enable the establishment of a life plan.
- Recognition of the inter-dependence of the older person in society.

Mutuality

Definition   The recognition of the others' values as being of equal importance in decision-making.

Description the nurse must believe in the inherent worth of the recipients of care and in their strengths and capabilities. Central to this notion of mutuality is the fundamental belief in the autonomy of the patient. Promoting individual autonomy should be a dynamic and interrelated partnership between nurse and patient. It should not be based on assumptions about what the person might want to do, or on the desire to protect the rights of individuals to do what they want. But it should be the effort to help persons become clear about what they want to do, by helping them discern their values in the situation (Gadow, 1990). It may only be through the confirmation of their values that a person's decision can be self-determined. Once the decision has been made, it is therefore the role of the nurse to provide the support necessary for the person to reach the desired goal(s). This calls for expertise in flexibility and creativity in nursing care. The nurse facilitates coping and reinforces normality in daily life through presencing (Benner, 1984) - the art of 'being with' a person without the need to be 'doing to' the person. A nurse, who thus allows herself to respond to the individuality of each person, will in some way allow herself to be a different nurse to each person. She will also find herself changing with time as expertise in facilitating decision-making grows and develops and in response to the changing needs of individuals. Central to this approach is the aim of providing a therapeutic environment.

Such an environment is not achieved by the emphasis on 'hygienic factors' alone (Miller and Gwynne, 1972). While the provision of comfortable and pleasant care conditions goes some way towards the creation of a therapeutic environment, the relationship between patient and carer can guarantee it. However this is not a one-way relationship, i.e. nurse to patient, but is indeed a reciprocal relationship where both parties grow as a result of the relationship. Growth through learning, challenge and the expression of emotions, aids the development of qualities of imagination, compassion and self-realisation in practice. This relationship establishes a personal-professional connection based on mutual respect and honesty (Genevay and Katz, 1990). It involves 'being with' and 'doing with', through the active participation of the patient in order to activate the potential within themselves.

Working with an older person in this way can be thought of as a mutual process of learning, or as Casement (1988) sees it - '*I as a nurse am learning from the patient*'. If a nurse can trust in the relationship she has with a patient, then it is all right to be led by the patient, not in a passive sense of being led but in a dynamic sense where the cues and nuances of the patient's behaviour direct the focus of the action that needs to be taken. The patient is thus given a real part to play in helping the nurse discover new ways of working and a real partnership is established. Fresh insights emerge and the tendency to fall back onto old ritualised practices is avoided. There are of course other times when firmness in approach has to be taken and sometimes without this firmness the person would feel insecure and at risk. However as long as the reasons for this are negotiated into the plan of care, partnership can still be maintained. Through mutuality, those who care and those who are cared for, don't have to relate to each other as strong and weak, but both can grow in each other's capacity to learn from each other as equals. Therefore the focus is on helping the older person to look at him/herself in the context of a *citizen*, rather than through the limited context of a patient.

Key Attributes;

- Patients' perceptions being of equal value to the perceptions of nurses and other health care workers.
- Respect for patients' subjective view of their lives, as presented through their historical accounts as central to negotiated care decisions.

- The expression of values by the nurse in order to complete the partial perspective held by the patient.
- The reinforcement of patients' decisions in a multidisciplinary context in order to reduce organisational constraints on autonomous decision-making.

Enabling Factors;

- A willingness to listen to and understand patients' expression of their values and to hold these central to decision-making.
- A willingness to work with the perceptions and understandings of family and significant others and to integrate these perceptions with those of the patient in establishing a plan of care.
- A willingness to suspend prior knowledge/understanding until the patient has told their 'story'.
- A willingness to learn from the relationship with the patient.

Transparency

Definition   The making explicit of intentions and motivations for action and the boundaries within which care decisions are set.

Description being transparent involves helping the person make sense out of what is happening to them in their world. The emphasis is on helping the person cope with threats to their identity and make the transition to their new world. It avoids making assumptions about the individual or the imposition of rules and regulations before the individual has established their own identity. The nurse, in being with the person, seeks to determine the personal meaning which the experience of illness, suffering or dying is to have for that individual (Gadow, 1980). Ultimately, the individual's self-determination means understanding the meaning of an experience, before decisions are reached about how best to respond practically to the experience. The experience of disability can create a dissonance between the person and the body. The nurse is in the unique position of bridging these extremes and creating harmony and integrity. The nurse can assist the individual to understand their body, accept it as their own and 'live it' instead of allowing it to remain alien. The nurse becomes a professional friend and the nurse-patient relationship assumes some of the qualities usually described as part of a socially meaningful relationship. Many usual nursing tasks remain important, as it is through these that the physical needs of the person are met. But, as a friend, the nurse needs to know herself, what she is able to give and when to draw the line. In knowing this, the nurse makes explicit the boundaries of decision-making and is explicit about the degree of risk that is possible in decisions and ways of minimising risk. Acceptance of individuality and ethical reflection are fundamental to being transparent in care decisions. When a nurse goes more by the older person's direction and less by her own particular agenda or that of the organisation, it becomes easier to notice when the person is feeling out of tune with what is being planned and the direction that he/she is being taken. Unquestioning acceptance of organisational constraints on individuality is no excuse for the erosion of the person's ability to exercise their full decision-making potential.

Key Attributes;

- An understanding of patients' expectations of health care/health care practitioners and working with these expectations to minimise constraints on autonomous action.
- An assessment of risks in decision-making and the limits beyond which risks cannot be taken.
- The explicit expression of values in care decisions.
- The balancing of nurses values with those of patients and their families/significant others.

Enabling Factors;

- An understanding of professional boundaries in decision-making.
- An understanding of responsibility and accountability in professional decision-making.
- A patient-centred approach to risk assessment and risk-taking.
- A willingness to make explicit intent and motivation for actions.
- A willingness to make explicit the conversation agenda.

Although the primary nurses in this study worked in clinical areas that espoused a philosophy of patient-centredness and the contemporary ideology of caring, there was little evidence of the nurse as a facilitator of authentic consciousness evidenced in the presentation of the data collected. In the focus group interview with expert gerontological nurses, participants expressed their concern at the lack of expertise demonstrated by the primary nurses who participated in the research. However, in their discussions, they considered these nurses to be typical of most nurses in their sphere of experience. Therefore, in presenting this framework as an approach to facilitating autonomy and older hospitalised people, it is necessary to consider ways in which the current context of practice needs to change in order to accommodate such an approach. To do this, the themes identified by the focus group of expert nurses will be used to identify future developments in practice.

Developing Potential for Facilitating Authentic Consciousness

A Cultural Shift in Philosophical Values

Expert Group Interview/Lines 2452-2468

EX4:   ... people need to be able to take on a different view of things and able to see a different kind of potential when the whole system is kind of set up in a particular way and how do you change it? Because you've got teachers and educators and you've got role models and supervisors and people in clinical settings who have all been socialised in this system and what I think it needs is actually a complete culture shift, a shift in philosophical values, to see people as people who have responsibility for their own health and come into a system that should not totally remove that, that kind of ownership.

The group of expert nurses was consistent in the view that there was a need for significant changes in nursing and health care practice if nurses are to value older peoples' potential for autonomous decision-making. Members of the group, to represent the changes that were needed used the theme, 'A Cultural Shift in Philosophical Values'. The focus of the required change is that of viewing older people as persons who have responsibility for their own health. The main barriers to achieving this were seen to be the organisation of services for older people and the socialisation of educators and leaders of services.

    Changes in the delivery of acute health care services for older people have been significant over the past ten years as identified in Chapter 2. As discussed in Chapter 2, the increasing demands on emergency services, reduction in the number of available hospital beds, shorter lengths of stay, increased throughput and the erosion of the Health Service's commitment to the provision of continuing health care have all impacted on the way health care services are provided and the practice of health care workers. In addition the prevailing culture of consumerism has enabled a shift away from society's collective responsibility for the provision of an equitable and just health care system to one that is based on individual responsibility.

The combined effects of the organisation of services and the preparation of nurses who work with older people for creative practice can be seen to have an impact on the ability of nurses to develop patient-centred approaches to practice. For many years there has been concern expressed regarding the appropriateness of education programmes for nursing practice with older people (Davis *et al*, 1997; Sills *et al*, 1988; Nolan, 1998). Research by Davis *et al* (1997) found that there was a lack of coherence and structure in curricula, little involvement of users in curriculum design, little evidence in established curricula of an emphasis on autonomy and independence and little explicit attention to practice implications. The focus group emphasised the need for changes in the educational preparation of nurses if the philosophy presented in this research was to be made a reality.

The expert group supported the approach to autonomy as presented in this research, i.e. an approach to autonomy based on an individual's values. They recognised that talking with patients and families about values and using the outcomes from these discussions as a means of evaluating how well an older person's autonomy was being respected was a useful vehicle for exploring the processes of care-giving as opposed to a focus on how well the care outcomes were achieved. For example, the focus on achieving a short length of stay may not always be consistent with the values of the patient or family. In such situations, without the nurse, patient and family clarifying their values base and its relationship to the goal of care, there was potential for conflict. In addition the group recognised that while families were often the people who had most knowledge about the values that the patient might hold, there was a danger of nurses not recognising that there may be a 'split in values' among family members:

Expert Group Interview/Lines 1876-1880

EX1:   Because ... the value shift has already occurred and there is a big chasm
       between what the older person might want and what the rest of the family
       wants and the family have moved apart, or the relatives or the carer ...
       They have moved apart too significantly to bring them together.

The importance of nurses having skill in recognising conflict among family
members was seen as crucial to nurses effectively facilitating an
individual's authentic consciousness.   Nurses need to be aware of the
particular approach that might be needed in particular care situations and
be able to adjust their interactional approach to suit that situation:

Expert Group Interview/Lines 1891-1902

EX2:   the number of times I see nurses walk into situations ... I pick up as an
       outsider, have picked up tensions and then say, 'what's going on' and and
       it's only later that they they think it's unavoidable. But it might have been
       avoidable if it had been handled ... sensing that there was that values
       clash.

The group recognised the skill involved in balancing a duty of care to the
patient while at the same time maintaining the involvement of relatives in
care decisions and without allowing the relatives' perceptions and views to
dominate the situation. For many of the group, the key to doing this is
maintaining '*the older person's identity*' as central to care decisions and
helping them to maintain that in the sense of who they are in the context of
their lives, i.e. their biography. Rather than removing them from their
biographies, an approach that held values as central to care decisions,
would determine actions based on what they want for their futures. The
alternative scenario and the one that the expert group felt dominated the
research data, was that of the older person being seen as a 'care thing', i.e.
an object. Holding values as central allowed a variety of possible 'futures'
to emerge:

Expert Group Interview/Lines 1942-1944

EX4:   ... your appreciating the uncertainties of that older person as well because
       there may be any number of futures to that older person in that situation.

The perceived barrier to nurses working in this way was that of *wanting a happy ending* (EX1/line 1950). By controlling the outcome of care, the group suggested that this prevented nurses from needing to face the many difficulties and challenges associated with working with the patient's agenda - for example balancing the need for early discharge in order to maintain throughput, with the actual needs of the patient. In addition, the group suggested that nurses often had an inability to appreciate the life skills that the person had because the patient was unable to demonstrate these skills in a hospital context, due to the attitudinal, organisational and socialisation constraints already identified in earlier discussions:

Expert Group Interview/Lines 1949-1967

EX4:   ... people don't seem to have a vision of what this person's like and also accept the reality of, yes well they do get along by hanging onto the sideboard and a pile of papers that's built up in the hall and that they don't mind that, that they can tolerate that or even they will tolerate it or they don't like it but they will tolerate it because it enables them to achieve a better hope or a better dream ...

The issue of nurses' inability to accept the potential choices that many older people might make, that is, if they had the choice to do so, is raised here. The group saw 'taking a risk' as one of the biggest challenges that nurses face in working in a patient centred way that valued the autonomy and the decision-making capacity of older people.

The challenge of this was described by one participant as the balancing of '*professional knowledge and competence versus personal knowledge and competence versus self care ability*' EX3/Line 2115. This nurse expressed the view that the challenge in accepting patient-centred risk assessment is that of balancing professional knowledge and personal knowledge, or, as described in earlier discussions, the softening of the professional with the personal. The group identified that nurses needed to be able to balance their technical competence and expertise and their professional caring roles with the patient's understanding of their own well-being and their potential futures. This supports the central tenet in this thesis, of autonomy being a shared concept between nurse and patient set within the context of an interconnected relationship. Earlier data identified the determination required by patients to sustain their capacity for autonomy because of the various constraints posed. In addition the expert group recognised the vulnerability of all patients in hospital and that reducing this vulnerability and enabling decision-making is one of the key roles of the nurse. This has already been identified in this thesis as a central component of the role of the nurse as a facilitator of authentic consciousness.

Unsticking

The expert group suggested that there are problems with the way nurses *'think'* about their practice. In addition they identified problems with nurses' inexperience in dealing with complex care situations and that many nurses seem *to 'get stuck'* in their practice:

Expert Group Interview/Lines 2344-2350

EX1:   I think it is thinking ... but I also feel that I don't think we can change that way of thinking but it's a process that nurses go through. But what happens if they get stuck in part of that process. There is something that's not there either in the basic or in their ongoing support and development when nurses qualify ...

The group identified that many nurses appear to get stuck in their practice, i.e. they adopt ritualistic and routinised approaches to practice. To them, this happens because of a failure to recognise alternative approaches and/or a failure of organisations to create a learning culture that supports the continuous development of staff competence and skill. Members of the group recognised that in developing their skill as facilitators of another's authentic consciousness, nurses would need to be able to explore their own values and beliefs. To do this, they suggested would be a *'painful journey'* for many and that without continuous support and development they would *'shut down'* because *'to change would cost not only in their professional life, but in their personal life'* (EX2/Line 2405). Another member of the group described this as being like *'standing on the edge of the cliff and they just can't jump ...they'd rather go back even though they know what they've got isn't good enough ...'* (EX5/Line 2420). However, another group member presented the corollary to that suggestion, which again emphasised the need for continuous professional development:

Expert Group Interview/Lines 2427-2429

EX1:   But imagine, imagine the nurse who was at the end of the cliff who wanted
to go across but there was nobody to lay a path out ...

Members of the group recognised that working in a patient-centred way
required both '*personal bravery*' (EX1/lLine 2434) and supported
development to make the necessary changes. The personal bravery arose
from individual recognition of the need for change and the organisational
structure that supported a learning culture.   Three elements were
considered to be essential to the development of such a culture - reflective
practice, clinical supervision and clinical leadership.   Each of these
elements is currently achieving a high profile in practice and organisational
development plans in health care settings.

Conclusions

This chapter has proposed a conceptual framework within which an older
person's authentic consciousness can be facilitated. While this framework
has been developed, problems have been identified by the expert group that
challenge the reality of making such a philosophy happen in practice.

The final chapter will explore the limitations of this research and
the potential implications of the work on future research, education and
practice development agendas. Options for taking the work forward will
be explored.

11 Limitations, Implications and Aspirations

Introduction

This book has identified the limitations of an individualistic understanding of the concept of autonomy and has outlined a conceptual framework for autonomy based on the theory of authentic consciousness. It has been argued that changes to the way gerontological nursing practice is conceptualised and conceived in practice are necessary if nurses are to facilitate an older person's authentic consciousness whilst in hospital. What is the practical reality of such a proposal? Any theory that calls for action to be transformed, must not only spell out those aspects that require changing, but it should also provide an action-plan indicating how and by whose action this change is to take place (Fay, 1987).

In suggesting that a reconceptualisation of gerontological nursing practice in hospitals is necessary or indeed possible, there is a danger of introducing an 'idealism' that Fay (1987) warns against. This chapter then, will explore some methodological limitations of this research. It will discuss these in relation to the decision to utilise an interpretive approach rather than one located in a Critical Social Science paradigm (Fay, 1987).

In considering these limitations, the chapter will discuss the potential for this research to be developed further through a critical social science framework. Should this work proceed in this way then the results of this research has many implications for the practice of gerontological nursing.

Implications of the research for clinical practice development, nurse education, user involvement in care decisions and research will be discussed. These will be presented within the context of current political and policy agendas. It is from the consideration of these that my aspirations for the further development of the outcomes of the research and areas that could benefit from further study will be explored. In particular, it will be suggested that the conceptual framework of autonomy as authentic consciousness provides a useful basis for the framing of practice developments in gerontological nursing practice.

283

Limitations

Heidegger (1990) suggests that the act of 'being' in the world naturally necessitates interpretation and re-interpretation in order to make sense of the lived world. At the outset of this research, I was conscious of the many manifestations of the concept of autonomy. For reasons outlined in chapters 1 to 3, the idea of autonomy as individualism appeared to offer little to the enhancement of the consumer rights of older hospitalised people. In addition, it was evident from my own practice as a nurse, those I worked with, and the limitations outlined in the research literature that the conceptualisation of autonomy as individualism, limits a person-centred approach to patient care, and practice that is focused on connected relationships. So if an individualistic conceptualisation of patient autonomy is unachievable for older people in hospital, then what conceptualisation of autonomy is achievable? This agenda was articulated through the research questions:

- What is the meaning of autonomy in a relationship between a professional nurse and an older patient?
- When working with older people, can the nurse promote the principle of patient autonomy while functioning as an autonomous practitioner?

The first question set out to explore and challenge existing concepts of autonomy and their philosophical underpinnings. The decision to adopt an interpretative approach to the research was derived from this research question. In addition, as outlined in earlier chapters, the 'language of autonomy' as exhibited in nurse-patient communication structures and patterns was considered to be a useful focus in understanding the meaning of autonomy. However, the danger of 'armchair theorising' (Hammersley, 1992) that did not reflect the realities of the current context of practice was a potential hazard in adopting this approach. The establishment of a critical dialogue with research participants, other nurses and patients minimised the impact of this and facilitated the emergence of insights in the analysis of the data that enabled the conceptualisation of autonomy as authentic consciousness. It further assisted with the design of the framework for nursing practice as a means of facilitating authentic consciousness and thus the answering of the second research question.

However, a number of criticisms are made of the interpretative approach that are relevant to this research and its ongoing development. These have been summarised by Schwandt (1994; 130) as:

- The problem of criteria.
- The lack of critical purchase.

The Problem of Criteria

What counts as an adequate account of intersubjective meanings?, that is, how does one make sense of a variety of subjective accounts? Essentially, critics of interpretative accounts (Crotty, 1996) argue that in the absence of a set of valid criteria for interpretation, accounts are either 'subjective idealism' (that is, only *my* account) or relativistic (that is, no right or wrong account, all accounts are equally good or bad). A number of actions were instigated in this research to minimise the impact of both of these claims.

Firstly, as outlined in Chapter 4, a structured approach to data analysis using conversation analysis techniques was adopted. This enabled the choosing of data sets based on their overall contribution to the area of interest rather than their 'worth' as judged by my individual preferences for particular data sets. In addition, research participants were provided with the opportunity to critique my initial descriptions of their interactions and to either provide alternative descriptions or explanations for actions. Thirdly, 'experts'; were used to challenge my initial descriptions of the data and to provide an interpretative framework from the identification of dominant themes in the research data. Older people who had experience as patients corroborated these themes. New themes generated by me were matched against those of the expert group. Finally, data sets to be included were chosen for their ability to illustrate the themes generated, that is, for their representativeness of all data in that theme.

At no time in this research have I chosen to hide the values that I hold as a gerontological nurse. Indeed, chapter one explicitly outlines these values and their impact on me as nurse, researcher and person. Throughout the work I have used reflection as a means of 'checking out' the fittingness (Koch, 1994) of the interpretations made and where appropriate have included these reflections in this book. Koch (1995) argues that many hermeneutic researchers manage the subjective-objective divide by standing 'outside of the hermeneutic circle of understanding'. She suggests that such researchers fail to appreciate the full impact of the hermeneutic circle and its ability to transform individual understanding. Koch suggests that unless the researcher's understanding develops alongside the understanding of the phenomena being studied, an incomplete understanding is achieved. My intention was not to treat the actions of participating nurses as 'object-like entities' (Packer, 1985) with my role as researcher being that of critiquing the effectiveness of particular actions. Rather, by maintaining my stance within the hermeneutic circle of understanding, a dialogue existed between the experience of participants and my experience as a researcher and nurse. To do otherwise would have removed the possibility of achieving a genuine comprehension of the phenomena being studied through shared understandings. In addition, by standing outside of the hermeneutic circle the dangers of me as researcher making 'judgemental interpretations' of the data could have arisen. By ensuring that my interpretations were either confirmed or challenged by participating nurses, nurse experts and older people themselves, I not only achieved a more rigorous understanding of the issues, but also of my own beliefs, values and prejudices.

In order to prevent subjective idealist and relativistic challenges, Guba and Lincoln's (1981) criteria for demonstrating rigour in qualitative research were used as my own benchmark for establishing rigour in the research process - credibility, fittingness, auditability and confirmability.

Credibility is enhanced when researchers describe and interpret their own experiences as researchers in relation to the behaviours and experiences of participants. This involves the researcher being 'self-aware' of motivations and values underpinning methodological decisions, and the potential impact on the analytical process and feelings in relation to participants' behaviours. In this research, this self-awareness was maintained through the use of a reflective diary. In addition the expert nurses' focus group and the patients' focus group both challenged and corroborated initial interpretations made. The expert nurse focus group also provided an appropriate venue for me to make explicit some of the feelings I held about the data and the practice of particular nurse participants. Members of the expert group provided appropriate challenge and insights concerning behaviours and enabled the transcendence of initial emotional reaction.

A research study meets the criterion of fittingness when its findings can fit into contexts outside the study situation and when its audience views its findings as meaningful and applicable in terms of their own experiences (Guba and Lincoln, 1981). In this work the context of the research has been described. An overview of the research sites (within the limits of anonymity) and biographical descriptions of nurse and patient participants have been provided. The provision of this context enables the reader to decide if the resulting interpretations are transferable to their practice and the context in which it occurs.

Auditability is the criterion for rigour in the consistency of the data (Guba and Lincoln, 1981). A study and its findings are auditable when another researcher can clearly follow the 'decision trail' used by the investigator in the study (Sandelowski, 1986). A decision trail involves the articulation of the decisions made by the researcher at each stage of the research design. The decision trail adopted in this research has been clearly outlined through each chapter of the book and in chapter 4 in particular. This includes a detailed account of my emerging interest in the subject matter; my beliefs and values; the aims of the study; the choice and role of participants; the relationship between me and the research participants; the methods of data collection and analysis and the categorisation of the data into themes, including approaches used to determine their 'truth value'.

Confirmability requires making explicit the way in which interpretations have been derived. Guba and Lincoln (1981) suggest that confirmability is achieved when credibility, fittingness and auditability have been established. Throughout the research, I have made my beliefs and values and 'prejudices' explicit, a detailed account of the context of the research has been provided. Chapter 4 describes each stage of decision-making.

The Lack of Critical Purchase

Interpretative accounts are sometimes considered to lack critical interest or the ability to critique the accounts produced (Denzin and Lincoln, 1994). Critics of interpretative methodologies (*for example*, Fay, 1987) argue that because the interpreter is necessarily distanced from the phenomena being investigated, then interpretivists cannot engage in an explicit critical evaluation of the social reality they seek to portray (Denzin and Lincoln, 1994). While I recognise the limited capacity for interpretive approaches to emancipate individuals from dominant repressive ideologies, like Elliott (1987), I am puzzled by the assertion that the process of interpretation does not enable the critique of power relationships in which practice is situated. The processes of interpretation utilised in this research provided opportunities for participants to critique the fittingness of the interpretations made and to consider opportunities for change. Individual nurse participants clearly recognised aspects of their practice that were ineffective, inappropriate or repressive. Through their engagement in reflective conversations, the process of interpretation itself was seen to raise to individual consciousness attitudes, beliefs and behaviours that were previously unconscious. This ability to interpret ones own practice is a central component of the reflective practitioner (Schön, 1991) and is central to the development of clinical expertise (Manley and McCormack, 1997). These reflective conversations and other anecdotal discussions with the nurses who participated in this research suggest that indeed participating in this work has had a positive impact on individual nurses' practice, in particular their use of language and communication with patients and their families. However, this is not to suggest that this process of raising individual nurses' consciousness of particular factors that inhibit the facilitation of an individual's authentic consciousness is enough to change dominant practice cultures. Cultural change is more complex than this.

However, the fact that these accounts of individual consciousness raising are 'anecdotal', identifies the primary limitation of the methodology adopted. This research has identified dominant power relationships and their impact on the relationship between nurses, patients, families and relatives and the health care team. While these factors have been identified, there has been little opportunity to change these power relationships and indeed it could be argued that the results of this research in themselves have little direct impact on practice.

It was from such a concern that 'Critical Social Theory' (Habermas, 1985; Fay, 1987; Carr and Kemmis, 1986) and the methodology of 'Critical Social Science' have been developed. Critical social science argues that an interpretive approach provides useful knowledge that is of 'practical interest' in understanding and clarifying the conditions for meaningful communication and action. Fay (1987) highlights the place of interpretation in a critical social theory when he suggests that for a social theory to be critical and practical, firstly there needs to be a recognition of 'crisis' in the social system and secondly that this crisis is in part caused by a 'false consciousness'. Interpretation forms the first stage of a critical social science endeavour. It does this through the provision of a systematic critique of participants' self-understandings and social practices. This critique acts as a precursor to deciding on the most appropriate approaches for changing prevailing power relationships. What Fay (1987) suggests is that clarifying the factors that comprise the prevailing system of domination, is the first stage of a critical social science methodology. This research makes a significant contribution to the clarification of factors that enhance and inhibit person-centredness in gerontological nursing practice. Individual nurse participants, nurse experts and older people themselves have corroborated these factors. In this way, this research can be seen to form stage one of a critical social science endeavour, i.e. clarifying a focus for change and development.

This is an important outcome of this research and later in this chapter, suggestions for ongoing research and development will be made for the development of gerontological nursing practice and older peoples' experiences of hospitalisation. The completion of this research comes at a time of significant change in the organisation of services for older people and therefore has the potential to impact on gerontological nursing practice and the experience of older people in hospital.

Implications

Current health and social policy impacts greatly on older people and their receipt of effective care services. Therefore, the potential for the results of this research to influence and shape the development of clinical practice and the principles underpinning the organisation of services for older people are great.

It is true that the process of ageing places greater demands on an individual's health status (*for example*, Grimley-Evans, 1991). As a result older people may need more support from health care resources. However, it has been argued in this book that longevity is not a central issue in the quality of life of older people. Instead the maximising of an individual's potential to live life to their full capacity is central. This is of equal importance for older hospitalised people, whom I have suggested experience systems of domination that limit their ability to fully participate in care decisions or to influence the basis on which decisions are reached. The use of the findings of this research in a practice development strategy, could enable older people to have their potential maximised and to have their voices heard in care decisions.

In the United Kingdom, the erosion of National Health Service continuing care services has coexisted with the reduction of secondary care facilities through an emphasis on a 'Primary Care Led NHS' and the loss of specialist gerontology units. Reduced lengths of stay, day case treatment and a focus on the effective management of medical emergencies has meant that secondary care facilities are more stringently targeted at acute care episodes and the expectation that follow up care would take place in a community based facility. For older people in particular, this policy has resulted in significant changes to the organisation of their care services. The clarification of issues raised in this research has been informed by theories first developed in the context of continuing care (*for example* Collopy, 1988; Agich, 1993). Other research into the autonomy of older people in continuing care services (Davis *et al*, 1997) suggests that the issues raised here in respect of older people in hospital are similar to those of older people in continuing care. There are significant opportunities for the results of this research to be applied in a continuing care context with the intention of developing a 'resident-centred' approach to practice based on the enhancement of the individual's authentic consciousness.

Nurses working with older people have always experienced difficulties in articulating the knowledge, skills and expertise underpinning their practice and their impact on patient outcome. Many problems exist in measuring effectiveness in nursing with older people that moves beyond symptom management, treatments and specific care inputs or therapies. Gerontological nursing balances the support of normal ageing processes with the management of disease and illness. It encompasses both health and social aspects of care, with a major component of gerontological nursing focusing on the support of the individual through life transition. To demonstrate effectiveness in this context, there is a need for a broad based definition of 'evidence' that encompasses not just results of treatments, but that also includes recognition of the older person's experiences of care. The adoption of a 'life plan' approach in establishing an individual's desired outcomes from care, can enable the collection of evidence from practice that is centred on articulating the achievement of patients' desired outcomes alongside intended outcomes determined from more 'objective' measurement.

The emphasis on the provision of dignified care for older hospitalised people that has arisen because of pressure from patient advocacy groups and the media provides many opportunities for the implementation and evaluation of the findings of this research. Research by 'The Health Advisory Service 2000' (HAS 2000) (Health Advisory Service 2000, 1998) highlighted the importance of communication, negotiation and respect for an individual's values in the assessment of care need and the establishment of care plans. The findings of the work of HAS 2000 are consistent with the findings of this research and therefore represent an opportunity for the testing in practice of the framework developed. The research by HAS 2000 emphasised in particular, the importance of ongoing education and development in gerontological practice. While, the appropriateness of pre-registration nurse education programmes are currently questioned, there is scope for the utilisation for the conceptual underpinnings of the framework developed in this research to act as an approach for ongoing life-long learning in gerontological nursing. However, the implications of this on the way gerontological education is provided are great. The expert group were clear that the philosophical basis of gerontological nurse education would need to be challenged, if an approach to practice such as that recommended in this research was to be adopted. The research challenges nurses to 'engage' with older people in a way that places them at the centre of all care decisions. Such an engagement would require nurses to adopt an approach to practice that does not see older people as 'problems', but instead as citizens with a right to make decisions about their needs, facilitated by an expert practitioner. It appears therefore, that if such a philosophical change is to occur, then older people themselves need to be involved in the planning of education programmes with nurses. Currently there is little evidence of older people being placed at the centre of planning in nurse education programmes or being viewed as partners in educational processes (Traynor and Rafferty, 1998). The approach to practice highlighted in this research would require a change in nursing attitudes, that views working with older people in partnership as a mutual process of growth and development.

However, the problems associated with getting evidence into practice and changing clinical practice has been well documented (Kitson *et al*, 1998). Gerontological nursing practice is no different to any other branch of nursing in this respect. While much innovative practices have been developed in settings for older people, there still exists, much ritualised and routinised approaches to the organisation and delivery of services. Therefore, my aspirations for this research do not lie in its dissemination through publications alone. Instead, there is much potential for the development of the research outcomes as a practice development framework set within a critical social science philosophy.

Aspirations

It would be 'easy' at this stage of the research to devise a list of recommendations to be addressed by educationalists, care providers, and practitioners. However, given the difficulties that exist in changing clinical nursing practice and the attitudinal and organisational barriers that hinder such changes, there is a need to consider this research in the context of future practice developments.

The conceptual framework of autonomy as authentic consciousness identifies five imperfect duties (sympathetic presence, informed flexibility, negotiation, transparency and mutuality), three 'stances' in which the care situation is located (engagement' partial disengagement and complete disengagement) and three contextual factors that enable this relationship to happen (patients' values history, context of the care environment and the nurses' values history, knowledge and experience). It is clear from these components of the framework that the implementation of this framework and the practice changes required, is beyond the responsibility of individual nurses. While individual nurses clearly have a responsibility for the quality of their practice and the way that practice develops, much organisational change is needed to realise the full potential of the proposed framework. Elsewhere, it has been suggested that for practice to develop in the way that this research proposes, changes in service delivery are required at individual, organisational and strategic levels (McCormack *et al*, 1999). The conceptual framework provides a basis for benchmarking existing practices and determining changes needed in order for practice to be based on principles of authentic consciousness. As articulated by the expert group in this research, an approach to life-long learning that enables practitioners to articulate their values, develop practice knowledge and take risks is needed. The facilitation of learning in practice through contracted learning is one such approach that would be appropriate.

'Experience' is a valuable source of knowledge and recognising the development of nurses' experience in a particular practice context can be an essential route towards the development of 'expertise' in practice. Every aspect of nursing - clinical, managerial or educational is predominantly practice focused. In order for experience to become learning, there needs to be a systematic approach in place to assist nurses to reflect on practice experience, critically review the elements of that practice, actively engage in developing/experimenting with practice and synthesising the learning gained from the process. Nurses are adult learners, and adult learning theory argues that learning is most effective when the learner is able to make sense of new knowledge in the context of their immediate life experience (Jarvis, 1983; Schön, 1990). An approach such as this would enable nurses to do what members of the expert group described as 'unsticking', which is, freeing themselves from unnecessary routines and rituals. It would be consistent with their desire for the establishment of organisational cultures that support the continuous development of staff competence and skill, facilitated by a 'critical companion' (Titchen, 2000). Titchen (2000) has described an approach to the facilitation of learning in practice by a critical companion who accompanies the learner on their learning journey and enables growth and development. It would be easy to underestimate the amount of support nurses need to clarify their values, and their impact on the lives of older people in hospital. The personal and professional challenges associated with engaging with such work are great. Having a critical companion who engages in 'skilled companionship' (Titchen, 2000) as a means of facilitating growth and understanding in practice would appear to be essential. It is my particular aspiration to develop the role of 'critical companion' in gerontological settings as a means of empowering nurses to facilitate a philosophy of authentic consciousness. In doing this, opportunities to 'test' the proposed framework can be maximised as well the potential to create significant changes in practice at patient, organisational and strategic levels. The anticipated benefits of adopting this approach would be:

... to Older Hospitalised People

- More effective practice because of more knowledgeable and person-centred approaches.
- Explicit recognition of their personhood.
- Engagement with staff in the development of their expertise in facilitating person-centred practice and thus creating a culture of 'reciprocity' in care services.
- An opportunity for older people to assist practitioners with their learning and professional development.

... to Nursing Staff

- Provides a framework for life-long learning and a systematic process for engaging with it.
- Provides a framework for continuous professional development.
- Engages staff with the continuous development of practice as an integral component of their roles.
- Creates an individual and organisational commitment to the development of creative and effective person-centred services.

... to Service Providers

- Introduces the concept of 'life-long learning' and engages staff in the process.
- Provides a model of learning and development that places the patient at the centre of educational aims and processes.
- Provides a framework for the continuous development of practice.
- Provides a framework for clinical supervision in practice.
- Acts as a means of developing clinical expertise.
- Acts as a means of continuous performance review.

... to Education Providers

- Operationalises a philosophy of systematic practice development, integrated with research, education and policy development.
- Makes learning in practice an explicit commitment of education institutions.
- Generates new knowledge from practice to inform the development of teaching and learning strategies.

... to the Research Community

- Provides opportunities to critically explore concepts of 'person-centredness' in practice.
- Provides a basis for the development of a 'person-centred' research agenda.
- Enables the evaluation of care inputs and their impact on person-centred outcomes.
- Assists with the utilisation of 'evidence' in practice.
- Generates inductively derived knowledge.
- Tests deductively derived knowledge.
- Contributes to the evaluation of the effectiveness of organisational systems in supporting person-centred practice.

Gerontological nursing continues to be criticised for its routinised and often institutionalised approach to practice. The adoption of this framework into practice and the ongoing facilitation of its implementation provide opportunities to change the dominant emphasis on 'problems' to one where the authenticity of older people is maximised and held central in care delivery.

Conclusions

A conceptual understanding of autonomy as authentic consciousness has been developed in this book. It is clear that conflicting interpretations of autonomy exist in the literature and that available interpretations of autonomy do not facilitate 'person-centred' practice. Universal moral principles are not being rejected in this research. Instead it is argued that autonomy as authentic consciousness enables the operationalisation of universal moral principles in the context of nurse-patient relationships that aim to promote uniqueness and individuality. Through the data analysis, it was evident that autonomy as individualism is not a viable option for many older hospitalised people. While there is an intention to promote choice and partnership in care decision-making, in reality this is not authentic choice. Instead, the choices available to older hospitalised people appear to be hindered by numerous contextual and attitudinal factors. By viewing autonomy as authentic consciousness an alternative perspective of autonomy can be achieved. A perspective that is not based on any one person being the 'final arbiter' of decisions, but which is instead set within a framework of negotiation based on an individual's values base. Gaining an understanding of an individual's values base is central to this way of working, and while it is acknowledged that the demands of everyday nursing practice can often work against this approach, it is also recognised that there is potential for much attitudinal and behavioural change that could enable this philosophy to be achieved. The nurse as a facilitator of an individual's authentic consciousness would appear to offer a way of regenerating gerontological nursing practice - a regeneration that identifies it as a process of dynamic caring that maintains autonomy at a time when an individual's sense of independence is under greatest threat. Through the facilitation of authentic consciousness, maintaining an outlook that is hopeful and bright can help the future for an older person whose sense of independence is under greatest threat. The importance of skilled, expert caring nursing practice can never be underestimated in the care of older people, because as Weinberg (1978) says:

> Each person has his own and unique life, his own memories, hopes, expectations, habits, and biases. Each has had a responsibility in the management of his own life ... Each has found support, reinforcement, guidance, and correction from loving and perceptive others; and each has suffered at the hands of others.

Older people should not 'suffer' because of the care they receive from nurses. The expert gerontological nurse tries to give the patient as many opportunities as possible to exercise freedom of choice, to express opinions, to make decisions, to talk while the nurse really listens and to have the opportunity to express their authentic self in a negotiated partnership with the nurse.

Bibliography

Abramson, J.S. (1990), 'Enhancing patient participation: clinical strategies in the discharge planning process', *Social Work in Health Care*, vol. 14, no. 4, pp. 53-71.

Abramson, J.S., Donnelly, J., King, M.A. and Mailick, M.D. (1993), 'Disagreement in discharge planning: a normative phenomenon', *Health and Social Work*, vol.18, no. 1, pp 57-64.

Abramson, L.Y., Seligman, M.E.P., Teasdale, J.D. (1982), 'Learned Helplessness', *Journal of Abnormal Psychology*, vol. 87, no. 1, pp. 49-74.

Agich, G.J. (1993), *Autonomy and Long-Term Care*, Oxford University Press, Oxford.

Anderson, D.C. (1979), 'Talking with Patients About Their Diet', in D.C. Anderson (ed.), *Health Education in Practice*, Croom Helm, London.

Atkinson, J.M. and Drew, P. (1979), *Order in Court: the Organisation of Verbal Interaction in Judicial Settings*, Macmillan, London.

Ayer, A.J. (1964), *The Concept of a Person and Other Essay*, Macmillan & Co Ltd, London.

Bailey, K.P. and Mayer, G.G. (1980), 'Evaluation of the implementation of primary nursing', *Nursing Dimensions*, vol. 7, no. 4, pp. 82-84.

Baker, D.E. (1978), *Attitudes of Nurses to the Care of the Elderly*, Unpublished PhD Thesis, University of Manchester.

Baldock, J. and Prior, D. (1981), 'Social Workers talking to clients: a study of verbal behaviour', *British Journal of Social Work*, vol. 11, pp. 19-38.

Baly, M. (1980), *Nursing and Social Change*, Heinemann, London.

Barker, E.M. (1991), 'Rethinking Family Loyalties', in N.S. Jecker (ed.) *Aging and Ethics*, Humana Press, Clifton, New Jersey.

Beauchamp, T.L. and Childress, J.F. (1983), *Principles of Biomedical Ethics*, Oxford University Press, Oxford.

Beck, L.W. (1956), *Kant: Critique of Practical Reason*, Macmillan, London.

Beiseker, A. and Beiseker, T. (1990), 'Patient information-seeking behaviours when communicating with doctors', *Medical Care*, vol. 28, pp. 19-28.

Benn, S.I. (1976), 'Freedom, autonomy and the concept of a person', *Proceedings of the Aristotelian Society*, vol. 76, pp. 109-130.

Benner, P. (1984), *From Novice to Expert: Excellence and Power in Clinical Nursing Practice*, Addison-Wesley, California.

Benner, P. (1994 [ii]), 'The Tradition And Skill Of Interpretive Phenomenology In Studying Health, Illness And Caring Practice', in P. Benner (ed.) *Interpretive Phenomenology: Embodiment, Caring and Ethics in Health and Illness*, Sage Publications, London.

Benner, P. and Wrubel, J. (1989), *The Primacy of Caring: Stress and Coping in Health and Illness*, Addison-Wesley Publishing Company, Wokingham.

Benner, P., Tanner, C. and Chesla, C. (1996), *Expertise in Nursing Practice: Caring, Clinical Judgement and Ethics*, Springer Publishing Company, New York.

Bergmann, F. (1977), *On Being Free*, University of Notre Dame Press, Notre Dame, Indianapolis.

Bergum, V. (1991), 'Being a Phenomenological Researcher', in J. Morse (ed.) *Qualitative Nursing Research: A Contemporary Dialogue*, Sage Publications, London.

Berlin, I. (1992), *Four Essays on Liberty*, Oxford University Press, Oxford.

Bernard, M. and Phillips, J. (1998), *The Social Policy of Old Age - Moving into the 21st Century*, Centre for Policy on Ageing, London.

Bertaux, D. (ed.) (1981), *Biography and Society: The Life History Approach in the Social Sciences*, Sage Publications, London.

Bhaskar, R. (1989), *Reclaiming Reality: A Critical Introduction to Contemporary Philosophy*, Verso, London.

Biggs, S., Phillipson, C. and Kingston, P. (1995), *Elder Abuse in Perspective*, Rethinking Ageing Series, Open University Press, Buckingham.

Binnie, A. (1988), *The Working Lives of Staff Nurses: a Sociological Perspective*, Unpublished Thesis, Warwick University.

Bishop, V. (1998), *Clinical Supervision in Practice. Some Questions, Answers and Guidelines*, Macmillan, Basingstoke.

Blanchard, C., Labrecque, M., Ruckdeschel, J., Blanchard, E. (1988), 'Information and decision-making preferences of hospitalized adult cancer patients', *Social Science and Medicine*, vol. 27, pp. 1139-1145.

Blegen, M.A., Goode, C., Johnson, M., Maas, M., Chen, L. and Moorhead, S. (1993), 'Preferences for decision-making autonomy', *IMAGE: Journal of Nursing Scholarship*, vol. 25, no. 4, pp. 339-343.

Blum, L.A. (1982), *Friendship, Altruism and Morality*, Routledge & Kegan Paul, London.

Bogoch, B. (1994), 'Power, distance and solidarity: models of professional-client interaction in an Israeli legal aid setting', *Discourse and Society*, vol. 5, no. 1, pp. 65-88.

Bornat, J. (ed.) (1994), *Reminiscence Reviewed: Evaluations, Achievements, Perspectives*, Open University Press, Milton Keynes.

Bowling, A. (1995), *Measuring Health: A Review of Quality of Life Measurement Scales*, Open University Press, Milton Keynes.

Boykin, A. and Schoenhofer, S. (1993), *Nursing as Caring: A Model for Transforming Practice*, National League for Nursing Press, New York.

Bradshaw, A. (1994), *Lighting the Lamp: The Spiritual Dimension of Nursing Care*, Scutari Press, London.

Bradshaw, A. (1995), 'What are nurses doing to patients? A review of theories of nursing past and present', *Journal of Clinical Nursing*, vol. 4, pp. 81-92.

Brewer, J.D., McBride, G. and Yearley, S. (1991), 'Orchestrating an encounter: a note on the talk of mentally handicapped children', *Sociology of Health and Illness*, vol. 13, no. 1, pp. 58-67

Bright, M. and Durham, M. (1997), 'Join our Campaign for the Old', *The Observer*, 5th October 1997.

Bristow-Ott, B. and Nieswiadomy, R.M. (1991), 'Support of patient autonomy in the do not resuscitate decision', *Heart & Lung*, vol. 20, no. 1, pp. 66-72.

British Gas (1991), *The British Gas Report on Attitudes to Ageing 1991*, British Gas, London.

British Medical Association and Royal College of Nursing (1995), *The Older Person: Consent and Care*, BMA Publishing, London.

Brody, H. (1978), 'The role of the family in medical decisions', *Theoretical Medicine*, vol. 8, pp. 253-257.

Brown, J., Kitson, A.L. and McKnight, T. (1992), *Challenges in Caring: Explorations in Nursing and Ethics*, Chapman and Hall, London.

Buchanan, A.E. and Brock, D.W. (1989), *Deciding For Others: The Ethics of Surrogate Decision Making*, Cambridge University Press, Cambridge.

Burnard, P. (1992), 'Some problems in understanding other people: analysing talk in research, counselling and psychotherapy', *Nurse Education Today*, vol. 12, pp. 130-136.

Burns, S. (1988), 'The role of the associate nurse', *The Professional Nurse*, vol. 18, pp. 20.

Bussis, A., Chittenden, E., Amarel, M. and Carini, P. (1978), *Educational Testing Service Data Integration Project*, Educational Testing Service, Princeton New Jersey.

Byrne, P.S. and Long, B.E.L. (1976), *Doctors Talking to Patients: a study of the verbal behaviour of general practitioners consulting in their surgeries*, HMSO, London.

Callahan, D. (1991), 'Limiting Health Care for the Old' in N.S. Jecker (ed.) *Aging & Ethics*, Humana Press, Clifton, New Jersey.

Campbell, A.V. (1984), *Moderated Love: A Theology of Professional Care*, SPCK, London.

Capitman, J. and Sciegaj, M. (1995), 'A contextual approach for understanding individual autonomy in managed community long-term care', *Gerontologist*, vol. 35, no. 4, pp. 533-540.

Carlsen, R.H. and Malley, J.D. (1981), 'Job satisfaction of staff registered nurses in primary and team nursing delivery system', *Research in Nursing and Health*, vol. 4, pp. 251-260.

Carlson, L., Crawford, N. and Contrades, S. (1989), 'Nursing student novice to expert: Benner's research applied to education', *Journal of Nursing Education*, vol. 28, no. 4, pp. 188-190.

Carper, B.A. (1978), 'Fundamental patterns of knowing in nursing', *Advances in Nursing Science*, vol. 1, no. 1, pp. 13-23.

Carr, W. and Kemmis, S. (1986), *Becoming Critical: Education, Knowledge and Action Research*, Falmer Press, Brighton.

Cartwright, T., Davson-Galle, P. and Holden, R.J. (1992), 'Moral philosophy and nursing curricula: indoctrination of the new breed', *Journal of Nursing Education*, vol. 31, no. 5, pp. 225-228.

Casement, P. (1988), *On Learning from the Patient*, Tavistock Publications, London.

Chervenak, F.A. and McCullough, L.B. (1991), 'Justified Limits on Refusing Intervention', in N. Daniels (ed.) *Duty to Treat or Right to Refuse?, Hastings Centre Report [Special Supplement]*, vol. 21, no. 2, pp. 12-18.

Chick, N. and Meleis, A.I. (1986), 'Transitions: A Nursing Concern', in P.L. Chinn (ed.), *Nursing Research Methodology - Issues and Implementation*, Aspen Publishers, Tunbridge Wells.

Childress, J.F. (1982), *Who Should Decide: Paternalism in Health Care*, Oxford University Press, Oxford.

Christensen, J. (1993), *Nursing Partnership: A Model for Nursing Practice*, Churchill Livingstone, London.

Christman, J. (1989), 'Introduction' in J. Christman (ed.), *The Inner Citadel: Essays on Individual Autonomy*, Oxford University Press, Oxford.

Clark, H. and Dyer, S. (1998), 'Equipped for going home from hospital', *Health Care in Later Life*, vol. 3, no. 1, pp. 35-45.

Clark, H., Dyer, S. and Hartman, L. (1996), *Going Home from Hospital: older people leaving hospital*, Policy Press, University of Bristol, Bristol.

Clinical Standards Advisory Group [CSAG] (1998), *Community Health Care for Elderly People*, Clinical Standards Advisory Group, London.

Coles, M. (1993), 'Pressure on the Professionals', *The Sunday Telegraph*, April 25.

Collopy, B.J. (1988), 'Autonomy and long term care: some crucial distinctions', *Gerontologist 28* (Supplement, June), pp. 10-17.

Collopy, B., Boyle, P. and Jennings, B. (1991), 'New Directions in Nursing Home Ethics', in N. Daniels (ed.) *Duty to Treat or Right to Refuse?, Hastings Centre Report [Special Supplement]*, vol. 21, no. 2, pp. 1-15.

Connelly, L.M., Keele, B.S., Kleinbeck, S.V.M., Schneider, K.J. and Cobb, A.K. (1993), 'A place to be yourself: empowerment from the client's perspective', *IMAGE: Journal of Nursing Scholarship*, vol. 25, no. 4, pp. 297-303.

Conway, J.E. (1996), *Nursing Expertise and Advanced Practice*, Quay Books, Dinton.

Cotter, A., Meyer, J. and Roberts, S. (1998), 'Humanity or bureaucracy? The transition from hospital to long-term continuing institutional care', *NT Research*, vol. 3, no. 4, pp. 247-256.

Coulton, C.J. (1990), 'Research in patient and family decision making regarding life sustaining and long term care', *Social Work in Health Care*, vol. 15, no. 1, pp. 63-78.

Coulton, C.J., Dunkle, R.E., Haug, M., Chow, J. and Vielhaber, D.P. (1989), 'Locus of control and decision making for posthospital care', *The Gerontologist*, vol. 29, no. 5, pp. 627-632.

Coupland, J., Coupland, N. and Granger, K. (1991), 'Intergenerational discourse', *Ageing and Society*, vol. 11, pp. 189-208.

Crawford, P., Nolan, P. and Brown, B. (1995), 'Linguistic entrapment: medico-nursing biographies as fictions', *Journal of Advanced Nursing*, vol. 22, pp. 1141-1148.

Crotty, M. (1996), *Phenomenology and Nursing Research*, Churchill Livingstone, Melbourne, Australia.

Cumming, E. and Henry, W.E. (1961), *Growing Old*, Basic Books, New York.

Curtin, L., Flaherty, M.J. (1982), *Nursing Ethics: Theories and Pragmatics*, Prentice-Hall International Editions, Englewood Cliffs.

Dalley, G. (1997), 'Health and Health Care', in G. Dalley, J. Falkingham, R. Hancock, J. Lewis, R. Means and C. Phillipson (1997), *Baby Boomers - Ageing in the 21st Century*, Age Concern England, London.

Dalley, G., Falkingham, J., Hancock, R., Lewis, J., Means, R. and Phillipson, C. (1997), *Baby Boomers - Ageing in the 21st Century*, Age Concern England, London.

Darton, R.A., Wright, K.G. (1993), 'Changes in the provision of long-stay care, 1970-1990', *Health and Social Care*, vol. 1, pp. 11-25.

Davies, C. (1976), 'Experience of dependency and control in work: the case of nurses', *Journal of Advanced Nursing*, vol. 1, pp. 273-282.

Davis, A. (1989), 'Clinical nurses' ethical decision making in situations of informed consent', *Advances in Nursing Science*, vol. 11, no. 3, pp. 63-69.

Davis, S., Ellis, L. and Lanker, S. (1997), *Promoting autonomy and independence among older people: an evaluation of educational programmes in nursing*, English National Board for Nursing, Midwifery and Health Visiting, London.

Denzin, N.K. and Lincoln, Y.S. (1994), *Handbook of Qualitative Research*, Sage Publishers, London.

Department of Health (1990), *The National Health Service and Community Care Act*, HMSO, London.

Department of Health (1991 [i]), *The Health of the Nation*, HMSO, London.

Department of Health (1991 [ii]), *The Patient's Charter*, HMSO, London.

Department of Health and Social Security (1984), DHSS Circular HC(84)13. *Health Services Management: Implementation of the NHS Management Inquiry*, HMSO, London.

Department of Health (1997), *The New NHS Modern and Dependable*, CM3807, December 1997, HMSO, London.

Dewing, J. (1994), *Caring - Women's Work?*, Conference Paper, Burford Clinical Nursing Conference on Human Caring, Keble College, Oxford.

Dex, S. (1991), 'Life and Work History Analysis', in S. Dex (ed.) *Life and Work History Analysis: Qualitative and Quantitative Developments*, Sociological Review Monograph 37, Routledge, London.

Dill, A.E.P. (1995), 'The ethics of discharge planning for older adults: an ethnographic analysis', *Social Science and Medicine*, vol. 41, no. 9, pp. 1289-1299.

Dingwall, R. (1980), 'Orchestrated encounters: an essay in the comparative analysis of speech-exchange systems', *Sociology of Health and Illness*, vol. 2, pp. 151-173.

Dingwall, R. and McIntosh, J. (eds.) (1978), *Readings in the Sociology of Nursing*, Churchill Livingstone, London.

Dingwall, R., Rafferty, A.M. and Webster, C. (1988), *An Introduction to the Social History of Nursing*, Routledge, London.

Downie, R.S. (1986), 'Professional ethics', *Journal of Medical Ethics*, vol. 12, pp. 64-65.

Doyle, L. (1993), 'On discovering the nature of knowledge in a world of relationships', in A.L. Kitson (ed.), *Nursing: Art and Science*, Chapman and Hall, London.

Drew, P. and Heritage, J. (1992), *Talk at Work: Interaction in Institutional Settings*, Cambridge University Press, Cambridge.

Dunne, J. (1993), *Back to the Rough Ground: 'Phronesis' and 'Techne' in Modern Philosophy and in Aristotle*, University of Notre Dame Press, London.

Dunning, A. (1995), *Citizen Advocacy With Older People: A Code of Good Practice*, Centre for Policy on Ageing, London.

Dworkin, G. (1989), 'The Concept of Autonomy', in J. Christman (ed.), *The Inner Citadel: Essays on Individual Autonomy*, Oxford University Press, Oxford.

Dworkin, G. (1991), *The Theory and Practice of Autonomy*, Cambridge University Press, Cambridge.

Ebersole, P. and Hess, P. (1990), *Toward Healthy Aging - Human needs and Nursing Response*, The CV Mosby Company, St. Louis.

Elliott, J. (1987), 'Educational theory, practical philosophy and action research', *British Journal of Educational Studies*, vol. xxxv, no. 2, pp. 149-169.

Ellul, J., Watkins, C. and Banes, D. (1993), 'Increasing patient engagement in rehabilitation activities', *Clinical Rehabilitation*, vol. 7, pp. 297-302.

Ely, M., Anzul, M., Friedman, T., Gardner, D. and McCormack Steinmetz, A. (1991), *Doing Qualitative Research: Circles Within Circles*, The Falmer Press, London.

Emanuel, E.J. (1991), *The Ends of Human Life - Medical Ethics In A Liberal Polity*, Harvard University Press, London.

Fairclough, N. (1989), *Language and Power*, Longman, London.

Falkingham, J. (1986), 'Dependency and ageing in Britain: A re-examination of the evidence', International *Social Policy*, vol. 18, no. 2, pp. 211-233.

Fay, B. (1987), *Critical Social Science: Liberation and its Limits*, Polity Press, Oxford.

Feinberg, J. (1989), 'Autonomy' in J. Christman (ed.) *The Inner Citadel: Essays on Individual Autonomy*, Oxford University Press, Oxford.

Field, P.A. and Morse, J.M. (1985), *Nursing Research: the application of qualitative approaches*, Croom Helm, London.

Ford, P. and McCormack, B. (1999), 'The contribution of expert gerontological nursing', *Nursing Standard*, vol. 13, no. 25, pp. 42-45.

Frankfurt, H.G. (1989), 'Freedom Of The Will And The Concept Of A Person' in J. Christman (ed.), *The Inner Citadel: Essays on Individual Autonomy*, Oxford University Press, Oxford.

Fried, T.R., Stein, M.D., O'Sullivan, P.S., Brock, D.W., Novack, D.H. (1993), 'Limits of patient autonomy: physicians attitudes and practices regarding life-sustaining treatments and euthanasia', *Archives of Internal Medicine*, vol. 153, pp. 722-728.

Fry, S. (1991), 'Health Care and Decision Making', in N. Jecker (ed.), *Aging and Ethics*, Humana Press, Clifton, New Jersey.

Fulford, K.W.M. (1996), 'The Definitions of Patient-Centred Care - Concepts of Disease and the Meaning of Patient-Centred Care', in K.W.M. Fulford, S. Ersser and T. Hope (eds.) *Essential Practice in Patient-Centred Care*, Blackwell Science, Oxford.

Fulford, K.W.M., Ersser, S. and Hope, T. (1996), *Essential Practice in Patient-Centred Care*, Blackwell Science, Oxford.

Gadamer, H.G. (1975), *Truth and Method*, Sheed & Ward, London.

Gadamer, H.G. (1993), *Truth and Method*, Sheed & Ward, London.

Gadow, S. (1980), 'Existential Advocacy: Philosophical Foundations Of Nursing', in S.F. Spicker and S. Gadow (1980), *Nursing: Images and Ideals - Opening Dialogue with the Humanities*, Springer, New York.

Gadow, S. (1990), 'Existential Advocacy: Philosophical Foundations Of Nursing', in T. Pence and J. Cantrell (eds.) *Ethics in Nursing: An Anthology*, National League for Nursing, New York.

Gadow, S (1991), 'Recovering the Body in Aging', in N.S. Jecker (ed.), *Aging and Ethics*, Humana Press, Clifton, New Jersey.

Garfinkel, H. (1967), *Studies in Ethnomethodology*, Prentice-Hall, Englewood Cliffs, New Jersey.

Genevay, B. and Katz, R.S. (1990), *Countertransference and Older Clients*, Sage, London.

Gilligan, C. (1977), 'In a different voice: women's conceptions of self and of morality', *Harvard Educational Review*, vol. 47, no. 4, pp. 481-517.

Gilligan, C. (1979), 'Woman's place in man's life cycle', *Harvard Educational Review*, vol. 49, no. 4, pp. 431-446.

Gilligan, C. (1982), *In a Different Voice: Psychological Theory and Women's Development*, Harvard University Press, Cambridge Massachusetts & London.

Goffman, E. (1959), *Presentation of Self in Everyday Life*, Doubleday, New York.

Goffman, E. (1961), *On the Characteristics of Total Institutions. First Essay in Asylums*, Penguin, Harmondsworth.

Golan, N. (1981), *Passing Through Transitions - a Guide for Practitioners*, Collier Macmillan Publishers, London.

Goldsmith, M. (1996), *Hearing the Voices of People with Dementia: Opportunities and Obstacles*, Jessica Kingsley Publishers, London.

Gorovirtz, H (1988) *Doctors' Dilemmas: Moral Conflict and Medical Care*, Oxford University Press, Oxford.

Gortner, S.R. and Zyzanski, S.J. (1988), 'Values in the choice of treatment: replication and refinement', *Nursing Research*, vol. 37, no. 4, pp. 240-244.

Graham, H. (1991), 'The concept of caring in feminist research: the case of domestic service', *Sociology*, vol. 25, pp. 61-78.

Greenwood, J. and King, M. (1995), 'Some surprising similarities in the clinical reasoning of 'expert' and 'novice' orthopaedic nurses: report of a study using verbal protocols and protocol analyses', *Journal of Advanced Nursing*, vol. 22, no. 5, pp. 907-913.

Grimley-Evans, J. (1991), 'Ageing and Rationing', *British Medical Journal*, vol. 303, pp. 869-870.

Grundy, S. (1982), 'Three modes of action research', *Curriculum Perspectives*, vol. 2, no. 3, pp. 23-34.

Guba, E.G. and Lincoln, Y.S. (1981), *Effective Evaluation*, Jossey-Bass, San Francisco.

Guba, E.G. and Lincoln, Y.S. (1994), 'Competing Paradigms in Qualitative Research', in N.K. Denzin and Y.S. Lincoln, *Handbook of Qualitative Research*, Sage Publishing, London.

Habermas, J. (1985), *The Theory of Communicative Action*, Beacon Press, Boston.

Hammersley, M. (1992), *What's Wrong With Ethnography?*, Routledge, London.

Handy, C.B. (1985), *Understanding Organisations*, Penguin Books, London.

Hardwig, J. (1984), 'Should Women Think in Terms of Rights', *Ethics*, vol. 94, pp. 441-455.

Hare, R.M. (1981), *Moral Thinking: It's Levels, Method and Point*, Oxford University Press, Oxford.

Haug, M.R. and Ory, M.G. (1987), 'Issues in elderly patient-provider interactions', *Research into Aging*, vol. 9, no. 1, pp. 3-44.

Health Advisory Service 2000 (1998), *"... Not Because They are Old ..."* - *an independent inquiry into the care of older people on acute wards in general hospitals*, The Health Advisory Service 2000, London.

Heath, C. (1981), 'The Opening Sequence In Doctor-Patient Interaction', in P. Atkinson and C. Heath (eds.) *Medical Work: Realities and Routines*, Gower, Aldershot.

Heath, C. (1986), *Body Movement and Speech in Medical Interaction*, Cambridge University Press, Cambridge.

Heidegger, M. (1990), *Being and Time*, Basil Blackwell, Oxford.

Heidrich, S.M. (1993), 'The relationship between physical health and psychological well-being in elderly women: a developmental perspective', *Research in Nursing and Health*, vol. 16, pp. 123-130.

Hekman, S. (1983), 'From epistemology to ontology: Gadamer's Hermeneutics and Wittgensteinian social science', *Human Studies*, vol. 6, pp. 205- 224.

Hennessy, C.H. (1989), 'Autonomy and risk: The role of client wishes in community-based long-term care', *The Gerontologist*, vol. 29, no. 5, pp. 633-639.

Heritage, J. (1984), 'A Change-Of-State Token And Aspects Of Its Sequential Placement', in J.M. Atkinson and J. Heritage (eds.), *Structures of Social Action: Studies in Conversation Analysis*, Cambridge University Press, Cambridge.

Heritage, J. (1988), 'Explanations as accounts: a conversation analytic perspective', in C. Antaki (1988), *Analysing Everyday Explanations: A Casebook of Methods*, Sage, London.

Heritage, J. (1991), 'On The Institutional Character Of Institutional Talk: The Case Of News Interviews', in D. Boden and D. Zimmerman (eds.) *Talk and Social Structure*, Polity Press, Cambridge.

Hertz, J.E. (1991), *The Perceived Enactment of Autonomy Scale: Measuring the Potential for Self-Care Action in the Elderly*, Unpublished PhD Thesis, University of Texas at Austin, Austin, Texas.

Hewstone, M., Stroebe, W., Codol, J.P. and Stephenson, M (1989), *Introduction to Social Psychology*, Basil Blackwell, Oxford.

High, D.M. (1991), 'A new myth about families of older people?', *The Gerontologist*, vol. 31, no. 5, pp. 611-617.

Holliday, I. (1992), *The NHS Transformed*, Baseline Books, Manchester.

Holmes, J. and Lindley, R. (1991), *The Values of Psychotherapy*, Oxford University Press, Oxford.

Holstein, J.A. and Gubrium, J.F. (1994), 'Phenomenology, Ethnomethodology, and Interpretive Practice', in N.K. Denzin and Y.S. Lincoln, *Handbook of Qualitative Research*, Sage Publishing, London.

Hope, T. (1992), 'The hedgehog and the Russian doll', *British Journal of Psychiatry Review of Books*, January 1992.

Hope, T. (1996), *Evidence-Based Patient Choice*, Kings Fund, London.

House of Commons Health Select Committee (1996), *Third Report, Long Term Care: Future Provision and Funding*, vol. 1, HSC 59-1, HMSO, London.

Howell, S. (1983), 'The Meaning Of Place In Old Age', in R. Rowles and R. Ohta (eds.) *Ageing and Milieu: Environmental Perspectives on Growing Old*, Academic Press, New York.

Hugman, R. (1991), *Power in Caring Professions*, The Macmillan Press Ltd., London.

Hulicka, I.M., Morganti, J.B. and Cataldo, J.F. (1975), 'Perceived latitude of choice of institutionalized and noninstitutionalized elderly women', *Experimental Aging Research*, vol. 1, pp. 27-39.

Hunter, D.J. (1993), 'To Market! To Market! a new dawn for community care', *Health and Social Care*, vol. 1, pp. 3-10.

Husserl, E. (1964), *The Idea of Phenomenology*, Martinus Nijhoff, The Hague.

Hutchinson, C.P. and Bahr, R.T. (1991), 'Types and meanings of caring behaviours among elderly nursing home residents', *Image: Journal of Nursing Scholarship*, vol. 23, no. 2, pp 85-88.

Jarvis, P. (1983), *Professional Education*, Croom Helm, London.

Jasper, M.A. (1994), 'Expert: a discussion of the implications of the concept as used in nursing', *Journal of Advanced Nursing*, vol. 20, pp. 769-776.

Jecker, N.S. (1991), 'The role of intimate others in medical decision making', in N.S. Jecker (ed.) *Aging and Ethics*, Humana Press, Clifton, New Jersey.

Jefferson, G. (1984), 'On The Organisation Of Laughter In Talk About Troubles', in J.M. Atkinson and J. Heritage (eds.) *Structures of Social Action: Studies in Conversation Analysis*, Cambridge University Press, Cambridge.

Jefferson, G. (1984), 'Caricature versus detail: on capturing the particulars of pronunciation in transcripts of conversational data', *Tilburg Papers on Language and Literature, No. 31*, University of Tilburg, The Netherlands.

Jefferson, G. (1988), 'On the sequential organisation of troubles talk in ordinary conversation', *Social Problems*, vol. 35, no. 4, pp. 418-441.

Jefferson, G. and Lee, J.R.E. (1981), 'The rejection of advice: managing the problematic convergence of a "troubles teller" and a "service encounter"', *Journal of Pragmatics*, vol. 5, pp. 399-422.

Jefferys, M. (1997), 'Inter-generational relationships: an autobiographical perspective', in A. Jamieson, S. Harper and C. Victor, *Critical Approaches to Ageing and Later Life*, Open University Press, Buckingham.

Jenny, J. and Logan, J. (1992), 'Knowing the Patient: one aspect of clinical knowledge', *Image: Journal of Nursing Scholarship*, vol. 24, no. 2, pp. 254-258.

Jirovec, M.M. and Maxwell, B.A. (1993), 'Nursing home residents functional ability and perceptions of choice', *Journal of Gerontological Nursing*, vol. 19, no. 9, pp.10-14.

Johns, C.C. (1989), *The Impact Of Introducing Primary Nursing On The Culture Of A Small Hospital*, Master of Nursing Thesis, University of Wales College of Medicine, Cardiff.

Johns, C. (1998), 'Opening the Doors of Perception', in C. Johns and D. Freshwater (eds.) *Transforming Nursing Through Reflective Practice*, Blackwell Science, Oxford.

Johns, C.C. (1991), *Becoming a Primary Nurse*, BNDU Publications, Burford, Oxon.

Johns, C.C. (1994), *The Burford NDU Model: Caring in Practice*, Blackwell Science, Oxford.

Johns, C.C. (1995), 'Achieving Effective Work As Professional Activity', in J.E. Schober and S.M. Hinchliff (eds.) *Towards Advanced Practice: Key concepts for health care*, Arnold, London.

Johns, C.C. (1997), *Becoming an Effective Practitioner through Guided Reflection*, Unpublished PhD thesis, Open University, Milton Keynes.

Johnson, M. (1976), 'That was Your Life: a biographical approach to later life', in J.M.A. Munnichs and W.J.A. Van der Heuvel (eds.) *Dependence and Interdependency in Old Age*, Martinus Nijhoff, The Hague.

Johnson, M. (1991), 'The Meaning of Old Age', in S.J. Redfern (ed.) *Nursing Elderly People*, Churchill Livingstone, Edinburgh.

Johnstone, M.J. (1989), *Bio Ethics - A Nursing Perspective*, WB Saunders, London.

Jones, L., Leneman, L., Maclean, U. (1987), *Consumer Feedback For The NHS: A literature review*, King Edward's Hospital Fund For London, London.

Judge, M. (1996), 'Perspectives on Patient-Centred Care - A Patient's Perspective', in K.W.M. Fulford, S. Ersser and T. Hope, *Essential Practice in Patient-Centred Care*, Blackwell Science, Oxford.

Kadushin, G. and Kulys, R. (1994), 'Patient and family involvement in discharge planning', *Journal of Gerontological Social Work*, vol. 22, no. 3-4, pp. 171-199.

Kastanbaum, R. (1983), 'Can the clinical milieu be therapeutic?', in G.D. Rowles, and R.J. Ohta (eds.) *Ageing and Milieu: Environmental Perspectives on Growing Old*, Academic Press, New York.

Katz, R.S. (1990), 'Using our Emotional Reactions to Older Clients: A Working Theory', in B. Genevay and R.S. Katz (eds.) *Countertransference and Older Clients*, Sage Publications, London.

Kemp-Smith, N. (1962), *Kant's Critique of Pure Reason*, Humanities Press, New Jersey.

Kenny, T. (1990), 'Erosion of individuality in care of elderly people in hospital - an alternative approach', *Journal of Advanced Nursing*, vol. 15, pp. 571-576.

Kitson, A.L. (1987), 'A comparative analysis of lay caring and professional (nursing) care relationships', *International Journal of Nursing Studies*, vol. 24, no. 2, pp. 155-165.

Kitson, A.L. (1993), 'Formalising concepts related to nursing and caring', in A.L. Kitson, *Nursing : Art and Science*, Chapman & Hall, London.

Kitson, A.L. (1996), 'Does nursing have a future?', *British Medical Journal*, vol. 313, pp. 1647-1651.

Kitson, A., Harvey, G. and McCormack, B. (1998), 'Approaches to Implementing Research in Practice', *Quality in Health Care*, vol. 7, no. 3, pp.149-159.

Kitwood, T. (1997), *Dementia Reconsidered: The Person Comes First*, Open University Press, Milton Keynes.

Klein, R. (1989), *The Politics of the National Health Service*, Longman, London and New York.

Koch, T. (1994), 'Establishing rigour in qualitative research: the decision trail', *Journal of Advanced Nursing*, vol. 19, pp. 976-986.

Koch, T. (1995), 'Interpretive approaches in nursing research: the influence of Husserl and Heidegger', *Journal of Advanced Nursing*, vol. 21, pp. 827-836.

Koch, T. and Webb, C. (1996), 'The biomedical construction of ageing: implications for nursing care of older people', *Journal of Advanced Nursing*, vol. 23, pp. 954-959.

Kohlberg, L. (1981), 'The Six Stages Of Moral Judgement', in L. Kohlberg (ed.), *Essays on Moral Development: The Philosophy of Moral Development*, Harper and Row, San Francisco.

Laing and Buisson Limited (1996), *Care of Elderly People Market Survey (Ninth Edition)*, Laing and Buisson, London.

Lanceley, A. (1985), 'Use of controlling language in the rehabilitation of the elderly', *Journal of Advanced Nursing*, vol. 10, pp. 125-135.

Langener, S.R. (1995), 'Finding meaning in caring for elderly relatives: Loss and personal growth', *Holistic Nursing Practice*, vol. 9, no. 3, pp. 75-84.

Langslow, A. (1992), 'Informed consent and self-determination', *The Australian Nurses Journal*, vol. 22, no. 2, pp. 29-31.

Latimer, J. (1997), 'Giving patients a future: the constituting of classes in an acute medical unit', *Sociology of Health and Illness*, vol. 19, pp. 160-185.

Lawler, J. (1991), *Behind the Screens: Nursing, Somology and the Problem of the Body*, Churchill Livingstone, London.

Leininger, M.M. (ed.) (1985), *Qualitative Research Methods in Nursing*, Harcourt Brace Jovanovich, New York.

Lewis, H. (1984), 'Self-determination: the aged client's autonomy in service encounters', *Journal of Gerontological Social Work*, vol. 7, no. 3, pp. 51-63.

Lidz, C.W. and Arnold, R.M. (1990), 'Institutional constraints on autonomy', *Generations*, vol. 14, [supplement], pp. 65-68.

Lindley, R. (1986), *Autonomy*, Macmillan, London.

Loxley, A. (1997), *Collaboration in Health and Welfare - Working with Difference*, Jessica Kingsley Publishers, London.

Luhmann, N. (1997), 'The Individuality Of The Individual: Historical Meanings and Contemporary Problems', in T.C. Heller, M. Sosna and D.E. Wellebery (1997), *Reconstructing Individualism: Autonomy, Individuality and the Self in Western Thought*, Stanford University Press, Stanford University, California.

Macleod-Clark, J. (1991), 'Communicating with Elderly People', in S.J. Redfern, *Nursing Elderly People*, Churchill Livingstone, London.

Macmillan, M.S. (1986), *Autonomy Shown in the Life Histories of Elderly People and a Nursing Response*, Unpublished PhD Thesis, University of Edinburgh, Edinburgh, Scotland.

Macmillan, M.S. (1994), 'Hospital staff's perceptions of risk associated with the discharge of elderly people from acute hospital care', *Journal of Advanced Nursing*, vol. 19, pp. 249-256.

Manley, K. and McCormack, B. (1997), *Exploring Expert Practice*, Masters in Nursing Distance Learning Module, Royal College of Nursing Institute, London.

Manthey, M. (1980), *The Practice of Primary Nursing*, Blackwell, Oxford.

Marchette, L., Box, N., Hennessy, M., Wasserlauf, M., Arnall, B., Copeland, D., Habib, K. (1993), 'Nurses' perceptions of the support of patient autonomy in do-not-resuscitate (DNR) decisions', *International Journal of Nursing Studies*, vol. 30, no. 1, pp. 37-49.

Mattiasson, A.C. and Anderson, L. (1995 [ii]), 'Organizational environment and the support of patient autonomy in nursing home care', *Journal of Advanced Nursing*, vol. 22, pp. 1149-1157.

May, C. (1995), "To call it work somehow demeans it': the social construction of talk in the care of terminally ill patients', *Journal of Advanced Nursing*, vol. 22, pp. 556-561.

Mayeroff, M. (1971), *On Caring*, Harper and Row, New York.

Meyers, D.T. (1989), *Self, Society and Personal Choice*, Columbia University Press, New York.

Miller, E. and Gwynne, G.A. (1972), *Life Apart. A Pilot Study of Residential Institutions for the Physically Handicapped and Young Sick*, Tavistock, London.

Moody, H.R. (1991), 'The Meaning of Life in Old Age', in N.S. Jecker, *Aging & Ethics*, Humana Press, New Jersey.

Morganti, J.B., Nehrke, M.F. and Hulicka, I.M. (1980), 'Resident and staff perceptions of latitude of choice in elderly institutionalized men', *Experimental Aging Research*, vol. 6, no. 4, pp. 367-384.

Morse, J.M. (1991) (ed.), *Qualitative Nursing Research: a contemporary dialogue*, Sage Publications, London.

Muetzel, P. (1988), 'Therapeutic Nursing', in A. Pearson (ed.), *Primary Nursing: Nursing in the Burford and Oxford Nursing Development Units*, Croom Helm, London.

Munhall, P.L. (1991), 'Institutional review of qualitative research proposals: a task of no small consequence', in J. Morse (ed.) *Qualitative Nursing Research: A Contemporary Dialogue*, Sage Publications, London.

MacGuire, J. (1989), 'An approach to evaluating the introduction of primary nursing in an acute medical unit for the elderly - Part 2: Operationalising the principles', *International Journal of Nursing Studies*, vol. 26, no. 3, pp. 253-260.

MacIntyre, A. (1992), *After Virtue - a study in moral theory*, Duckworth, London.

MacLeod, M. (1994), 'It's the little things that count': the hidden complexity of everyday clinical nursing practice', *Journal of Clinical Nursing*, vol. 3, no. 6, pp. 361-368.

McCormack, B. (1992), 'A case study identifying nursing staffs' perceptions of the delivery method of nursing care in practice on a particular ward', *Journal of Advanced Nursing*, vol. 17, pp. 187-197.

McCormack, B. and Ford, P. (1999), 'The contribution of expert gerontological nursing', *Nursing Standard*, vol. 13, no. 25, pp.42-45.

McCormack, M. and Whitehead, A. (1981), 'The effects of providing recreational activities on the engagement levels of long-stay geriatric patients', *Age and Ageing*, vol. 10, pp. 287-291.

McCormack, B., Manley, K., Titchen, A., Kitson, A. and Harvey, G. (1999), 'Towards Practice Development: A vision in reality or a reality without vision', *Journal of Nursing Management*, vol. 7, pp.255-264.

McKinstry, B. (1992), 'Paternalism and the doctor-patient relationship in general practice', *British Journal of General Practice*, vol. 42, pp. 340-342.

McWilliam, C.L., Belle-Brown, J., Carmichael, J.L. and Lehman, J.M. (1994), 'A new perspective on threatened autonomy in elderly persons: the disempowering process', *Social Science and Medicine*, vol. 38, no. 2, pp.327-338.

Newman, M.A. (1994), *Health as Expanding Consciousness (2nd edition)*, National League for Nursing Press, New York.

Noddings, N. (1984), *Caring: a Feminine Approach to Ethics and Moral Education*, University of California Press, Berkeley California.

Nolan, M. (1998), 'Gerontological nursing: professional priority or eternal Cinderella?', *Ageing and Society*, vol. 17, no. 4, pp. 447-460.

Norman, R. (1993), *'I Did it My Way': Some Thoughts on Autonomy'*, Conference paper, Philosophy of education society of Great Britain, New College, Oxford.

Norton, D., McLaren, R. and Exton-Smith, A.N. (1975), *An Investigation of Geriatric Nursing Problems in Hospital*, Churchill Livingstone, Edinburgh.

Nozick, R. (1974), *Anarchy, State and Utopia*, Basic Books, New York.

Oddi, L.F. (1994), 'Enhancing patients' autonomy', *Dimensions of Critical care Nursing*, vol. 13, no. 2, pp. 60-68.

Orem, D.E. (1980), *Nursing: Concepts of Practice*, (2nd edn.) McGraw-Hill, New York.

Pankratz, L. and Pankratz, D. (1974), 'Nursing autonomy and patients' rights: development of a nursing attitude scale', *Journal of Health and Social Behaviour*, vol. 15, pp. 211-216.

Parsons, T. (1954), 'The Professions And Social Structure', *Essays in Sociological Theory*, Free press, Illinois.

Parsons, T. (1968), *The Structure of Social Action*, Free Press, New York.

Partridge, C. and Johnston, M. (1989), 'Perceived control of recovery from physical disability: measurement and prediction', *British Journal of Clinical Psychology*, vol. 28, pp. 53-59.

Paterson, J.G. and Zderad, L.T. (1976), *Humanistic Nursing*, Wiley, New York.

Paton, H.J. (1964), *Groundwork of the Metaphysics of Morals*, Harper & Row, New York.

Pearson, A. (1985), *The Effects Of Introducing New Norms In A Nursing Unit And An Analysis Of The Process Of Change*, Doctoral Thesis, Goldsmith College, University of London.

Pellegrino, E.D. (1979), 'Toward a reconstruction of medical morality: the primacy of the act of profession and the fact of illness', *The Journal of Medicine and Philosophy*, vol. 4, no. 1, pp. 32-56.

Penticuff, J.H. (1991), 'Conceptual issues in nursing ethics research', *The Journal of Medicine and Philosophy*, vol. 16, pp. 235-252.

Peplau, H. (1952), *Interpersonal Relations in Nursing*, G P Putnam's Sons, New York.

Pinch, W.J. (1985), 'Ethical dilemmas in nursing: the role of the nurse and perceptions of autonomy', *Journal of Nursing Education*, vol. 24, no. 9, pp. 372-376.

Pinch, W.J. and Parsons, M.E. (1993), 'The ethics of treatment decision making: the elderly patient's perspective', *Geriatric Nursing*, vol. 14, no. 6, pp. 289-293.

Polit, D.F. and Hungler, B.P. (1987), *Nursing Research: principles and methods*, JB Lippincott Company, Philadelphia.

Pollard, B.J. (1993), 'Autonomy and paternalism in medicine', *The Medical Journal of Australia*, vol. 159, pp. 797-802.

Porter, S. (1992), 'The poverty of professionalisation: a critical analysis of strategies for the occupational advancement of nurses', *Journal of Advanced Nursing*, vol. 17, pp. 720-726.

Porter, S. (1994), 'New nursing: the road to freedom', *Journal of Advanced Nursing*, vol. 20, pp. 269-274.

Porter, S. (1996), 'Contra-Foucault: soldiers, nurses and power', *Sociology*, vol. 30, no. 1, pp. 59-78.

Powers, B.A. (1992), 'The roles staff play in the social networks of elderly institutionalized people', *Social Science and Medicine*, vol. 34, no. 12, pp. 1335-1343.

Raps, C.S., Peterson, C., Jonas, M. and Seligman, M.E.P. (1982), 'Patient behaviour in hospitals: helplessness, reactance, or both?', *Journal of Personality and Social Psychology*, vol. 42, no. 6, pp. 1036-1041.

Rawls, J. (1971), *A Theory of Justice*, Oxford University Press, Oxford.

Rawls, J. (1992), *A Theory of Justice*, Oxford University Press, Oxford.

Richards, D.A.J. (1989), 'Rights and Autonomy', in J Christman, *The Inner Citadel: Essays on Individual Autonomy*, Oxford University Press, Oxford.

Ricoeur, P. (1977), 'The Model of the Text', in F. Dallmayr and T. McCarthy (eds.) *Understanding and Social Inquiry*, University of Notre Dame Press, Notre Dame, Indiana.

Ridley, B. (1989), 'Tom's Story: a quadriplegic who refused rehabilitation', *Rehabilitation Nursing*, vol. 14, no. 5, pp. 250-255.

Robbins, D.A. (1996), *Ethical and Legal Issues in Home Health and Long-Term Care: Challenges and Solutions*, Aspen Publishers, Inc., Maryland.

Robertson, I. (1986), 'Learned helplessness', *Nursing Times and Nursing Mirror*, vol. 82, 17th December, pp. 28-30.

Robinson, K.S.M. (1986), *The Social Construction of Health Visiting*, Unpublished PhD Thesis, Department of Nursing and Community Health Studies, Polytechnic of South Bank, London.

Rogers, C. (1961), *On Becoming a Person*, Houghton Mifflin Co., Boston.

Royal College of Nursing (1993), *Older People and Continuing Care - The Skill and Value of the Nurse*, RCN London.

Royal College of Nursing (1994), *The Skill and Value of Nurses Work with Older People*, RCN, London.

Royal College of Nursing (1995), *Nursing Homes: Nursing Values*, RCN, London.

Royal College of Nursing (1997), *What A Difference A Nurse Makes: An RCN Report On The Benefits Of Expert Nursing To The Clinical Outcomes In The Continuing Care Of Older People*, RCN, London..

Royal Commission on Long Term Care (1999), *Rights and Responsibilities. With Respect to Old Age*, The Stationary Office, London.

Ryden, M.B. (1985), 'Environmental support for autonomy in the institutionalized elderly', *Research in Nursing and Health*, vol. 8, pp. 363-371.

Sacks, H., Schegloff, E.A. and Jefferson, G. (1974), 'A simplest systematics for the organization of turn-taking for conversation', *Language*, vol. 50, no. 4, pp. 696-735.

Sacks, O. (1991), *A Leg to Stand On*, Pan Books, London.

Salvage, J. (1990), 'The theory and practice of 'new nursing'', Occasional Paper, *Nursing Times*, vol. 84, no. 4, pp. 42-45.

Sandelowski, M. (1986), 'The problem of rigour in qualitative research', *Advances in Nursing Science*, vol. 8, no. 3, pp. 27-37.

Saup, W. (1986), 'Lack of autonomy in old-age homes: a stress and coping study', *Journal of Housing for the Elderly*, vol. 4, no. 1, pp. 21-36.

Savage, J. (1995), *Nursing Intimacy - An Ethnographic Approach to Nurse-Patient Interaction*, Scutari Press, London.

Schegloff, E.A. (1992), 'Repair after next turn: the last structurally provided defence of intersubjectivity in conversation', *American Journal of Sociology*, vol. 97, pp. 1295-1345.

Schofield, I. (1994), 'An historical approach to care', *Elderly Care*, vol. 6, no. 6, pp. 14-15.

Schön, D.A. (1990), *Educating the Reflective Practitioner*, Jossey Bass, Oxford.

Schön, D.A. (1991), *The Reflective Practitioner: How Professionals Think in Action*, Avebury, Aldershot.

Schutz, A. (1967), *The Phenomenology of the Social World*, Northwestern University Press, Evanston.

Schwandt, T.A. (1994), 'Constructivist, Interpretivist Approaches to Human Inquiry', in N.K. Denzin and Y.S. Lincoln, *Handbook of Qualitative Research*, Sage Publishers, London.

Schwartz, H.I. and Blank, K. (1986), 'Shifting competency during hospitalization: a model for informed consent decisions', *Hospital and Community Psychiatry*, vol. 37, no. 12, pp. 1256-1260.

Scoccia, D. (1990), 'Paternalism and respect for autonomy', *Ethics*, vol. 100, January 1990, pp. 318-334.

Scott, M.B. and Lyman, S.M. (1968), 'Accounts', *American Sociological Review*, vol. 33, pp. 46-62.

Seedhouse, D. (1986), *Health - the Foundations of Achievement*, John Wiley & Sons, Chichester.

Seedhouse, D. (1988), *Ethics: The Heart of Health Care*, John Wiley & Sons, Chichester.

Seedhouse, D. (1992), 'Picturing limits to medicine', *Critical Public Health*, vol. 3, no. 2, pp. 36-42.

Seedhouse, D. and Cribb, A. (eds.) (1989), *Changing Ideas in Health Care*, John Wiley & Sons, Chichester.

Sefi, S. (1988), 'Health Visitors talking to mothers', *Health Visitor*, vol. 61, pp.7-10.

Selder, F. (1989), 'Life transition theory: the resolution of uncertainty', *Nursing and Health Care*, vol. 10, no. 8, pp. 437-451.

Siegler, M. (1977), 'Critical illness: the limits of autonomy', *The Hastings Centre Report*, 7 October, pp. 12-15.

Sills, P., Redfern, S.J., Kenny, W.T., Harrington, M. and Clarke, M. (1988), 'Services for the elderly by the year 2000: education and training issues', *Journal of Advanced Nursing*, vol. 13, pp. 416-424.

Silverman, D. (1993), *Qualitative Methodology and Sociology*, Gower, Aldershot.

Singleton, E.K. and Nail, F.C. (1984), 'Autonomy in nursing', *Nursing Forum*, vol. xxi, no. 3, pp. 123-130.

Slater, R. (1995), *The Psychology of Growing Old - looking forward*, Rethinking Ageing Series, Open University Press, Buckingham.

Smits, M. (1984), *The Structure And Organisation Of Nurse Patient Conversations - An Alternative Perspective*, Unpublished MSc Research Dissertation, University of Surrey, Guildford, Surrey.

Snowball, J. (1996), 'Asking nurses about advocating for patients: 'reactive' and 'proactive' accounts', *Journal of Advanced Nursing*, vol. 24, pp. 67-75.

Stockwell, F. (1972), *The Unpopular Patient*, Royal College of Nursing, London.

Strong, P.M. (1979), *The Ceremonial Order of the Clinic: Parents, Doctors and Medical Bureaucracies*, Routledge and Kegan Paul, London.

Strong, P.M. and Davis, A.G. (1977), 'Roles, role formats and medical encounters: a cross-cultural analysis of staff-client relationships in children's clinics', *Sociological Review*, vol. 25, no. 4, pp. 775-800.

Sullivan, R.J. (1990), *Immanuel Kant's Moral Theory*, Cambridge University Press, Cambridge.

Svensson, R. (1996), 'The interplay between doctors and nurses - a negotiated order perspective', *Sociology of Health and Illness*, vol. 18, no. 3, pp. 379-398.

Szasz, T. and Hollander, M. (1956), '*A contribution to the philosophy of medicine: Three basic models of the doctor-patient relationship*', *Archives of Internal Medicine*, vol .97, pp. 585-592.

Tanner, C.A., Benner, P., Chesla, C. and Gordon, D.R. (1993), 'The phenomenology of knowing the patient', *Image: Journal of Nursing Scholarship*, vol. 25, no. 4, pp. 273-280.

Taylor, A. (1993), *Older Than Time*, Harper Collins Publishers, London.

Taylor, B.J. (1992), 'From helper to human: a reconceptualization of the nurse as person', *Journal of Advanced Nursing*, vol. 17, pp. 1042-1049.

Taylor, S. (1979), 'Hospital patient behaviour: reactance, helplessness or control?', *Journal of Social Issues*, vol. 35, no. 1, pp. 156-184.

Teasdale, K. and Kent, G. (1995), 'The use of deception in nursing', *Journal of Medical Ethics*, vol. 21, pp.77-81.

Thalberg, I. (1989), 'Hierarchical Analysis of Unfree Action', in J. Christman, *The Inner Citadel: Essays on Individual Autonomy*, Oxford University Press, Oxford.

Titchen, A. (2000), *Professional Craft Knowledge in Patient-Centred Nursing and the Facilitation of its Development*, Ashdale Press, Kidlington, Oxon.

Townsend, P. (1974), 'Inequality and the Health Service', *The Lancet*, 15 June 1974, pp. 1179-89.

Traynor, M. (1996), 'A literary approach to managerial discourse after the NHS reforms', *Sociology of Health & Illness*, vol. 18, no. 3, pp. 315-340.

Traynor, M. and Rafferty, A.M. (1998), *Nursing Research and the Higher Education Context: A Research Working Paper*, Centre for Policy in Nursing Research, London.

Tronto, J.C. (1993), *Moral Boundaries: a political argument for an ethic of care*, Routledge, London.

Trygstad, L. (1986), 'Professional Friends: the inclusion of the personal into the professional', *Cancer Nursing*, vol. 9, no. 6, pp. 326-332.

Turner, P. (1993), 'Activity nursing and the changes in the quality of life of elderly patients: a semi-quantitative study', *Journal of Advanced Nursing*, vol. 19, pp. 239-248.

Uhlmann, R.F., Pearlman, R.A. and Cain, K.C. (1988), 'Physicians' and spouses' predictions of elderly patients' resuscitation preferences', *Journal of Gerontology*, vol. 43, pp. M115-M121.

United Kingdom Central Council for Nursing, Midwifery and Health Visiting (1992) *The Code of Professional Conduct*, UKCC, London.

Van Hooft, S. (1990), 'Moral education for nursing decisions', *Journal of Advanced Nursing*, vol. 15, pp. 210-215.

Victor, C.R. (1991), *Health and Health Care in Later Life*, Open University Press, Milton Keynes.

Wade, B. (1983), 'Different models of care for the elderly', *Nursing Times*, vol. 79, no. 12, pp. 33-36.

Wainwright, P. (1997), 'A new paradigm for nursing: the potential of realism', *Journal of Advanced Nursing*, vol. 26, pp. 1262-1271.

Waters, K.R. and Luker, K.A. (1996), 'Staff perspectives on the role of the nurse in rehabilitation wards for elderly people', *Journal of Clinical Nursing*, vol. 5, pp. 105-114.

Waterworth, A. and Luker, K. (1990), 'Reluctant collaborators: do patients want to be involved in decisions concerning care?', *Journal of Advanced Nursing*, vol. 15, no. 8, pp. 971-976.

Watkins, J., Drury, L., Preddy, D. (1992), *From Evolution to Revolution - The pressure on professional life in the 1990's*, University of Bristol, Bristol.

Watson, G. (1989), 'Free Agency', in J. Christman, *The Inner Citadel: Essays on Individual Autonomy*, Oxford University Press, Oxford.

Watson, J. (1988), *Nursing: Human Science and Human Care. A Theory of Nursing*, National League for Nursing, New York.

Weinberg, J. (1978), 'On adding insight to injury, Part 1', *Gerontologist*, vol. 16, pp. 4-10.

Weiss, G.B. (1985), 'Paternalism modernised', *Journal of Medical Ethics*, vol. 11, pp. 184-187.

Wells, T. (1980), *Problems in Geriatric Nursing Care*, Churchill-Livingstone, Edinburgh.

White Beck, L. (1956), *Kant: Critique of Practical Reason*, Macmillan, London.

Willcocks, D., Peace, S. and Kellaher, L. (1987), *Private Lives in Public Places: a research-based critique of residential life in local authority old people's homes*, Tavistock Publications, London.

Wilson, J. (1963), *Thinking with Concepts*, Cambridge University Press, Cambridge.

Wood, J.E., Tiedje, L.B., Abraham, I.L. (1986), 'Practising autonomously: a comparison of nurses', *Public Health Nursing*, vol. 3, pp. 130-139.

Wright, S.G. (1990), *My Patient-My Nurse: The Practice of Primary Nursing*, Scutari Press, London.

Yarling, R.R. and McEelmurry, B.J. (1990), 'The Moral Foundation of Nursing', in T. Pence and J. Cantrell (eds.), *Ethics in Nursing: An Anthology*, National League for Nursing, New York.

Young, R. (1980), 'Autonomy and the "Inner Self"', *American Philosophical Quarterly*, vol. 17, no. 1. Pp. 35-43.

Zimmerman, D.H. and West, C. (1975), 'Sex Roles, Interruptions And Silences In Conversation', in B. Thorne and N. Henley (eds.), *Language and Sex: Difference and Dominance*, Newbury House, Mass.

Zimmerman, D.H. and Wieder, D.L. (1970), 'Ethnomethodology and the Problem of Order', in J. Douglas (ed.), *Understanding Everyday Life*, Aldine, Chicago.

Zweibel, N.R. and Cassel, C.K. (1989), 'Treatment choices at the end of life: A comparison of decisions by older patients and their physician-selected proxies', *The Gerontologist*, vol. 29, pp. 615-621.